In Pursuit of Healthy Environi

In Pursuit of Healthy Environments brings temporal depth to a highly topical issue: the interaction between health and the environment. By means of a rich set of historical case studies from the Americas to Europe and from the tropics to the Arctic, the volume demonstrates that the concern for creating and finding healthy environments is not a new one, shows how the link between the environment and health has been perceived at different times and in different cultures and discusses the practical implications of these conceptualizations.

The book, written by scholars from architecture, cultural anthropology, history, Indigenous Studies, media studies and sociology, will be of interest to a reader interested in the historical roots of today's health-related environmental issues. It discusses the spatiality and materiality of the conceptions of health and the practices of nurture in colonial and post-colonial environments and shows how greatly indigenous and colonial mindsets have differed during the last 300 years.

It also investigates how certain environments have become labelled as healthy and life-preserving while others are stigmatized by death and disease and how fluctuating these notions can be. Finally, it analyses the materialities and immaterialities, as well as the transgenerational and transboundary characters of environmental and medical knowledge.

Esa Ruuskanen is a Senior Research Fellow and the person responsible for the minor in Environmental Humanities at the University of Oulu, Finland. His research interests include the environmental history of Western and Northern European peatlands, energy histories and the environment-technology interaction.

Heini Hakosalo works as a Senior Research Fellow at the University of Oulu, Finland. She specializes in modern and contemporary history of medicine. Her research interests include the history of brain sciences in late nineteenth-century Europe, the beginnings of women's medical education in Finland and Sweden, the history of tuberculosis in twentieth-century Finland, and the history of birth cohort studies after the Second World War.

Routledge Studies in Environment, Culture, and Society

Series editors: Bernhard Glaeser and Heike Egner

This series opens up a forum for advances in environmental studies relating to society and its social, cultural, and economic underpinnings. The underlying assumption guiding this series is that there is an important, and so far little-explored, interaction between societal as well as cultural givens and the ways in which societies both create and respond to environmental issues. As such, this series encourages the exploration of the links between prevalent practices, beliefs and values, as differentially manifested in diverse societies, and the distinct ways in which those societies confront the environment.

Learning and Calamities
Practices, Interpretations, Patterns
Edited by Heike Egner, Marén Schorch, and Martin Voss

Trading Environments
Frontiers, Commercial Knowledge, and Environmental Transformation, 1750–1990
Edited by Gordon M. Winder and Andreas Dix

Transdisciplinary Research and Sustainability
Collaboration, Innovation and Transformation
Edited by Martina Padmanabhan

Global Change in Marine Systems
Integrating Natural, Social and Governing Responses
Edited by Patrice Guillotreau, Alida Bundy and Ian Perry

In Pursuit of Healthy Environments
Historical Cases on the Environment–Health Nexus
Edited by Esa Ruuskanen and Heini Hakosalo

For more information, please visit: www.routledge.com/Routledge-Studies-in-Environment-Culture-and-Society/book-series/RSECS

In Pursuit of Healthy Environments

Historical Cases on the Environment–Health Nexus

Edited by Esa Ruuskanen and Heini Hakosalo

Routledge
Taylor & Francis Group

LONDON AND NEW YORK

First published 2021
by Routledge
2 Park Square, Milton Park, Abingdon, Oxon OX14 4RN

and by Routledge
605 Third Avenue, New York, NY 10017

First issued in paperback 2022

Routledge is an imprint of the Taylor & Francis Group, an informa business

British Library Cataloguing-in-Publication Data
A catalogue record for this book is available from the British Library

Library of Congress Cataloging-in-Publication Data
Names: Ruuskanen, Esa, editor. | Hakosalo, Heini, editor.
Title: In pursuit of healthy environments : historical cases on the environment–health nexus / edited by Esa Ruuskanen and Heini Hakosalo.
Description: Abingdon, Oxon; New York, NY : Routledge, 2021. |
Series: Routledge studies in environment, culture, and society |
Includes bibliographical references and index.
Identifiers: LCCN 2020023746 (print) | LCCN 2020023747 (ebook) |
ISBN 9780367259051 (hardback) | ISBN 9780367259099 (ebook)
Subjects: LCSH: Environmental health–History. |
Environmental health–History–Case studies.
Classification: LCC RA565 .I55 2021 (print) |
LCC RA565 (ebook) | DDC 362.1–dc23
LC record available at https://lccn.loc.gov/2020023746
LC ebook record available at https://lccn.loc.gov/2020023747

ISBN 13: 978-0-367-61624-3 (pbk)
ISBN 13: 978-0-367-25905-1 (hbk)
ISBN 13: 978-0-367-25909-9 (ebk)

DOI: 10.4324/9780367259099

Typeset in Times New Roman
by Newgen Publishing UK

Contents

Illustrations

Figures

Table

Contributors

Min Bae worked as a dentist in South Korea (DDS, Yonsei University; and Master of Clinical Dentistry in Clinical Orthodontics, Hallym University), but after changing his career (BA, Hongik University in History Education), he has worked as a history teacher (Soongeui Girls' High School, Seoul). After receiving his second master's degree in 2014 (in Medical Humanities and History of Medicine, Seoul National University), he is currently a PhD student in Modern History at the University of St Andrews, UK. His academic interest areas are medical professionalism, intellectual history of medicine, and the medical market.

Laura Pérez Gil is a Professor in Anthropology at the Federal University of Paraná (Brazil) and Director of the Archaeology and Ethnology Museum of the same university. Her recent publications concern the transformation of Amazonian indigenous shamanic systems in contemporary contexts, as well as the connection between shamanism and violence. She also conducts research on ethnographic collections of Amazonian indigenous peoples in museums.

Heini Hakosalo works as a Senior Research Fellow (History of Sciences and Ideas) at the University of Oulu, Finland. She specializes in the history of medicine and health during the 19th and 20th centuries. Her major research projects have dealt with Foucauldian histories of medicine and psychiatry, the history of brain sciences in late nineteenth-century Europe, the beginnings of women's medical education in Finland and Sweden and the history of tuberculosis in twentieth-century Finland. She is the principal investigator of the research project *Lives over Time: Birth Cohort Studies as a Form of Knowledge-Production, from the Second World War to the Present*, funded by the Academy of Finland.

Marcel Hartwig is an Assistant Professor in English and American Studies at the University of Siegen. He has contributed research papers in edited volumes and international journals in the fields of media studies, television studies, literary criticism, gender studies, and popular culture. Currently, he is finalizing his post-doctoral project in the field of transatlantic studies entitled "Transit Cultures: 18th Century Medical Discourses and Knowledge Media in the North American Colonies". He is co-editor of *Media Economies: Perspectives on American Cultural Practices* (2014), the Rock Music Studies special issue on *American Rock Journalism* (2017), and the forthcoming reader *Canonizing David Lynch: Audiovisual Aesthetics and Shocking Standards* (2020).

Mikko Jauho has a background in Sociology and is a Senior Researcher at the Centre for Consumer Society Research at the Faculty of Social Sciences, University of Helsinki. He works at the intersections of science & technology studies, governmentality studies, sociology of health and illness, and consumer studies, focusing on the various ways knowledge is deployed in the government of health and illness, and utilizing both contemporary and historical approaches and materials. He is presently finishing a project charting the historical emergence, political and practical deployment and current understanding of the notion of lifestyle risk in public health policy and personal health care, using risks associated with cardiovascular diseases as the empirical case.

Dolly Jørgensen is a Professor of History at the University of Stavanger, Norway, and the co-founder of Greenhouse, an environmental humanities initiative at UiS. Her research spans from medieval to contemporary environmental issues. Her primary areas of interest are human–animal relations, the urban environment, and environmental policymaking. She is an active participant on the Editorial Boards of the journals *Agricultural History* and *Environment and History*.

Kalle Kananoja is a research fellow at the University of Oulu, Finland, working on the history of slavery and medicine in the early modern Atlantic world. His recent and forthcoming publications include a co-edited volume *Healers and Empires in Global History: Healing as Hybrid and Contested Knowledge* (2019) and *Healing Knowledge in Atlantic Africa: Medical Encounters 1500–1850* (2020).

Ritva Kylli is a Senior Lecturer in the Faculty of Humanities at the University of Oulu. She specializes in the study of the Arctic and northern food history. Recently, she has focused on food, health, and environmental history of the Sámi in a multidisciplinary research project funded by the Finnish Cultural Foundation.

Petteri Pietikäinen is a Professor of the History of Sciences and Ideas at the University of Oulu, Finland. His research interests include the history of madness and mental health; the history of evolutionary theories; the history of Utopian thought; and relations between the human sciences and society. His major publications include *Alchemists of Human*

Nature: Psychological Utopianism in Gross, Jung, Reich and Fromm (2007), *Madness: A History* (2015) and *Social Class and Mental Illness in Northern Europe*, co-edited with Jesper Vaczy Kragh (2019).

Otto Pipatti is a sociologist and currently studying the history of Westermarckian evolutionary sociology and anthropology between 1890s and 1950s. His first book, *Morality Made Visible: Edward Westermarck's Moral and Social Theory*, was published in 2019. Pipatti works as a post-doctoral researcher at the Department of Social Research, University of Helsinki, Finland.

Esa Ruuskanen is a Senior Research Fellow and the person responsible for the minor in Environmental Humanities at the University of Oulu, where he has been a faculty member since 2011. His research interests include the environmental history of Western and Northern European peatlands, energy histories and the environment-technology interaction. He has published several articles and book chapters on post-war Finnish energy policies (2015 and 2019), the changing valuation and uses of peat bogs in the Nordic countries, Baltic region and Ireland (e.g. 2016, 2018 and 2019) and the theory of environmental history (2017).

Anu Soikkeli, DSc, PhD, is a professor at the Oulu University School of Architecture. Her research interests include the heritage and conservation of traditional wooden buildings; reconstruction period housing architecture and building projects, and the human–environment relationships in the Arctic region. Soikkeli has been a PI in several European and national research projects and has published over 160 articles.

Pirjo Kristiina Virtanen is an Assistant Professor in Indigenous Studies at the University of Helsinki. Her publications include *Indigenous Youth in Brazilian Amazonia* (2012) and *Creating Dialogues: Indigenous Perceptions and Changing Forms of Leadership in Amazonia* (2017), as well as several publications on mobility, Amazonian biocultural landscapes, Amazonian indigenous onto-epistemologies, Arawak history, and decolonizing research methods. She has carried out extensive fieldwork in Southwestern Amazonia.

Michael Zeheter is a Lecturer and Research Associate at the University of Trier (Germany). Dr Zeheter received his PhD from the University of Konstanz in 2015. His current research project focuses on the cultural history of mineral water consumption in Europe from the 1830s onwards. His major publications include *Epidemics, Empire and Environment: Cholera in Madras and Quebec City 1818–1910* (2015) and *Die Ordnung der Fischer. Fischerei und Nachhaltigkeit am Bodensee 1350–1900* (2014). His research interests lie in environmental history, history of consumption, history of science, and medical history.

Panagiotis Zestanakis works as a Post Doc at the University of Hamburg, Germany. He earned his PhD in contemporary European history from the University of Crete in 2017. His research interests revolve around the history of everyday life in post-dictatorship Greece, the history of media and representations and the uses of contemporary history in participative web cultures. His work has appeared in several international journals such as *Film, Fashion and Consumption, Transfers, Journal of Greek Media* and *Culture and Journal of Consumer Culture*.

Acknowledgements

This volume sprang from the workshop "Environment and health in history", organized by the editors, which took place at the University of Oulu in November 2016. The workshop was supported by the Faculty of Humanities, University of Oulu, and we wish to thank Dean Paula Rossi for her support. The workshop was also supported and funded by the Academy of Finland, for which we thank the Research Council for Culture and Society. We are grateful for the fascinating presentations and exchanges of ideas during the workshop, including those participants whose work is not published in this volume. Here we would especially like to thank Daniel Blackie, Markku Hokkanen, Antti Häkkinen and Marianne Junila. Special thanks also go to Emily Briggs, Elena Chiu and Lakshita Joshi who helped to compose and format the manuscript. We would also thank the series editors Bernhard Glaeser and Heike Egner for their interest in publishing the volume and their foreword to the book, and the staff at Routledge for accomplishing our project. Finally, we thank the authors of the chapters for their enthusiasm and dedication to this volume.

Esa Ruuskanen and Heini Hakosalo
Oulu, 2020

Introduction

Heini Hakosalo and Esa Ruuskanen

Despite their apparent affinity, there has been surprisingly little interaction between the fields of environmental and health history before the late 2010s. We think that these fields should be natural partners, considering how many similar interests they share. Often, it is not even meaningful to separate environmental and health issues from each other. Take, for example, malaria. Ancient people had bound the birth and spread of the disease to certain landscapes, especially to swamps and marshes. To avoid the deathly grip of malaria, humans located their settlements on mountains and in the highlands and, as scientific-technological systems evolved, began to envisage how they could transform these disease-infected areas into healthy and affluent surroundings. The valuation of landscape was not only about economy but also about a complicated set of notions about health and beauty – in other words, about existential and aesthetic values and beliefs.

Historical famines are another case in point. These have typically been triggered by agricultural failures linked to climatic conditions and have often been aggravated by technological or social factors such as poor infrastructure, the unequal distribution of goods or inefficient relief measures. More often than not, prolonged malnourishment and hunger have been accompanied by disease, and it has often been impossible to ascertain how much of the overall famine mortality is due to disease and how much to hunger. Similarly, the countermeasures that have been taken to control the damage, to alleviate suffering or to prevent similar crises from happening again are guided by conceptions concerning both health and the environment (as well as by a tangle of political, social and economic concerns).

Environmental history is relative newcomer as a well-defined historical subfield. While medical history has a long institutional history, it has remained relatively isolated from the historical mainstream, partly because of its traditional affiliation with medical faculties. During the past two decades or so, both subfields have moved closer to the historical mainstream and have come to play a more prominent role in academic debate. They have also grown increasingly conscious of their shared interests. Publications, conferences, courses and study programmes, as well as the establishment of the network

"H-EnviroHealth,"[1] can be taken as evidence of the increasing collaboration between the two historical sub-fields. Medical history journals are increasingly likely to discuss environmental issues, and journals like *Environmental History* often include papers that are highly relevant from the point of view of the history of health.[2] The same goes for book series that publish case studies on environmental and medical history, respectively. However, so far, there have been few deliberate attempts to bring the two together in the same volume. The most notable exception is *Environment, Health and History*, edited by Martin Gorsky and Virginia Berridge (2011).[3]

This being said, a retrospective look reveals that both medical and environmental historians have, for a long time, dealt with topics that are also relevant to the other subfield. For instance, British environmental history, which partly sprouted from research on urban and industrial history, has shown an interest in the environmental effects of urbanization and industrialization from the 1980s onwards.[4] Peter Brimblecombe,[5] Bill Luckin,[6] Stephen Mosley,[7] Daniel Schneider[8] and Peter Thorsheim,[9] to name but a few, represent this research orientation. The history of pollution, the theme they deal with, has usually looked at the development of modern sewage systems on the one hand, and the public response to air pollution caused by the use of fossil fuels on the other. Both involved the accumulation of knowledge through medical research and studies at the chemistry-biology interface, various solutions based on new technologies, and issues of control through policies and regulations.

In his award-winning book *Hybrid Nature*, Daniel Schneider explores late nineteenth-century sewage treatment plants as hybrid ecosystems that incorporate elements of nature and industry. These ecosystems, as Schneider shows, are biophysical in nature and rely on the ability of communities of organisms – from bacteria to animals – to degrade sewage and recycle various substances back to the environment. Biological sewage treatment plants developed into a crucial tool for protecting health and the environment.[10] The same applies to smoke-prevention technologies which, as Stephen Mosley shows, were often utilized in inapt ways in late nineteenth-century industrial Manchester.[11] These technologies became more commonly used only after the introduction of binding legislation and more effective pollution control. Overall, sewage systems and pollution control devices manifest assemblages which stemmed from the growing concern surrounding health-related and environmental risks.

Risks related to toxic and hazardous discharges and waste appear to be a fruitful basis for a fusion of the histories of the environment, health and medicine. For example, Susanna Rankin Bohme,[12] Jessica van Horssen,[13] Melanie Kiechle,[14] Nancy Langston[15] and Richard Newman[16] have carried out research on the theme in question. By analysing the use of synthetic oestrogen diethylstilbestrol (DES), a hormone disruptor, in the US during the mid-twentieth century and showing how human bodies and the environment can become saturated with synthetic chemicals, Langston tells a story of risks. As does Bohme, whose book *Toxic Injustice* illustrates how irrevocably the use of a pesticide – in this case dibromochloropropane, known as DBCP – may become enmeshed in cumulating risks and tangible harms related to environmental health. Kiechle, in turn, writes a multi-sensory urban history by focusing on the shifting smellscapes of nineteenth-century American cities, when the old miasmatic theory which thought diseases were caused by bad air still held. As Kiechle acknowledges, sensory knowing is subjective. The sense of smell, which was the best and often the only way to measure smells at that time, was interwoven with issues of social justice, social control and urban development.

Another theme that brings the two fields together is "ecological imperialism," a theme introduced by American environmental historian Alfred Crosby in the mid-1980s. In a way, Crosby started a new way of looking at global history as a complicated set of social, cultural, environmental and biological factors by analysing the impact of Old World crops, weeds, livestock, people and pathogens on previously isolated communities in the Americas and the Pacific. He suggested that the success of sixteenth- and seventeenth-century European colonies was partly due to non-human forces.[17] Crosby's argument is not without its critics, and he has sometimes been labelled an environmental determinist – unfairly so, since he also emphasizes the impact of military and economic incursions on the subjugation of the Indigenous peoples of the Americas.

Crosby's claims were subjected to thorough re-examination by, for instance, Paul Kelton, who studied the biological processes involved in the colonization of North America in *Epidemics and Enslavement* (2009) and *Cherokee Medicine, Colonial Germs* (2015). Kelton argues that not only European diseases, but also long-continuing raids, enslavement and the trauma caused by them made some Indigenous nations powerless in the face of colonization. Kelton shows how some Indigenous nations tried to adapt to the turbulent times and the spread of European diseases with the help of various cultural practices, from healing ceremonies to patient isolation.[18] As for the impact of the "Columbian exchange," it may have been even greater than Crosby assumed. Koch at al. (2019) have recently suggested that the huge depopulation in the Americas, caused mainly by European-imported pathogens, led to massive changes in land use: massive enough to cause a marked decline in the global atmospheric CO_2 concentration and a drop in global temperatures. "These changes," the authors conclude, "show that human actions had a global impact on the Earth's system in the centuries prior to the Industrial Revolution."[19]

The environment broadly conceived – natural, built and social – has always been present in the history of diseases. More specifically, the role of the natural environment has been prominent in some strands of medical history. One of these strands is historical epidemiology, concerned with mapping historical epidemics, explaining their outlook with reference to natural, climatic and social conditions, and relating environmental changes to patterns of mortality and morbidity. As epidemics have often come with major demographic, social and economic consequences, it has not been too difficult to convince political, social and economic historians of the relevance of studying them. However, whereas the representatives of more traditional history of epidemics were prone to regard "the disease itself" as a constant, the eye of the storm as it were, around which the human and social drama unfolded, contemporary health historians are more likely to regard disease as a historical phenomenon, albeit one with its own rhythm of change, which can differ considerably from the cycles of political history or medical thought. For instance, Kelton's works show that the history of epidemics continues, under new guises, to provide a meeting ground for both histories of medicine and the environment.[20]

Another fertile meeting point for environmental and medical points of view has been the history of public health. Closely connected to the history of epidemics, the history of public health has been about the search for effective means of preventing disease in the population. If the focus of epidemiology has been in identifying the environmental and other factors that explain epidemic disease, a focus of public health efforts has been in finding ways to change the environment (natural, built, social) so as to make it inhospitable to disease. For a long time, the major threat to the health of the populations, and thus the major motivation behind the development of public health, were outbreaks of infectious diseases. That changed with the mid-twentieth century epidemiological transition, after which the focus of both epidemiological research and public health efforts shifted towards chronic disease, at least in the developed countries. These changes are, to an extent, also reflected in the historiography of public health. While there is no shortage of historical research on specific aspects of public health, historians have been less eager tackle its general development, as indicated by the fact that George Rosen's *A History of Public Health,* originally published in 1958, was reprinted in 2015.[21]

Inquiries into the relationship between health and place have various points of contact with environmental history. From the 1990s onwards, broad medical geographies have increasingly given way to studies on health in place.[22] For instance, historians and geographers have studied how and why certain loci became invested with healing qualities and how local communities have relied on the natural environment for food and medication (for much of human history, it is difficult or impossible to tell the two strictly apart). The vast majority of drugs, of course, originate in the natural environment – mainly in the vegetable and animal kingdoms. For instance, penicillin and streptomycin, which are among the most potent modern drugs, were initially natural substances, discovered in mould and soil, respectively. Apart from specific food and medical substances, people have attributed health-inducing powers to vegetation, air and water and other environmental features over which humans have little short-term control. They have travelled far and wide in search of reputedly health-inducing destinations. Some of these places have been "purely" natural, with few man-made elements, others have been entangled with the built environment. Hospital planning made use of health-inducing environmental factors – for instance, sunlight or fresh air – until the early twentieth century, and the architecture used for tuberculosis sanatoria even longer.[23]

The interaction between humans and micro-organisms provides another meeting point for historians of health and the environment. Speculation about the existence of disease-causing animacula go back to antiquity, but these remained decidedly marginal in medical thought until the late nineteenth century, when the rise of bacteriology made microscopic organisms visible and established their role in the causation of disease. The rise of bacteriology indeed led to the boundaries of "nature" being partially redrawn. The 1930–1940s saw the introduction of a series of efficient antibacterial drugs. The golden age of antibiotics coincided with the epidemiological transition, which quickly reduced the burden of contagious disease and thereby boosted medical optimism. During this period, the interaction between humans and micro-organisms was typically conceptualized as a battle, and a battle that humans were destined to win in the near future. Now that antibiotic drug development has stagnated and the rise of drug-resistant strains of bacteria have seriously undermined such optimism, it seems that we would have been better served by a more environmentally orientated conceptualizations, with bacteria regarded as part of the natural environment and indeed as part of the human body rather than external enemies to be defeated.

Medico-environmental history is problem-based rather than discipline-based, and thus open to interdisciplinary collaboration. There are many points of contact with neighbouring disciplines. For instance, anthropological and oral historical inquiries underline the relevance of indigenous and lay knowledge and practice, helping medical and environmental histories to enrich and adjust their traditionally expert-orientated point of view. Health geographers and historians are both interested in place and landscapes of health, although their source materials and methods differ. Archaeological investigations have provided a new take on the Neolithic Revolution, including the emergence and role of zoonotic diseases. Science, Technology, Society (STS) scholars show a great deal of interest in human–microbe interaction and human–animal interaction.

In the medical field, every now and then, voices are raised calling for more integrative ways to regard human disease and health. Integrative approaches often provide openings for interdisciplinary co-operation. One such effort was the biopsychosocial model, introduced in the 1970s by George Engel (1913–1999), an American internist and psychiatrist. Inspired by the system theoretical approach, Engel sought to challenge the prevailing biomedical reductionism and dualism and replace it with a model that explained disease with reference not only to the psyche *or* to the soma, but both, and also to the environment. Engel, and people inspired by his approach, usually perceive "the environment" as the social environment, although there is nothing in the model as such which precludes a broader interpretation of the environment.[24] A more recent integrative effort is the "One Health" approach, which stresses the need to view human health in relation to animal and plant health.[25] Other recent developments in medicine also call attention to the environment. The rise of epigenetics has highlighted the impact of environmental factors on human heredity and transgenerational health, and the study of human microbiome demonstrates the permeability of the boundary between humans and non-humans.

One further way in which the history of health and medicine and environmental history can balance and complement each other has more to do with their general disciplinary profiles or "styles" than with individual themes of interest. The history of medicine has its disciplinary roots in early twentieth-century medical schools, although it is now predominantly conducted outside medical faculties. Reflecting these historical origins, and despite critical self-reflection and forceful counterdiscourses since the 1980s, the historiography of medicine has sometimes carried teleological and progressivist, even celebratory, undertones. In contrast, environmental history came into being during and as a response to environmental crises and has been characterized as "declensionist."[26] Although environmental history is not all about decline and catastrophe, and medical history is not all about the triumphal procession of (modern) medicine, both still stand to gain from being confronted with a somewhat different take on the *longue durée*.

As the examples above show, environmental and health historians are often dealing with highly complex issues. When health and the environment are explored side by side, cultural, social and technological realms become enmeshed in biological and ecological realms, and vice versa. The concept of interaction emerges as the focus of attention instead of traditional causal determinism or understanding of the meanings linked to the goals: humans and their surroundings, culture and nature, human bodies and microorganisms are components of an intricate interplay process. Both parties are active agents, and the outcome of the action is difficult to predict, unlike the outcome of rule-based causal processes. Contingency, coincidence and chaos play a bigger role than when examining natural or cultural processes as such, separated from each other.[27]

In Pursuit of Healthy Environments: Historical Cases on the Environment–Health Nexus brings temporal depth to a highly topical issue: the interaction between health and the environment. By means of a rich set of historical case studies, the volume explores the changing relationship between health and the environment, and historically changing understandings of them and their interaction. It demonstrates that the concern for creating and finding healthy environments is not a new one, exemplifies how the link between the environment and health has been perceived at different times and in different cultures, and discusses the practical implications of these conceptualizations.

The book approaches the subject from three interrelated thematic angles. In Part I, Dolly Jørgensen, Michael Zeheter, Panagiotis Zestanakis and Heini Hakosalo contemplate how certain landscapes and ecosystems have come to be labelled as healthy and life-preserving while others have become stigmatized by death and disease, and how fluctuating these notions can be. The foci they investigate incorporate such dissimilar material embodiments of environment–health interconnections as medieval waste products, mineral water bottles, smog over Athens, and tuberculosis sanatoria.

In Part II, Marcel Hartwig, Ritva Kylli, Anu Soikkeli, Pirjo Kristiina Virtanen and Laura Pérez Gil trace the spatialities and materialities related to the conceptions of health and well-being and the practices of nurture and hygiene in colonial, as well as post-colonial environments. Their chapters, spanning from mid-eighteenth century colonial British America to mid-twentieth century Arctic Lapland to present-day Brazilian and Peruvian Amazonia, show how greatly indigenous and colonial and post-colonial mindsets have differed both conceptually and in practice.

Lastly, in Part III, Kalle Kananoja, Min Bae, Mikko Jauho, Petteri Pietikäinen and Otto Pipatti look at the formation of environmental and medical knowledge in different historical contexts. Their chapters shed light on the question of how medical and environmental knowledge has become interwoven and how this process has articulated visions of social futures, of both risk and benefit to society, from the mid-eighteenth century onwards.

Notes

1 See https://networks.h-net.org/h-envirohealth. Accessed 28 November 2019.
2 In April 2020, the two most read articles in *Environmental History* dealt with disease (polio and animal diseases in the 1870s, respectively). See https://academic.oup.com/envhis. Accessed 22 April 2020. The most-read article in *Medical History* handled lead poisoning and Bath water, i.e. environmental pollutants.
3 Gorsky and Berridge 2011.
4 Ruuskanen and Väyrynen 2017, 467.
5 Brimblecombe 1988.
6 Luckin 1986; Luckin 2015.
7 Mosley 2001.
8 Schneider 2011.
9 Thorsheim 2006.
10 Schneider 2011, xv–xvi.
11 Mosley 2001.
12 Bohme 2014.
13 van Horssen 2016.
14 Kiechle 2017.
15 Langston 2011.

16 Newman 2016.
17 Crosby 2004.
18 Kelton 2007; Kelton 2015.
19 Koch et al. 2019, 30.
20 There is no shortage of studies (and popular expositions) on the history of specific epidemic diseases, on specific outbreaks of contagious diseases, and on specific local and national responses to epidemic disease. Perhaps because of the vastness of the topic, it is more difficult to find studies on the general history of epidemics. Exceptions include Kiple 1993, Byrne 2008 and Snowden 2019. For a synoptic view on the intellectual history of epidemiology, see Susser and Stein 2009.
21 Rosen 2015 [1958]. Another general history is Dorothy Porter's *Health, Civilization and the State* (1999). *New Public Health,* a handbook now in its fourth edition, although not specifically historical, contains helpful insights into the history and development of the discipline (Baum 2016).
22 Foley 2010, 3.
23 Kisacky 2017, 167, 177.
24 Engel 1977. On Engel's influence in medicine, see Guillemin and Barnard 2015. On the historical context of his model, see Tanner 2019, 284–97.
25 Zinsstag, Jakob et al. 2015.
26 Fleming and Johnson 2014, ix.
27 Ruuskanen and Väyrynen 2017, 469–70.

Bibliography

Bohme, Susanna. 2014. *Toxic Injustice: A Transnational History of Exposure and Struggle*. Berkeley CA: California University Press.
Brimblecombe, Peter. 1988. *The Big Smoke: A History of Air Pollution in London since Medieval Times*. London: Methuen.
Baum, Fran, ed. 2016. *The New Public Health*. 4th edition. Oxford: Oxford University Press.
Byrne, J.P., ed. 2008. *Encyclopedia of Pestilence, Pandemics, and Plagues*. 2 vols. Westport, CT: Greenwood.
Crosby, Alfred. 2004 [1986]. *Ecological Imperialism: The Biological Expansion of Europe, 900–1900*. Studies in Environment and History. 2nd edition. New York: Cambridge University Press.
Engel, Georg. 1977. "The Need for a New Medical Model: A Challenge for Biomedical Science." *Science* 196: 126–29.
Fleming, James Rodger and Ann Johnson, eds. 2014. *Toxic Airs: Body, Place, Planet in Historical Perspective*. Pittsburgh: University of Pittsburgh Press.
Foley, Ronan. 2010. *Healing Waters: Therapeutic Landscapes in Historic and Contemporary Ireland*. Farnham, UK: Ashgate.
Gorsky, Martin and Virginia Berridge, eds. 2011. *Environment, Health and History*. Basingstoke: Palgrave Macmillan.
Guillemin, Marilys and Emma Barnard. 2015. "George Libman Engel: The Biopsychosocial Model and the Construction of Medical Practice." In *The Palgrave Handbook of Social Theory in Health, Illness and Medicine*, edited by Fran Collyer, 236–50. London: Palgrave Macmillan.

Horssen, Jessica van. 2016. *A Town Called Asbestos: Environmental Contamination, Health, and Resilience in a Resource Community*. Vancouver: UBC Press.

Kelton, Paul. 2007. *Epidemics and Enslavement: Biological Catastrophe in the Native Southeast, 1492–1715*. Lincoln: University of Nebraska Press.

Kelton, Paul. 2015. *Cherokee Medicine, Colonial Germs: An Indigenous Nation's Fight against Smallpox, 1518–1824*. Norman OK: University of Oklahoma Press.

Kiechle, Melanie. 2017. *Smell Detectives: An Olfactory History of Nineteenth-Century Urban America*. Seattle: University of Washington Press.

Kiple, K.F., ed. 1993. *The Cambridge World History of Human Disease*. Cambridge: Cambridge University Press.

Kisacky, Jeanne. 2017. *Rise of the Modern Hospital: An Architectural History of Health and Healing, 1870–1940*. University of Pittsburgh Press.

Koch, Alexander, Chris Brierley, Mark M. Maslin, and Simon L. Lewis. 2019. "Earth System Impacts of the European Arrival and Great Dying in the Americas after 1492." *Quaternary Science Reviews* 207: 13–36.

Langston, Nancy. 2011. *Toxic Bodies: Hormone Disruptors and the Legacy of DES*. New Haven: Yale University Press.

Luckin, Bill. 1986. *Pollution and Control: A Social History of the Thames in the Nineteenth Century*. London: CRC Press.

Luckin, Bill. 2015. *Death and Survival in Urban Britain: Disease, Pollution and Environment 1800–1950*. London: I.B. Tauris.

Mosley, Stephen. 2001. *The Chimney of the World: A History of Smoke Pollution in Victorian and Edwardian Manchester*. Cambridge: White Horse Press.

Newman, Richard. 2016. *Love Canal: A Toxic History from Colonial Times to the Present*. New York: Oxford University Press.

Rosen, George. 2015 [1958]. *A History of Public Health*. Revised and expanded edition. Baltimore: Johns Hopkins University Press.

Ruuskanen, Esa and Kari Väyrynen. 2017. "Theory and prospects of environmental history." *Rethinking History* 21(4): 456–73.

Schneider, Daniel. 2011. *Sewage Treatment and the Contradictions of the Industrial Ecosystem*. Cambridge, MA: MIT Press.

Snowden, Frank. 2019. *Epidemics and Society: From the Black Death to the Present*. Yale University Press.

Susser, Mervyn and Zena Stein. 2009. *Eras in Epidemiology. The Evolution of Ideas*. Oxford New York: University Press.

Tann, Jakob. 2019. "Die kontroverse Karriere der Kybernetik." In *Auf der Suche nach einer anderen Medizin. Psychosomatik im 20. Jahrhundert*, eds. Alexa Geisthövel and Bettina Hitzer. Berlin: Suhrkamp.

Thorsheim, Peter. 2006. *Inventing Pollution: Coal Smoke and Culture in Britain since 1800*. Athens, OH: Ohio University Press.

Voyles, Traci Brynne. 2015. *Wastelanding: Legacies of Uranium Mining in Navajo Country*. Minneapolis: University of Minnesota Press.

Zinsstag, Jakob, Esther Schelling, David Waltner-Toews, Maxine Whittaker and Marcel Tanner, eds. *One Health: The Theory and Practice of Integrated Health Approaches*. CABI, 2015.

Part I

Healthy and unhealthy environments

Chapter 1

Crafts and cleanliness

The regulation of noxious business activity in English towns during the fourteenth to sixteenth centuries

Dolly Jørgensen

Introduction

In their plan for cleaning the River Wensum in 1532, Norwich town council identified the businesses that should be charged more than the average resident for river cleaning operations because their trades had a more significant effect on the river's quality: "barkers, dyers, calaundrers, parchementmakers, tewers, sadelers, brewers, wasshers of shepe, and all suche great noyers of the same rever tobe ffurder charged than other persons shalbe...."[1] Twenty years later, Norwich town council reiterated their stance on polluting industries – "dyers, calendrers, tanners, glovers, parchemyn makers, brewers and encrochers of the river" – as annoyances in the town because of pollution.[2]

Norwich's list of polluters is quite comprehensive: textile manufacturing (launderers, washers of sheep skins, dyers), leather working (barkers, tawyers, saddlers, tanners, glovers, and parchment-makers) and brewers. These particular trades consumed significant quantities of water and often generated noxious wastes which contaminated water sources. *Noxious* here connotes both harmful and unpleasant which, as this chapter will show, was the case with these crafts' by-products. Norwich councilmen therefore felt justified in levying higher environmental taxes on these businesses. The Norwich lists provide a starting point for a more general inquiry into the environmental aspect of the relationship between late medieval/early modern business and boroughs in England.

Before delving into the sanitary controls placed onto these crafts, we need to recognize their importance in the premodern urban milieu. From English lists of taxpayers and citizens, historians have reconstructed the general employment scene in various cities.[3] A detailed study of Norwich's economy from 1275 to 1348 showed that almost half of the working population was in manufacturing, a quarter provided food and drink, 15% were merchants and traders and the remainder provided services, worked in the building trades, or were artists. Leather and cloth working were the largest manufacturing industries in Norwich.[4] Records for Coventry show a similar picture: of the 739 persons named in fourteenth- and early fifteenth-century records, there were 211 (29%) in the cloth trades, 132 (18%) merchants, 108 (15%) metal workers, 80 (11%) in the production of food and drink and 79 (11%) in leather and fur trades. The cloth trades, therefore, dominated the town economy, although metal and leather working were also significant. Members of the leading crafts were influential in local government: by 1450, the guilds of the drapers, dyers, smiths, shoemakers, and whittawers (white tanners) all had members who had held town offices.[5] Textile manufacturing in the late fourteenth century likewise dominated York, with about 28% of the freemen involved in the industry. It appears, however, that the textile crafts suffered decline and contraction in the fifteenth century.[6] These figures reveal the significance of crafts to the medieval urban economy. Of particular importance for this study, we see that cloth working, leatherworking, and victualing comprised high proportions of the working population in the English towns.

Location also plays an important role in the discussion of environmental effect of each industry. In the Middle Ages, businesses of the same type tended to be located together in specific parts of town. Modern streets with names such as Fishmongers Row and Shambles Street are legacies of this practice. Historians often identify where the different trades operated in some cities based on property records, naming evidence and archaeological finds.

The regulation of businesses for product quality is well-known to medieval historians. Local government officials actively monitored the freshness of meats and fish and the quality of goods such as cloth sold in the marketplace. Guilds, which organized the craftspeople, managed the output of their individual members to maintain industry standards. Guild regulations, which were approved and enacted by local authorities, covered the quality of input materials, the types of permitted processing, final goods standards, and labour organization. Governments monitored the production of food and drink to ensure the health and well-being of residents; butchers, for example, were often condemned in local ordinances for selling rotten meat.[7]

As this chapter will show, in addition to market-focused economic measures, local government also regulated craft businesses with an eye on their output to the environment that could have detrimental health effects. The trades listed in the Norwich documents – textile manufacturing, leather working, and brewing – were the target of environmental urban laws. Although industry was vital to the urban economy, premodern local governments were unwilling to overlook the environmental consequences of many craft operations. The authorities recognized potential polluters and created environmental laws to limit damage to both property and residents. The sections below present the environmental effects of each craft type called out in the Norwich list and identify the ways in which English local governments attempted to regulate their activities to promote cleanliness.

Textile manufacture

The technology of medieval textile manufacturing involved heavy use of water, which during the course of the processing steps, became contaminated with oils, fibres and bacteria. Textile manufacturers in northern Europe primarily worked with wool or linen (made from flax or hemp). Wool was prepared by carding (using a board with teeth to separate the fibres), spinning, weaving, and then fulling. In the fulling process, the wool cloth was trampled under-foot while submerged in water. The fuller added clay, known as fullers' earth, to the water to remove the wool oils and speed the matting process. Cloth was fulled in a tub of water or directly in a water body. The processing of flax and hemp included removing the seeds and soaking the steams in water (called "retting") to soften the fibre by bacterial action. After the stems were washed and dried, they were beaten and scraped to remove the outside fibres. After being woven, the linen cloth was washed again and then bleached in the sun.[8] Cloth preparation thus resulted in the release of oils, seeds, stems, and loose fibres to the water. In addition, the process of retting created foul-smelling, noxious effluent.[9]

Town governments identified these textile production outputs as a menace to cleanliness and acted to control this source of water pollution. In Norwich, a complaint against the Dutch and Walloon textile workers charged that they were cleaning their wool processing equipment on the banks of the river to "the greate infeccion of the same." In addition, the workers combed wool in their open shops and poured out the wash water from their shop floors into the gutters. Because the water contained combing fibres and the workers did not pour supplemental clean water into the gutter to wash the residue downstream, it "reasteth in the gutters and breade the greate infeccions ..."[10] Norwich council responded by banning the washing of wool equipment at the river and ordered that wool combing must not take place near the street. This kind of regulation was nothing new – according to the York Civic Ordinances of 1301, canvas and linen were not permitted in the gutters.[11] In addition, the Norwich regulations required the wool workers to throw out scouring water only at night and to cast additional clean water after it so that the wool particles and contaminated water would "passe to the cockeyes under the grownde withoute the hurte of anye parson."[12] Water pollution from cloth working was clearly identified in this passage as the cause of health problems.

Blocked water drains and washwater would become stagnant and create odours, which, at the time, were linked to disease.[13] Thus, local governments worked hard to maintain free-flowing waterways.[14] Although the flax and wool cloth-processing activities had economic benefits for the town, the councils were not willing to sacrifice sanitation to support the cloth industry. Because of Coventry's significant cloth working industry, retting in the River Sherbourne appears to have been enough of a problem that in 1554, the council ordered that no one was allowed to place any hemp or flax in the river.[15] They also banned the washing of cloth from looms at the drinking water conduit because this would have caused contamination of the drinking water source.[16] Common business practices in the textile industry required town council intervention.

Although the raw fabric itself had environmental consequences, the most visible and harmful effects of the textile process came from dyeing. Dyers could add colour at any stage in the process from raw material to finished cloth. Dyers primarily relied on cultivated plants, such as madder for red and woad for blue, to make their dyes. In order to fix most dyes to the cloth, the fibre had to be first dipped in a mordant, typically ferrous sulphate or alum. Woad required the addition of an alkali substance such as potash to make the dye soluble. The dye bath was typically heated in a cauldron and the cloth dipped into it.[17] The dyeing liquors were both caustic, because of the additives, and odoriferous, making them unpleasant to work with. A drawing in the fifteenth century Italian silk dyer's manual *Trattato dell' Arte della Seta* even shows a dyer pinching his nose while stirring a hot pot of red dye.[18] Because unpleasant organic smells were linked to disease and uncleanliness, dyeing was considered to create unhealthy air.

A significant water supply was necessary during the dyeing processes, leading most dyers to choose a location next to a stream or river. The water also needed to be relatively clean in order to avoid the introduction of impurities that could adversely affect the dyes, leading many dyers to position their businesses near the river's entrance into the town. Excavations in Norwich uncovered a complete fifteenth-century dyer's workshop on the banks of the River Wensum, including furnaces, hearths, a water storage pit and a drain to take effluent to the river.[19] Evidence from Norwich indicates that most of the dyers located their shops along the River Wensum northwest (and upstream) of the city centre. The street names in this section of town reveal the heavy emphasis on cloth production: Shearing Cross, Fullers' Hole, Maddermarket, etc. One group of dyers operated on a small tributary of the Wensum in the west section of town, while the fullers were located near the most central dyers on the river.

Coventry's dyers also located their shops near the river at the two far ends of town. The dyers' water supply came via wooden channels ("waterlades") from the river and tributary brooks, but this posed a problem because the channels blocked the watercourse and increased the threat of flooding. The council ordered dyers to remove their waterlades unless the mayor and the council granted an easement for the channel and the dyer paid a yearly fee. Even the permitted waterlades had to be drawn up every night in order to avoid the "perell of ffloodes fallyng in nyghttyme."[20]

Because the dyers' shops were located upstream of the city centre in order to procure clean river water for their process, any wastes they subsequently ejected into the water would make its way downstream. Cloth processing generated solid and liquid refuse (cinders, paste, alkaline water, grease, etc.)

which required disposal. Dyers often appear to have disposed of corrosive waste dye liquids from the dye-vats and cinders from the heating operations into the river. According to archaeological finds in Bristol, England, dyers apparently dumped madder and weld at the wharf in fourteenth century.[21] These dyes probably discoloured the water where the material was dumped. Visible signs of pollution (colour and particulate matter in the water) as well as the effect on the taste of the water may have concerned residents and the councilmen. Cities attempted to deal with this issue by regulating where dyers could dispose of their waste. For example, in 1421, Coventry's mayor commanded that no dyer put fat or filth in the river.[22] This regulation of dyer waste was part of a series of medieval environmental laws in the Mayor's Proclamation, alongside restrictions on sweeping the streets while it was raining to get rid of waste, throwing filth into the local river, and disposing of waste in the town ditch.

Court records of Norwich show that improper dyer waste disposal was punished: the local court fined three dyers in 1390–91 for inappropriate disposal of craft wastes. First, they fined John Wake 20s. for throwing cinders, paste, and other dyer wastes into the river. Second, they found John Long guilty of placing muck, cinders and other refuse by the stakes on the banks of the river. He was fined 6s.8d. Third, the court fined another dyer, John Lymmes, 2s. for disposing of muck and paste in the road under the wall of St. Martin's churchyard.[23] The entries in the Norwich court records indicate that the government treated the disposal dyer craft waste similarly to other solid wastes. When dyers threw these solid (cinders) and semi-solid (paste) wastes from the dyeing process into the river or the streets, the court officials fined them. Officials demanded that craftspeople managed their waste to minimize uncleanliness.

In Nottingham, it appears that the biggest problem was the dumping of liquid and semi-liquid wastes from the dye vats into the streets and gutters. In the court records of Nottingham for 1395, a jury found that all the dyers of the town, naming specifically the seven worst culprits, "stifle the common people with the stench from the residues of their waters dropping and falling on the King's highway." The jury said that dye waters caused "corruption of the whole people passing."[24] In 1407, the same jury found Robert Chesterfield guilty of injuring "the neighbors with dye-water."[25] Robert had been one of the offending dyers named in 1395, indicating that although he had been previously warned and fined he continued the practice. Robert likely did not modify his behaviour both because of both the real need to get rid of the water somewhere and the convenience of the street gutters. Other named offenders in 1395, however, do not show up again, meaning that they may have found alternate disposal methods (probably discharging the dye water directly into the river instead of the street). In 1512, a little over 100 years later, four dyers were again fined for causing uncleanliness: "for corupte water of ther occupacion corrupting the stretes."[26] These court records demonstrate that dyer waste was considered to be a health hazard, something which "corrupted" the air with stenches that directly affected passers-by. The town governments thus diligently attempted to control the disposal of those wastes in order to promote town cleanliness.

Leather working

The second group of craftsmen that local governments considered to be an environmental hazard worked with hides. Leather, the preserved hides of animals, was one of the primary materials used for medieval clothing, animal harnesses and military equipment. In order to make animal hides durable, leather creation included numerous chemical and biological processes, most of which generated noxious by-products.

The first step was to clean the hides of blood, dung, and salt left over from the butchering process. The tanner then allowed the hairs on the skin to rot, sometimes sprinkling the hair side with urine or soaking the skins in lime in order to loosen the hairs for removal. After the hairs were removed, the tanner treated the skins to make them flexible. This was done either through alkaline bating, which involved immersion in bird guano or dog dung, or acidic drenching, which required treatment in fermenting barley or rye. After all this preparatory work, the hides were tanned in a liquor typically made from oak bark. Hides often stayed in the tanning liquor for a year before removal and final washing. The tawyer followed a similar process of preparing hides except that, instead of using oak bark, the tawyer treated the skins with a paste of alum and oil.[27] Tanning and tawying were foul-smelling processes that required hazardous strong acidic or basic liquors. The fluids included ingredients such as lime, dung, urine, and one-year-old soaked oak bark. No wonder tanning was considered an environmental danger!

Like dyeing, the tanning process required significant amounts of water and generated highly noxious effluent. For this reason, most tanneries were located on a river or stream, although some may have used well water. Just as in the case of dyers, tanners needed clean incoming water to create their tanning liquors and wash skins. A study of the property owners in fourteenth-century Norwich shows that tanners operated on several of the river tributaries (cockeys) upstream of the town centre, mainly on the opposite side of the river.[28] By being located across the river, the tanners minimized the nuisance created by smells from the tanning process, but their upstream location also meant that all wastewater would flow right through the central urban area. The location of this main group of Norwich tanneries made their by-products and impact on the river visible to the town's inhabitants. Two other groups of tanners were located on cockeys downstream of the urban centre, so they would not have caused such obvious problems.

In Coventry, tanning operations took place on the west side of town just outside the walls. Two groups of tanners have been identified in the records: one on Well Street near Radford Brook (the tributary entering the Sherbourne from the north) and the other on Spon Street near the Sherbourne River. Just as in Norwich, the Coventry tanners, were located upstream of the city centre in order to get clean water for their process. It appears that some skinners used water from the town's drinking water supply system instead of the river. According to a property lease of 1564, four skinners leased four washing houses, called "the Skyners houses," and obtained permission to use water supplied via the town conduit system for washing skins.[29]

In the processing steps, wastewater contaminated with blood, pieces of flesh, lime, and tannins would require disposal and this would all flow downstream. The town residents would have sensed the physical contamination from tanning operations – the water stank, it tasted strange, and discarded flesh and fat floated on top of it. Some local governments found that they needed to control these industrial pollutants because of downstream uses of the water, particularly in food preparation.

In York, the contamination of water by the tanning crafts came to the fore. The York government issued legislation aimed at tanners several times. York's leatherworking industry followed the same pattern as Norwich and Coventry: tanners located their shops upstream of the city centre, in this case on the Ouse River near its entrance into the town. The placement of the tanners in this part of town is also attested by the name of the street Tanners Row and the fact that the tanners' guild leased a large piece of land in the area.[30] The river turned out to be a convenient resource for tanners – they began washing skins directly in the river. This activity was expressly forbidden by the council because of concerns that it would cause food contamination. The York council forbade tanners from washing skins between the waterfront monastic property and a pier where butchers washed entrails, as well as any place on either side of the river where water was drawn for brewing or baking.[31] The pier was known as The Pudding Holes – it served as a public washing place where, among other things, the entrails of beasts used to make black pudding were cleaned (thus the source of its name). The local government therefore determined that it was important to keep the water at Pudding Holes clean.[32] York's council stated that tanners were not to lie, cast, or wash limed skins or leather in the water above Pudding Holes because of "corrupcion of the water of Ouse."[33] The problem with this mandate was that the tanners had deliberately located themselves upstream in order to obtain clean water. By forcing them downstream of Pudding Holes, they would have to be located downstream of the city centre. It is interesting to note, however, that saddlers and skinners appeared to have already been located downstream of the bridge. These restrictions clearly demonstrate that York council recognized that washing leather contaminated the water, making it unfit for use in food or drink preparation. The council sought to render the water safe for consumption through its control of the leatherworking industry.

Parchment-makers posed the same environmental problems as tanners. The parchmenter first thoroughly washed skins bought from a butcher and, following the same practice as tanners, let the hide rot so that the hair could be removed. But instead of tanning the hide, the parchmenter stretched the skin over a frame and allowed it to dry. He then vigorously scraped the hide, generating a pile of shavings, to create parchment often as thin as tissue paper. The parchment-maker's process thus created dirty water, hair, and scrapings which required disposal.[34] Because these wastes are quite similar to the tanners, it is easy to see why the Norwich council identified parchmenters and tanners as river polluters.

Norwich's list of troublesome trades also included two leather-working trades: glovers and saddlers. These trades could also create water pollution. Glovers and saddlers moulded leather supplied by tanners. In order to work the leather into objects such as armour and saddles, the material was soaked in cold water until thoroughly saturated. This allowed the leather to be moulded and decorated by stamping or punching. After completing the ornamentation of the leather surface, the leatherworker often decorated the object with stain, dyes or tempera paint.[35] The guild ordinances of Worchester, England issued in 1467, specifically restricted the leather-dressing activities of saddlers and glovers in the local river: the workers were required to shave and wash skins in very specific places and they were not to cast animal waste into the river.[36] The craftsmen in these trades clearly shaved and washed leather, generating scrap flesh and contaminated water, and therefore, these activities needed to be limited to certain areas of the water course.

Overall, tanning businesses posed a paradoxical problem for local officials concerned about the environment. Tanning operations required significant amounts of relatively clean water to produce well-tanned leather. This meant that tanners preferred to locate upstream of the city centre. Yet the process also generated noxious wastewaters which required disposal. Since contaminated water (whether generated in tanning vats or from direct contact with skins washed in the river) would have to enter the main watercourse, local officials wanted this activity downstream of other industries requiring clean water, particularly food services, as seen in the case of York. There was thus a tension between the needs of industry and those of urban residents who wanted clean water.

Brewing

Brewers were the last of the three groups of craftsmen mentioned in the Norwich document as posing problems for the river water. Brewing generated some semi-solid waste. After the fermentation process, impurities and unprocessed vegetable matter remained in the beer. To collect this matter, medieval brewers hung bags filled with items that would attract the residue, including oxen and pigs' feet, fish membranes, and oak bark. In addition, the brewer could filter the beer to remove the dregs. Straw was often used as a filter and became impregnated with yeast.[37]

Brewers' waste materials required disposal and it is possible that the Norwich mention of brewers as causing environmental problems refers to their waste disposal practices. Yet, specific entries dealing with pollution from brewers are rare. One of the few is a record of a beer brewer in Lincoln named Hodshone, who was also an elected alderman of the town, being fined for allowing his brewing waste to flow into the river in 1584.[38] The court record noted that both his craft wastes and dung from his pigsty was entering the river.

This connection of brewers with pigs is not incidental. Brewers dregs made good fodder for swine. A Northampton ordinance from 1549 singled out brewers and bakers as owning many swine – they were permitted to send six pigs out with the common swineherd, whereas others were allowed only four.[39] Keeping pigs meant that brewers would have raised them in backyard pens. In the court records of Ramsey, brewers were fined several times for having pigsties that did not meet the town's cleanliness standards or allowing pigs to run loose.[40]

The most regulated part of the brewer's craft was its main ingredient: water. As might be expected, town governments demanded that brewers produce beer that was clean. In 1305, the brewers of Oxford were told to draw water only from places where the water was fresh and pure, rather than using water collected near sewers, which had been the practice previously. This dirty water subsequently made the beer "not as wholesome and as nourishing as it ought to be" and was a "detriment to health."[41] The beer brewers of Northampton were likewise ordered to only sell beer that was "wholesome for a man's body."[42]

Acquiring clean water could, however, come into conflict with other uses for the water. This happened in Coventry, who turned to regulating brewers' use of drinking water. Coventry inhabitants obtained drinking water from underground sources because the local surface water was not potable.[43] In the Middle Ages, Coventry had an extensive network of water conduits to distribute well water. The town government and local philanthropists invested significant funds in the conduits and intended the water for personal use. In 1444, the Coventry council issued the first restriction against industrial use of the conduits in the records, stipulating that brewers could not use the water for brewing, but only to prepare food. The mayor and the warden split the fine of 40d. (3s. 2d.).[44] The ban on brewers was reissued several times over a span of 100 years and the fine was eventually raised to 20s. beginning in 1497.[45] Brewers wanted to use the water to steep the barley, but this was not permitted without a special licence. In 1493, the council made a list of all brewers permitted to use conduit water for brewing and steeping because they paid annually to the conduit repair fund. Each of them paid a fee of 6s. 8d., which had been mandated in 1483. Two persons paid double the normal rate (13s. 4d.), which might mean that they used twice as much water as normal brewers.[46] However, according to a 1450 proclamation, the council did permit brewers and malters to use conduit water for the dressing of mead.[47] Coventry's restrictions on the use of conduit water in the brewing process shows that crafts and cleanliness required oversight. The government had invested significant amounts to supply the population with drinking water and although brewers required water for making beer, drinking water superceded brewers' needs.

Conclusion

Medieval crafts such as dyeing, tanning and brewing were the backbone of the urban economy, but the environmental consequences of many craft operations could not be overlooked. Even in the Middle Ages, authorities recognized potential polluters and created environmental laws to limit their effect on property and persons. In spite of the economic importance of these crafts, councils expressed concerns about the water contamination associated with them. To combat these detrimental practices, the councils issued legislation specifying where certain crafts could take place and where they were forbidden, and how their waste products should be disposed of. This chapter has demonstrated the active involvement of English town governments in pursuing healthy environments by regulating urban craft operations from the fourteenth to the sixteenth centuries.

As the craft descriptions reveal, the physical environmental damage of many medieval crafting businesses was highly visible and odoriferous. The most regulated trades of cloth and leatherworking had this trait in common: they generated large quantities of pungent waste products, whether liquid or solid, that required disposal either directly into water bodies or onto the land. These noxious materials, both unpleasant and harmful to health, were targeted by the town authorities. This means that crafts which generate non-odoriferous wastes, including metalworkers and building trades such as brick makers, masons, and glass workers, were considered to be clean. Modern science tells us that metal waste is, in fact, highly toxic especially through ingestion, but because metal wastes are non-volatile and disposed of in onsite pits, they were neither as visible nor as smelly as the wastes generated by tanners, dyers, and brewers. Visibility and odour, then, were key factors in English urban environmental law.

Notes

1   Hudson and Tingey 1906, vol. 2, 115–16. Much of the content of this chapter was explored earlier in my unpublished PhD dissertation (Jørgensen 2008).
2   Hudson and Tingey 1906, vol. 2, 129.

3 This is a notoriously labor-intensive and difficult process. Many of the reconstructions are made by looking through property transactions, city tax lists and other city council records for persons with identified trades. The problem with such an approach is that we typically get only property holders or free citizens in the records. Even the most complete records, we only have a listing of 10–15% of the urban population. Women (when not identified in a trade), children and the elderly are absent from the counts. In addition, non-citizens, including servants and apprentices, are typically not included. Because almost all households had at least one servant and most craftsmen had at least one apprentice, these populations are quite significant. However, these figures still give an indication of the relative importance of different trades in the medieval city.

4 Rutledge 2004, 160.

5 Stephens 1969, 151–57. The occupational structure is confirmed in a list of crafts and their members (603 persons) contributing armour for the defence of the city in 1450: 40% cloth industry, 20% metal, 14% leather and fur, and 10% food and drink.

6 Tillot 1961, 84–91.

7 See, for example, the discussion of guilds in Tillott 1961, 91–97 and in Stephens 1969, 157–62.

8 Description of cloth working processes from Walton 1991, 319–54.

9 This is because the bacterial concentrations lowered the dissolved oxygen content in the water, creating a situation similar to a stagnant pool where algae grow. There has been some archeological work into water contamination, or lack thereof, associated with retting. Mark Robinson found that flax retting in Saxon times did not cause significant water pollution in the Rivers Nene and Thames. However, he notes that these are larger water bodies with significant flow and smaller channels would have been more severely affected. See Robinson 2003, 141–42.

10 Hudson and Tingey 1906, 335.

11 Prestwich 1976, 1301.

12 Hudson and Tingey 1906, 335–36.

13 I explore the link in the Middle Ages between odours of waste and ideas of cleanliness in a forthcoming chapter: Jørgensen, "Environment. Managing urban sanitation for sanitas."

14 For a discussion of town river management to keep the waterways clear of waste and silt in the period, see Jørgensen 2010.

15 Harris 1907–13, pt. 3, 810–11.

16 Ibid., pt. 2, 338.

17 Description of dyeing processes from Walton 1991.

18 The image is in the manuscript Plut. 89 sup. Cod. 117, Biblioteca Laurenziana which has been printed as a facsimile in *Trattato dell'arte della seta in Firenze*.

19 Ayers 2006, 32.

20 Harris 1907–13, pt. 1, 28 and 31–32.

21 Walton 1991, 337.

22 Harris 1907–13, pt. 1, 32.

23 Hudson 1892, 70, 73, and 75. In the first case, the court specifically identified these wastes as being from his craft, "de arte sua." Fines are given in shillings (s.) and pence (d.); there are 12 pence in a shilling.

24 Markham 1898, Roll of Presentments of the Mickletorn Jury, 275 and 273. The entry on page 273 was a general finding of fault with all dyers for "ejection of

the waters of their art." This finding was actually stricken from the roll because of the later entry which named specific individuals.

25 Stephenson, vol. 2, Roll of Presentments of the Mickletorn Jury, 41. Later Nottingham collected a 4 pence fine from the dyer John Hawys for disposing of water in the street in 1512: Stephenson, vol. 3, 339.
26 Stephenson 1885, vol. 3, 339.
27 Description of tannery process from Cherry 1991, 295–318.
28 Tannery locations from diagram in Rutledge 2004, 162.
29 Coventry City Archives, BA/C/12/1/4, 24 February 1564.
30 Attreed 1991, 31–33.
31 Sellers 1991 and 1915, 15.
32 Raine 1955, 224–25. York's council also required fish cleaning to take place down-stream of Pudding Holes rather than above it in 1580 and forbade the disposal of dung and filth at the location. Interestingly, Coventry had a quite different problem with washing entrails for pudding. In that case, butchers had been washing entrails in the conduit water reserved for drinking. The council outlawed the practice and set a 40d. fine for violators. See Harris 1907–13, pt. 1, 208.
33 Sellers 1991 and 1915, Part II, 247.
34 de Hamel 1992, 8–12.
35 Cherry 1991, 304.
36 Smith 1870, Section LI. The ordinance also applied to butchers and bakers. It is interesting to note that tanners are not listed, so the saddlers and glovers may have been performing some or all of the tanning processes as well as working the leather into final goods.
37 Unger 2004, 151–52.
38 Historical Manuscripts Commission, *The Manuscripts of Lincoln*, 69.
39 Markham 1898, Vol. 1, 341.
40 DeWindt 2009, entries in 1335, 1358, and 1459.
41 Salter 1920, 11.
42 Markham 1898, Vol. 1, 347.
43 Lapworth 1925.
44 Harris 1907–13, pt. 1, 208
45 Ibid., pt. 1, 232 and 255; pt. 2, 338 and 517; pt. 3, 584, 788, 808–9 and 812.
46 Ibid., pt. 2, 548–549.
47 Ibid., pt. 1, 255. Reiterated in 1497: pt. 3, 584.

Bibliography

Attreed, Lorraine C., ed. 1991. *The York House Books 1461–1490*, 2 vols. Wolfeboro Falls, NH: Alan Sutton.
Ayers, Brian. 2006. "Craft Industry in Norwich from the 12th to the 18th century." In *Lübecker Kolloquium zur Stadtarchäologie im Hanseraum V: Das Handwerk*, edited by Manfred Gläser, 27–46. Lübeck: Schmidt-Römhild.
Cherry, John. 1991. "Leather." In *English Medieval Industries*, edited by John Blair and Nigel Ramsay, 295–318. London and New York: Hambledon and London.
de Hamel, Christopher. *Scribes and Illuminators*. Toronto: University of Toronto Press, 1992.

DeWindt, Edwin Brezette, ed. 2009. *The Court Rolls of Ramsey, Hepmangrove and Bury, 1258–1600*. Ann Arbor, MI: MPublishing, University of Michigan Library.

Harris, Mary Dormer, ed. 1907–1913. *The Coventry Leet Book: or Mayor's Register, Containing the Records of the City Court Leet or View of Frankpledge, A.D. 1420– 1555, with Divers other Matters*, 4 parts. London: Kegan Paul, Trench, Trübner & Co.

Historical Manuscripts Commission. 1895. *The Manuscripts of Lincoln, Bury St. Edmund's and Great Grimsby Corporations*. London, HMSO.

Hudson, W., ed. 1892. *Leet Jurisdiction in the City of Norwich During the XIIIth and XIVth Centuries*. London: Bernard Quaritch.

Hudson, W. and J.C. Tingey, eds. 1906, 1910. *The Records of the City of Norwich*, 2 vols. London: Jarrold & Sons.

Jørgensen, Dolly. "Environment. Managing Urban Sanitation for Sanitas." In *A Cultural History of Medicine in the Middle Ages*, edited by Iona McCleery. London: Bloomsbury Academic, forthcoming.

Jørgensen, Dolly. 2010. "Local government responses to urban river pollution in late medieval England." *Water History* 2(1): 35–52.

Jørgensen, Dolly [Dolores]. 2008. "Private Need, Public Order: Urban Sanitation in Late Medieval England and Scandinavia." Unpublished PhD dissertation. University of Virginia.

Lapworth, Herbert. "City of Coventry, Report on Water Supply," 12 November 1925, presented to the Chairman and Members of the Waterworks Committee of the Council of the City of Coventry, City of Coventry Archives.

Markham, Christopher A., ed. 1898. *The Records of the Borough of Northampton*, vol. 1. Northampton: Corporation of the County Borough of Northampton.

Prestwich, Michael. 1976. *York Civic Ordinances, 1301*. Borthwick Papers, No. 49. York: University of York.

Raine, Angelo. 1955. *Medieval York: A Topographical Survey Based on Original Sources*. London: John Murray.

Robinson, Mark. 2003. "Saxon Flax Retting in River Channels and the Apparent Lack of Water Pollution." In *The Environmental Archaeology of Industry*, edited by Peter Murphy and Patricia E.J. Wiltshire, 141–42. Oxford: Oxbow Books.

Rutledge, Elizabeth. 2004. "Economic Life." In *Medieval Norwich*, edited by Carole Rawcliffe and Richard Wilson, 157–88. London: Hambledon and London.

Salter, H.E., ed. 1920. *Munimenta Civitatis Oxonie*. Devizes: George Simpson & Co.

Sellers, Maud, ed. 1912, 1915. *York Memorandum Book, lettered A/Y in the Guidhall Muniment Room*, 2 parts. Durham, UK: Andrews & Co.

Smith, Joshua Toulmin, ed. 1870. *English gilds: the original ordinances of more than one hundred early English gilds: together with The olde Usages of the cite of Wynchestre; the Ordinances of Worcester; the Office of the Mayor of Bristol; and the Costomary of the Manor of Tettenhall-Regis: from manuscripts of the fourteenth and fifteenth centuries*. London: Published for the Early English Text Society by the Oxford University Press.

Stephens, W.B., ed. 1969. *A History of the County of Warwick, volume 8: The City of Coventry and Borough of Warwick*. London: Victoria County History.

Stephenson, W.H., ed. 1882–1885. *Records of the Borough of Nottingham being a series of extracts from the archives of the corporation of Nottingham*, vols 1–3. Nottingham: Corporation of Nottingham.

Tillott, P.M., ed. 1961. *A History of the County of Yorkshire: The City of York.* London: Victoria County History.

Trattato dell'arte della seta in Firenze, vol. 1. 1980. Florence: Cassa di risparmio di Firenze.

Unger, Richard. 2004. *Beer in the Middle Ages and the Renaissance.* Philadelphia: University of Pennsylvania Press.

Walton, Penelope. 1991. "Textiles." In *English Medieval Industries*, edited by John Blair and Nigel Ramsay, 319–54. London and New York: Hambledon and London.

Chapter 2

Healthy nature in a bottle?

The contested naturalness of mineral water

Michael Zeheter

Introduction

If Europeans buy and drink bottled water today, the chance is very high that they are consuming natural mineral water. According to the European Federation of Bottled Waters, the federation of the continent's trade associations, in the middle of the 2010s 83 per cent of the 52 billion litres of packaged water consumed in the European Union were natural mineral water.[1] This is an enormous market share, especially when considering the fact that the actual differences between different types of bottled water are actually quite small. If it is labelled "natural mineral water", "spring water" or "table water", the product invariably contains more than 99 per cent H_2O plus miniscule amounts of minerals, trace elements and sometimes dissolved gas.

Why do European consumers prefer one type of bottled water to another and what characteristics make natural mineral water preferable in their eyes? It is quite difficult to give a general answer to this question due to a lack of available consumer surveys covering Europe as a whole. There are, however, some market research reports that can give us some hints. In Germany, market research conducted by several firms for the *Verband Deutscher Mineralbrunnen*, the German trade association of natural mineral water producers, has consistently shown that consumers perceive mineral water as a healthy and natural product. Both these characteristics are closely connected in the eyes of those German consumers who were interviewed. They think that mineral water is healthy because it contains valuable minerals but no calories, and that, crucially, those minerals have not been put into the water using an industrial process. In the eyes of German consumers, natural mineral water is a special product because it is pristine.[2]

This image of mineral water as a naturally healthy beverage is, of course, not accidental. Producers have emphasized both characteristics consistently for decades. Advertisements in Germany, France, Switzerland and many other countries show mineral water as originating in a natural landscape untouched by human influence; mineral water has been provided by Mother Nature's specifically for the benefit of humankind.[3] According to this image, the producers of mineral waters are barely involved facilitators, who only provide access to this natural resource.

This image of mineral water as a pure, natural and healthy product is, of course, not uncontested. Everyone who has had the opportunity to visit a bottling facility can testify to the highly engineered way in which producers turn ground water into a commodity. The bottled water business is a highly profitable global industry with detrimental effects on the environment and in some instances on local societies. The list of issues that journalists, academics as well as environmental and social justice activists across the globe have raised is long. This includes the exploitation of a public resource by private for-profit companies, the denigration of the quality of tap water by the bottled water industry, the difference in price between bottled and tap water and the fuel used to transport bottled water from its source to the consumer.[4]

The most prominent issue, however, is probably the packaging in the form of convenient, yet disposable, PET bottles. From their production from petroleum, the alleged contamination of their contents with dangerous hormones, to the pollution of land and sea after consumption in the absence of effective recycling systems in large parts of the world, water bottles have become a symbol for the excesses of global capitalism.[5] While critics rarely make an explicit distinction between mineral and other kinds of bottled water, Europe's mineral water industry has to deal with the same allegations as the global bottled water industry, using public relations campaigns to establish a more favourable counter-narrative. This is apparently successful. Despite all the environmental concerns, consumers continue to buy and drink bottled water across the globe, including mineral water in Europe.[6]

It is not just the packaging and other environmental issues that are casting doubt on the naturalness of mineral water. The water itself is not necessarily as pristine as the advertising might suggest. According to the European Community's Directive 80/777/EEC, which in 1980 defined natural mineral water for the first time for all the Member States and is the legal foundation for the product category across the continent to this day, producers can legally manipulate natural mineral waters. Article 4, section 1 clearly states "that unstable elements, such as iron and sulphur" can be removed and that the content of carbon dioxide can be reduced or increased. The directive, however, explicitly prohibits other forms of manipulation such as antibacterial sterilization.[7] If some forms of manipulation conform to the label "natural" while others do not, this poses the question what the label "natural" actually means and how the criteria for distinguishing "natural" and "artificial" mineral waters developed.

A gift of nature reproduced?

The idea that mineral waters are a gift from Nature – or God – is not new, but a recurring theme that can be traced through the centuries. Since the resurgence of balneology as a form of medical treatment in the Renaissance, medical practitioners have stressed humankind's good fortune that such a powerful and beneficial remedy was readily available for all who could be bothered to come to Europe's many thermal or highly mineralized springs. While the dominant form of consumption of those waters changed over the course of the early modern age – from bathing in thermal waters over bathing in cold mineralized waters to drinking cold or (more rarely) hot mineralized waters – the notion of the special healing properties bestowed by nature on a limited number of springs remained an important and convincing argument.[8] Spa towns across the continent employed it to attract visitors with increasing success. Especially during the nineteenth century, taking the waters at one of the prominent spas became a common way for the upper and middle classes to improve their health and spend a few pleasant weeks away from daily business. Thus, in the middle of the nineteenth century, hundreds of thousands of Europeans travelled each spring and summer to one of the many spa towns to enjoy the medical benefits of their naturally healthy waters and the beautiful natural landscapes in which they were located.[9]

From the late seventeenth century onwards, the medical properties of mineral waters increasingly fascinated not only balneologists but also chemists. For the emerging science of chemistry, mineral waters were a particularly intriguing subject of research. How could solid particles be solved in a translucent liquid or how gases were contained in a liquid and under which circumstances they were released fascinated generations of chemists who developed new methods of analysis in order to study and better understand those phenomena.[10] During the eighteenth century, the question also arose if it was possible to emulate natural mineral waters in the laboratory. By the end of the century, chemists had achieved such a level of progress in this regard that it became increasingly difficult to discern between natural and artificial mineral waters using laboratory tests. Subsequent improvements in production processes made viable the mass production of artificial mineral waters in the first decades of the nineteenth century.[11]

The entrepreneur who used this new technology in the most successful way was probably Friedrich Adolph August Struve, a Saxon physician and apothecary who perfected the production of artificial mineral waters on a larger scale. He managed to reproduce exact copies of the waters of some Europe's most famous spa towns such as Vichy, Spa, Carlsbad, Marienbad, Pyrmont, Ems or Selters and sold them to eager customers at his drinking pavilions. From his headquarters in Dresden, Struve established drinking pavilions in major European cities such as Berlin, Cologne, Moscow, Riga and Saint Petersburg, and in the fashionable seaside resort of Brighton in the United Kingdom. His targeted customers, the urban upper middle class, could thus enjoy the taste and health benefits of some of the most celebrated medicinal waters of Europe at a much cheaper price, out of season and without the inconvenience of travelling great distances.[12]

Struve was not alone, but he was the most celebrated and successful producer of artificial mineral waters for medical purposes. During the nineteenth century, dozens of producers of artificial mineral waters established businesses in big cities and small towns.[13] The emergence of artificial mineral waters was not a major threat to the spa town's business success and social standing. People visited them for medical reasons, but there were other cultural and social incentives to go there that Struve's pavilions could not provide. The situation was far more serious for those spa towns who bottled their product and shipped it to urban customers. In the first half of the nineteenth century, numerous medicinal waters were available in larger cities. Patients who were unwilling or unable to travel to a spa town or wanted to continue their drinking cure beyond the traditional spring and summer season could find an adequate alternative in pharmacies or in certain merchants.[14]

For those bottlers of natural mineral waters, the emergence of an alternative on the urban markets was of great concern for two reasons. First, it was far cheaper to produce artificial mineral waters at the place of consumption than to transport them over long distances. Second, the reputation of many bottled natural mineral waters suffered from the perception that the bottling process and the lengthy transportation process diminished their medical efficiency, the latter point especially was a serious threat to the bottlers' business. Even if they could claim that their natural product was superior at the spring, it was far more difficult to argue the same at the place of consumption. There, those depleted natural mineral waters faced competition from freshly prepared artificial mineral waters that claimed to be exact copies, but of the original state at the source. Thus, producers of artificial waters offered an alternative that promised the identical medical benefits, but with better therapeutic effects and at a lower price.[15]

What followed was a long and protracted debate among experts about the respective virtues of artificial and natural mineral waters. Proponents of the superiority of natural mineral waters made two different arguments to support their opinion. First, they claimed that the artificial imitations of natural mineral waters were not as accurate as their producers claimed. Either they had missed out some minerals or had neglected the particular circumstances of the waters' genesis such as temperature, pressure, magnetism or – in the late nineteenth or early twentieth century – radioactivity. While they did not deny that artificial waters could have some therapeutic value, they insisted on the clear superiority of natural waters.[16] The second argument was based on the long-established assertion that they had a special quality that made them more than the sum of their chemical parts. This mysterious property distinguished natural mineral waters which had medicinal effects from simple ground water, which also happened to contain some minerals and gases, or from the even more mineralized seawater. The intangible quality of natural mineral waters was the contribution of nature, a certain characteristic of a water's place of origin that was impossible to reproduce in a laboratory or factory.[17]

The producers tried to counter this argument with experiments and observation. Struve, for example, did concede that imperfect copies of medicinal waters could have negative consequences for the drinker. Therefore, it was vital to restrict these reproductions not only to the dominant chemical contents, but to also pay attention to those that appeared only in minor concentration. Only if the reproduction was accurate, could an artificial water have the desired effect. The evidence that they indeed materialized, was collected by observing the effects of those artificial waters on patients who underwent a drinking cure. Well-known physicians and professors of medicine observed their patients' reactions to the artificial waters and recorded them for Struve. They concluded that the medical effect of his artificial waters showed no discernible difference from natural waters.[18]

Since neither side of the argument was able to produce any overwhelming evidence for their position, the dispute continued throughout the nineteenth and into the twentieth century.[19] In the end, it lost its urgency due to the decreased importance of the drinking cure as medical practice during the last decades of the nineteenth century. By this time, the dispute about the superiority of natural mineral waters had shifted to another arena due to a change in consumer preference.

Regulating and classifying bottled water

During the final third of the nineteenth century, there was a remarkable shift in the consumption of mineral waters. While the drinking cure for medical purposes was still of great importance for the numerous European spa towns, the public increasingly developed a taste for lightly mineralized waters. They were no longer consumed primarily for medical purposes, but as a healthy and refreshing beverage in restaurants, cafés, at refreshment stands or at home. Thus, mineral water found a place both at the table, accompanying wine or food, and as part of mixed drinks such as whisky soda.[20]

The highly mineralized waters of most spa towns had far too intense a taste to be fit for those purposes. For the producers of artificial mineral waters it was easy to satisfy this new demand. The production process was identical and required only an adjustment of the amounts of carbon dioxide and minerals. Combined with improvements in the bottling process such as the mass manufacturing of glass bottles, bottling machines and bottle washing machines, producers of artificial mineral waters started to cater to the urban mass market at a price that was also affordable for the lower middle and working classes. If required, producers could easily adjust the recipe for water according to the customers' wishes; they quickly discovered that there was also a lucrative mass market for lemonade, ginger ale and tonic water. Artificial mineral waters became so successful in the United Kingdom and Germany, that the term "mineral water" was increasingly associated with their product, not with the natural medicinal waters consumed in the spa towns.[21]

For the producers of bottled natural mineral waters this shift was a challenge as well as an opportunity. If they wanted to compete with artificial mineral waters, they had to offer a product that would satisfy the consumers' expectations in terms of both taste and price. The traditional spa towns could not compete in either department, as a large and noisy steam-powered bottling facility would have compromised their function as a leisure and health resort. They continued to confine themselves to the relatively small market of natural medicinal waters for which patients would be happy to pay a higher price.[22]

From the 1870s onwards, a host of new producers of natural mineral waters emerged to fill the niche in the market that the established spa towns could not. Some exploited previously known springs that had not been used commercially before; others had been recently discovered accidentally or purposefully struck by drilling. Most of these new producers were located far away from the established spa towns or urban centres, but the expansion of the rail network into more remote areas connected them to their customers and ensured a fast and cheap mode of transportation. Combined with the use of modern bottling technologies, these new producers of light and often sparkling natural mineral waters quickly gained a foothold in urban markets, where they competed against the locally produced artificial mineral waters.[23]

To do so successfully, many producers of natural mineral waters began to resort to those methods of manipulating their water introduced by the producers of artificial mineral waters. Since the natural mineral waters rarely contained the right amount of carbon dioxide, they resorted to artificially reintroducing the gas that had escaped at the well or even adding gas that they bought from elsewhere. They also used chemical methods to remove iron and sulphur from the water. The former usually oxidized after bottling, forming an unappetizing sediment at the bottom of the bottle. This had been an issue for a long time, but now chemical techniques allowed for its complete elimination. Sulphur did not impair a water's optics, but its smell and taste and was unwelcome.[24]

By introducing such methods of manipulation, these producers of natural mineral waters tried to balance the demands of their customers with the natural properties of the resource they were exploiting. At the same time, they opened themselves up to attacks both from the producers of artificial mineral waters who could now claim that artificial and natural mineral waters were not that different and from those producers of natural mineral waters who did not resort to such manipulation who could now claim that such altered waters should not be considered natural. In 1899, for example, Siemens and Co, the company leasing the famous mineral waters of Niederselters from the Kingdom of Prussia at the time, sued Nassauer Selterser Mineralbrunnen, the owner of the less-famous neighbouring mineral waters of Oberselters, because the latter sold their product as natural mineral water despite adding carbon dioxide before bottling. Siemens and Co accused their neighbours of gaining an unfair advantage. They alleged that their competitor misled its customers by wrongly claiming that their water had same status as the water from Niederselters.[25]

In the end, the local district court at Camberg rejected the lawsuit, not because the accusation had proven to be false, but because of a precedent. It noted that Apollinaris, which was at the time involved in a similar lawsuit, removed salt and added carbon dioxide to its water, but it was still sold as natural mineral water.[26] This example shows how muddled things had become at the turn of the twentieth century. Both producers of artificial and natural mineral waters now used similar methods to create a product that tried to satisfy the tastes of its consumers. Whether the producers started from a source of mineralized water or from distilled water was apparently little more than a technicality.

Around the turn of the century, the producers of bottled waters faced a situation in which one of the central categories for distinguishing different kinds of products was fundamentally disputed. Was a "natural" mineral water completely unchanged during the bottling process, was some manipulation admissible to retain that label or could it be extended to artificial waters that emulated natural ones? For the producers of natural mineral waters this was an existential question. Their business success depended on the consumers' willingness to pay more for a supposedly higher-quality product; while their claim to higher quality rested solely on the naturalness of their waters. They were, however, also competitors and the fact that some of them manipulated their water in order to please their customers added an additional fault line.

Yet, despite those conflicts and divisions, the producers of natural mineral waters in some European countries managed to act and curb the threat to their status and their claim to producing a natural product. Some of their reactions were located at the company level; others required collective action and depended on their respective national governments or the courts.

One way to deal with the problem was by paying close attention to their labels. Since most consumers did not obtain their mineral water directly from the producer but from merchants or shopkeepers, the label on the bottle was the only way to identify the contents. Signs of origin were almost as old as bottled mineral waters themselves. In the seventeenth century, bottlers had marked earthenware vessels with their symbol, a practice that continued until glass bottles became the new standard in the late nineteenth century.[27] Although glass bottles often had the name of the company embossed on them, producers also made sure that their labels highlighted not only the name of the well as a brand name and a registered trademark, but also their mineral content and that they were a natural water.[28]

Labels, however, were not immune to fraudulent behaviour and the best way to stamp out such practices was through legislation or jurisdiction. Around the turn of the century, some European countries passed legislation regulating the sale of different kinds of mineral waters by establishing different categories of bottled waters and clear regulations for their production and labelling. In other countries, the producers themselves tried to establish industry standards and hoped that the courts would accept them.

First, there was an attempt to distinguish between medicinal waters and table waters. While the former were the direct descendants of the waters consumed in the spa towns, the latter category contained natural, as well as artificial refreshing beverages that had come to dominate the market since the 1870s. In France and Spain, medicinal waters had been legally defined in the early nineteenth century as part of the governments' drive to regulate the medical marketplace and improve public health. Since all medical remedies had to be centrally authorized and registered, this also applied to mineral waters consumed for medical purposes either at a spa town or after bottling at home.[29] In Europe, this was a rather rare arrangement. While government officials might inspect spa towns and control bottled medicinal waters, as in the Grand Duchy of Baden, and mineral waters were taxed as medical remedies, as in the United Kingdom, there was no comparable regulation.[30]

The success of natural mineral waters as a refreshing beverage posed a challenge to both the established forms of regulation in France and Spain as well as the *laissez-faire* in the rest of the continent. The emergence of new producers of bottled waters who did not originate from established and officially recognized spa towns posed a new regulatory challenge to the authorities. France tried to establish a distinction between registered medicinal (*eaux minérales*) and unregistered table waters (*eaux de table*) from 1878 onwards. Spain followed suit a few years later, but the matter proved to be intractable. How to decide into which category a water belonged was far from straightforward. Should it be the prerogative of the medical profession, based on the waters' chemical composition or the practices of consumption? Numerous attempts to follow these possible avenues failed because the many stakeholders with diverging interests could not agree on common criteria and standards, including the status of artificial and natural water. Physicians argued for the prohibition of the manipulation of medicinal waters, while pharmacists insisted on the medical value of artificial waters. Even after legislation in 1910 that disallowed the manipulation of medicinal waters, the classification as medicinal water remained arbitrary and producers simply ignored the law.[31]

In order to achieve some form of unity and greater political influence, the producers of the different kinds of bottled waters formed trade associations in several European countries. The Alliance of Mineral Water Manufacturers' Association in the United Kingdom, which comprised producers of natural as well as artificial waters, but was dominated by the latter, was a reaction to new trademark legislation in 1888, a topic that dominated the first volume of the organization's trade journal.[32] In Germany, the *Allgemeiner Verband Deutscher Mineralwasser-Fabrikanten* (General Association of German Mineral Water Producers) formed in 1898 to lobby against the liberalization of the German market for artificial mineral waters and pushed for higher regulatory standards.[33] The German producers of natural mineral waters, fewer in number and with less economic heft, but more prestige, founded their own association (*Deutscher Mineralbrunnen-Verband*) a few years later in 1904. This was a reaction both to the artificial producers' actions and to the aforementioned lawsuit against Apollinaris, which had profound consequences for the industry.[34]

After a protracted legal battle over several levels of jurisdiction, the Imperial Court in Leipzig finally decided, in December 1900, that Apollinaris could no longer declare their mineral water to be natural, since it removed salt and added carbon dioxide before bottling. The plaintiffs were both producers of artificial and natural mineral waters who sought clarification from the courts in the absence of relevant and clear legislation.[35] The ruling instigated a series of meetings between experts and producers of natural mineral waters in Gera (1901), Frankfort (1905) and Bad Nauheim (1911) with the aim of establishing industry standards for the declaration of different types of bottled waters not only in Germany, but also Switzerland and Austria-Hungary. The resulting Bad Nauheim Resolutions were a compromise and established several categories for bottled waters, acknowledging the complex situation. Medicinal waters had to remain completely unaltered. Iron could be removed and carbon dioxide could be added or removed from mineral waters without forfeiting the categorization as "natural" as long as the manipulation was noted on the label and the water contained 1,000 mg in dissolved minerals or 250 mg of carbon dioxide. Natural waters with a lower mineral content were categorized as natural spring waters. Waters that had been manipulated in another way were automatically classified as artificial.[36]

Although the Bad Nauheim Resolutions were only industry standards, agreed by producers with the help of experts, the German, Swiss and Austrian-Hungarian courts accepted them as binding in the many lawsuits that challenged them in the following years. Thereby, natural mineral water became a protected designation for a certain kind of bottled water. Its superiority was indirectly given official approval even without legislation and its producers profited from this label. Natural food, fashion and living became a lifestyle choice for many in the German-speaking countries and the "life reform movement" discovered natural mineral water as a healthy alternative to other beverages.[37]

This was, however, mostly a Central European phenomenon. Neither France, in Spain or Italy had attached similar importance to the label "natural" before the First World War. In the United Kingdom, there was no legislation regarding the classification of bottled waters and where the producers of artificial mineral waters dominated the trade. Market sales of artificial mineral waters dwarfed those of natural waters, most of which were imported from Germany or France. The fact that they were natural was apparently not a clear advantage in the British market.[38]

Contesting naturalness

What does it mean when producers of a product such as mineral water claim it is "natural"? They certainly cannot argue that the water they sell is untouched by human activity. Even if their water was bottled directly and as it came from the ground, the bottling process itself would be difficult to characterize as "natural". Their claim to "naturalness" is necessarily partial, a biased interpretation of the properties of their product that emphasizes certain aspects and neglects others.

The history of artificial and natural mineral waters during the nineteenth century suggests that the claim of being "natural" was the result of a long process of negotiation between different actors and stakeholders. What "natural" meant was never clear but constantly contested. The lines of conflict divided not only producers of artificial and natural waters but also producers of natural waters using different production techniques. In different European countries, the authorities came to different conclusions regarding the importance of "naturalness". In the United Kingdom, it was not an important category at all, while the German-speaking countries of Central Europe followed the arguments of the producers of natural waters after they had come to an internal compromise and put a premium on naturalness. Yet, as the French example shows, government intervention did not necessarily have binding consequences for the producers, if they chose to ignore it.

Thus, mineral water being "natural" is not natural. It is an attribution, not an essential property. If consumers associate "natural" with "healthy", they are perpetuating a centuries-old connection, but with a modern twist. As mineral waters began to lose their medicinal properties during the last third of the nineteenth century, their connection to their consumers' health changed. They were no longer supposed to restore the chronically ill and cure disease, as had been the expectation for those visiting the spa towns or undergoing a drinking cure at home. Instead, consumers increasingly preferred a kind of mineral water that would no longer heal but would maintain health if drunk regularly. For many consumers, the claim to healthiness was based on the naturalness of the product. That the manipulation of many natural mineral waters did not sever this connection between naturalness and healthiness at first appears surprising. Yet, maybe, it is just an acknowledgement, that the label "natural" is not only contested, but also rather meaningless.

Notes

1   European Federation of Bottled Water 2015, 3.
2   Marketingforschung Oppermann, Marktpsychologische Positionsanalyse 1984. Mineralwasser (Limonade); Marketingforschung Oppermann, Marktpsychologische Positionsanalyse. Mineralwasser (Heilwasser), 1988; Marketingforschung Oppermann, Marktpsychologische Positionsanalyse. Mineralwasser/Heilwasser, 1993; Marketingforschung Oppermann, Marktpsychologische Positionsanalyse

Mineralwasser/Heilwasser, 1996; Rheingold, Ergebnispräsentation Qualitative Marktanalyse Mineralwasser, 2001, all in Verband Deutscher Mineralbrunnen archive, Bonn-Bad Godesberg.

3 Advertisement for Gerolsteiner Sprudel, "Geschmack der aus der Tiefe kommt", 1978, Gerolsteiner Brunnen GmbH & Co. KG, company archive; Brochure by Volvic, 1978; Advertisement for Cristalp, in *La Capsule* 14 (1997), 2, both in Henniez company archive, Henniez.

4 Olson 1999; Ferrier 2001; Clarke 2004; Wanktin 2006; Royte 2008; Gleick 2010.

5 Hawkins, Potter and Race 2015, 3–4.

6 *L'eau minérale* 2008.

7 European Community, Council Directive 80/777/EEC, 15 July 1980, in: Official Journal of the European Communities No L 229/1.

8 Bitz 1989, 62–68, 81–94; Probst 1971, 28–34; Gerbod 2004, 35–56.

9 Blackbourn 2002; Fuhs 1992; Steward 2002; Gerbod 2004, 59–113; Mackaman 1998; Penez 2004.

10 Littleton 2003; Eklund 1976; Coley 1979, 1982, 1990; Taiani 1991, 83–86.

11 Coley 1984.

12 Struve 1824; Franz 1842; Eisenbach 2004, 128–29. Another successful entrepreneur in the artificial mineral water business was Jacob Schweppe. Back, Landa and Meeks 1995, 607; Simmons 1983.

13 Lersch 1863, 226; Brinkmann 1991.

14 Eisenbach 1982; Schneider 2000, 2004, 2005, 2011.

15 Kreysig 1825, 1–3.

16 Lee 1841, 110–13; Macpherson 1869, 294–97; Mitchell 1913, 78–81.

17 Taiani 1991, 86–95; Lee 1841, 111–13.

18 Struve 1824; Kreysig 1825; King 1826; Franz 1842, 12–13.

19 That the dispute was still undecided at the end of the nineteenth century is shown by the existence of Popper's *Die Heilquellen und ihr Werth* (1893). The book consists of a collection of answers of eminent physicians to questions regarding the usefulness of the drinking cure and the superiority of natural waters over artificial ones.

20 Posner 1905; Marty 2013, 43–49.

21 Marty 2013, 27–32; Teuteberg 2004, 130–33; Eisenbach 2004, 186–87. Telling is the number of handbooks covering the different aspects of the production of artificial mineral waters published from the 1860s onwards. Some German examples: Hager 1860; Goldberg 1892; Evers 1917; Luhmann 1922; Kühles 1938.

22 Marty 2013, 37; Teuteberg 2004, 136. That the consumption of medicinal waters was still considered to require professional guidance is demonstrated by Simon 1912.

23 Among those producers that emerged in the late nineteenth century are some of today's best-known brands such as Apollinaris, Gerolsteiner, Perrier, Rosbacher or Vittel. While a few such as Vittel had a comparatively short history as a successful spa town, the production of bottled water soon eclipsed the income made from visitors: Eisenbach 2004, 132–69; Marty 2005, 15–35; Contal 1982. The variety of natural mineral waters available on the European market is demonstrated by the trading catalogue of mineral water merchants Ingram and Royle of London (Ingram and Royle 1911).

24 Marty 2013, 98–100; Eisenbach 2004, 181.

25 Private lawsuit Siemens and Co against Nassauer Selterser Mineralquellen, 4 January 1899, Hessisches Wirtschaftsarchiv Darmstadt, 101/105.
26 District Court Camberg, Rejection of Lawsuit by Siemens and Co against Nassauer Selterser Mineralquellen, 13 March 1899, Hessisches Wirtschaftsarchiv, Darmstadt, 101/105. On the Apollinaris lawsuit, see Marty 2013, 103–05; Eisenbach 2004, 193.
27 Schneider 2004; Serly 2007, 103–06; Eisenbach 2004, 170–75.
28 On the importance of labels for the different waters from Vichy see Chambriard 1999, 153–56. Examples for labels from the late nineteenth and early twentieth centuries can be found in Eisenbach 2004, 146, 50, 61, 65, 69; Jung 2005, 25; Finamore 1984, 61; Chambriard 1999, 153.
29 Marty 2013, 75–82.
30 Ibid., 85–87.
31 Ibid., 90–100.
32 See numerous articles in *The British and Colonial Mineral Water Trade Journal* 1 (1888).
33 Marty 2013, 102.
34 Eisenbach 2004, 190–91; Marty 2013, 103–04.
35 Eisenbach, 191–92; Marty, 104–05.
36 Eisenbach, 194–95; Marty, 105–06.
37 Eisenbach, 195; Teuteberg 2004, 144–45.
38 Marty 2013, 107–14.

References

Unpublished sources

Gerolsteiner Brunnen GmbH & Co. KG, company archive
Henniez company archive, Henniez
Hessisches Wirtschaftsarchiv Darmstadt
Verband Deutscher Mineralbrunnen archive, Bonn-Bad Godesberg

Published sources

Back, William, Edward R. Landa and Lisa Meeks. 1995. "Bottled Water, Spas, and Early Years of Water Chemistry." *Ground Water* 33: 605–14.
Bitz, Matthias. 1989. *Badewesen in Südwestdeutschland 1550 bis 1840*. Idstein: Schulz-Kirchner.
Blackbourn, David. 2002. "Fashionable Spa Towns in Nineteenth-Century Europe." In *Water, Leisure and Culture: European Historical Perspectives*, edited by Susan C. Anderson and Bruce H. Tabb, 9–21. Oxford: Berg.
Brinkmann, Bernd. 1991. "Die künstliche Mineralwasser- und Badeanstalt in Köln." In *Wasserlust. Mineralquellen und Heilbäder im Rheinland*, edited by Silke Engel, 154–63. Köln: Rheinland-Verlag.
Chambriard, Pascal. 1999. *Aux sources de Vichy: naissance et développement d'un bassin thermal XIXe-XXe siècle*. Saint-Pourçain-sur-Sioule: Bleu autour.
Clarke, Tony. 2004. *Inside the Bottle: Exposing the Bottled Water Industry*. Ottawa, ON: Polaris Institute.

Coley, Noel G. 1979. "'Cures without Care': 'Chymical Physicians' and Mineral Waters in Seventeenth-Century English Medicine." *Medical History* 23: 191–214.

Coley, Noel G. 1982. "Physicians and the Chemical Analysis of Mineral Waters in Eighteenth-Century England." *Medical History* 26: 123–44.

Coley, Noel G. 1990. "Physicians, Chemists and the Analysis of Mineral Waters: 'The Most Difficult Part of Chemistry'." In *The Medical History of Waters and Spas*, edited by Roy Porter, 56–66. London: Wellcome Institute.

Coley, Noel G. 1984. "The Preparation and Uses of Artificial Mineral Waters (ca. 1680–1825)." *AMBIX* 31: 32–48.

Contal, Marie Hélène, ed. 1982. *Vittel, 1854–1936: création d'une ville thermale*. Paris: Moniteur.

L'eau minérale: Un produit naturel et protégé, une industrie responsable, un emballage recyclable. 2008. Paris: Chambre Syndicale des Eaux Minérales. At http://eaumineralenaturelle.fr/wp-content/uploads/2014/12/LIVRE_BLANC.pdf (accessed 23 February 2020).

Eisenbach, Ulrich. 2004. *Mineralwasser. Vom Ursprung rein bis heute. Kultur- und Wirtschaftsgeschichte der deutschen Mineralbrunnen*. Bonn: Verband Deutscher Mineralbrunnen.

Eisenbach, Ulrich. 1982. *Wirtschafts- und Sozialgeschichte des Niederselterser Brunnenbetriebs bis zum Ende des Herzogtums Nassau*. Wiesbaden: Historische Kommission für Nassau.

Eklund, Jon. 1976. "Of the Spirit in the Water: Some Early Ideas on the Aerial Dimension." *Isis* 67: 527–50.

European Federation of Bottled Water. 2015. "Industry Report." Brussels.

Evers, Friedrich. 1917. *Der Praktische Mineralwasser-Fabrikant. Auskunfts- und Vorschriftenbuch für die Mineralwasser-Fabrikation und deren Nebenzweige Fruchtsaft-, Fruchtessenzen-, Limonaden- und Alkoholfreie Getränke-Industrie.*

Ferrier, Catherine. 2001. "Bottled Water: Understanding a Social Phenomenon." A discussion paper. WWF. At www.ircwash.org/sites/default/files/Ferrier-2001-Bottled.pdf (accessed 23 February 2020).

Finamore, Roy, ed. 1984. *Perrier: And Now the Book*. Tokyo: Toppan.

Franz, J.H.A. 1842. *A Treatise on Mineral Waters, with Reference to Those Prepared at the Royal German Spa, at Brighton*. London: Churchill.

Fuhs, Burkhard. 1992. *Mondäne Orte einer vornehmen Gesellschaft. Kultur und Geschichte der Kurstädte 1700–1900*. Hildesheim: Olms.

Gerbod, Paul. 2004. *Loisirs et santé: les thermalismes en Europe des origines à nos jours*. Paris: Honoré Champion.

Gleick, Peter, H. 2010. *Bottled & Sold: The Story Behind Our Obsession with Bottled Water*. Washington, DC: Island Press.

Goldberg, Alwin. 1892. *Die natürlichen und künstlichen Mineralwässer. Ein Handbuch enthaltend eine kurze Zusammenfassung der wichtigsten Kapitel der Mineralquellenlehre und Darlegung der Prinzipien der Herstellung künstlicher Mineralwässer, insbesondere der Nachbildung natürlicher Mineralwässer*. Weimar: Bernhard Friedrich Voigt.

Hager, Hermann. 1860. *Vollständige Anleitung zur Fabrikation künstlicher Mineralwässer, sowie Beschreibung der dazu erforderlichen Apparate und Maschinen*. Berlin: Lissa.

Hawkins, Gay, Emily Potter, and Kane Race. 2015. *Plastic Water: The Social and Material Life of Bottled Water*. Cambridge, MA: MIT Press.

Ingram and Royle. 1911. *Natural Mineral Waters: Their Properties and Uses.* 12th edn. London: Ingram & Royle.

Jung, Heinz R. 2005. *Geschichte des Selters-Sprudels an der Lahn, 1887–2004.* Löhnberg: Selters Mineralquelle Augusta Victoria GmbH.

King, W. 1826. *Observations on the Artificial Mineral Waters of Dr. Struve, of Dresden, Prepared at Brighton.* Brighton: C. and B. Sickelmore.

Kreysig, Friedrich Ludwig. 1825. *Über den Gebrauch der natürlichen und künstlichen Mineralwässer von Karlsbad, Embs, Marienbad, Eger, Pyrmont und Spaa.* Leipzig: Brockhaus.

Kühles, Rudolf. 1938. *Handbuch der Mineralwasserindustrie. Hand- und Lehrbuch für die Praxis der gesamten Mineralwasser- und Limonaden-Industrie, Mineralbrunnen-, Mineralwasser- und Limonaden-Herstellungsbetriebe.* Lübeck: Charles Coleman.

Lee, Edwin. 1841. *The Mineral Springs of England and Their Curative Efficacy, with Remarks on Bathing and on Artificial Mineral Waters.* London: Whittaker.

Lersch, B. M. 1863. *Geschichte der Balneologie, Hydroposie und Pegologie oder des Gebrauchs des Wassers zu religiösen, diätetischen und medicinischen Zwecken.* Würzburg: Stahel'sche Buch- und Kunsthandlung.

Littleton, Charles. 2003. "Elite Science and Popular Pleasures: Robert Boyle, Chemical Analysis, and the 'Islington Waters'." In *Bäder und Kuren in der Aufklärung. Medizinaldiskurs und Freizeitvergnügen*, edited by Raingard Eßer and Thomas Fuchs, 161–83. Berlin: Berliner Wissenschafts-Verlag.

Luhmann, E. 1922. *Die Fabrikation der moussierenden Getränke. Praktische Anleitung zur Fabrikation aller moussierenden Wässer, Limonaden, Weine etc. und gründliche Beschreibung der hiezu nötigen Apparate.* Wien: A. Hartleben's Verlag.

Mackaman, Douglas Peter. 1998. *Leisure Settings: Bourgeois Culture, Medicine, and the Spa in Modern France.* Chicago: University of Chicago Press.

Macpherson, John. 1869. *The Spas and Wells of Europe, Their Action and Uses with Hints on Change of Air and Diet Cures.* London: Macmillan.

Marty, Nicolas. 2013. *L'invention de l'eau embouteillée: qualités, normes et marchés de l'eau en bouteille en Europe, XIXe-XXe sciècles.* Brussels: Peter Lang.

Marty, Nicolas. 2005. *Perrier, c'est nous! Histoire de la source Perrier et de son personnel.* Paris: Éditions de l'Atelier.

Mitchell, C. Ainsworth. 1913. *Mineral and Aerated Waters.* London: Constable & Company.

Olson, Eric D. 1999. *Bottled Water: Pure Drink or Pure Hype.* New York: National Resources Defense Council.

Penez, Jérôme. 2004. *Histoire du thermalisme en France au XIXe siècle: eau, médecine et loisires.* Paris: Economica.

Popper, Julius, ed. 1893. *Die Heilquellen und ihr Werth. Was die Aerzte denken! Ein balneologisches Hand- und Nachschlage-Buch für Publicum und Aerzte.* Wien: Adolph W. Künast.

Posner, L. 1905. "Gebrauch und Missbrauch von Tafelwässern." *Die Gesundheit in Wort und Bild* 7: 381–86.

Probst, Irmgard. 1971. "Die Balneologie des 16. Jahrhunderts im Spiegel der deutschen Badeschriften." PhD thesis. Münster.

Royte, Elizabeth. 2008. *Bottlemania: How Water Went on Sale and Why We Bought It.* New York: Bloomsbury.

Schneider, Konrad. 2011. "Das Geschäft mit dem Heil- und Tafelwasser. Zum Mineralwasserhandel in Frankfurt a. M. bis zur Einführung der Gewerbefreiheit (1864)." *Nassauische Annalen* 122: 157–81.

Schneider, Konrad. 2005. "'Stets in Guter Füllung'. Zur Mineralwasserabfüllung vom 16. Jahrhundert bis in die Zeit des industriellen Füllbetriebs." *Jahrbuch für Westdeutsche Landesgeschichte* 31: 203–55.

Schneider, Konrad. 2004. "Der Mineralwasserversand aus Bad Soden a. Ts. Milchbrunnen, Champagnerbrunnen und Wilhelmsbrunnen." *Nassauische Annalen* 115: 353–70.

Schneider, Konrad. 2000. *Der Mineralwasserversand und seine Gefässproduktion im rheinisch-hessischen Raum vom 17. bis zum Ende des 19. Jahrhunderts.* Koblenz: Forneck.

Serly, Petra. 2007. "Mineralwasser und Verpackung. Von der Keramik zum Kunststoff. Zu der Konkurrenz der Materialien bei der Abfüllung und dem Versand." *Bayerisches Jahrbuch für Volkskunde*: 103–12.

Simmons, Douglas A. 1983. *Schweppes: The First Two Hundred Years.* London: Springwood.

Simon, Oscar. 1912. *Die Karlsbader Kur im Hause. Ihre Indikation und ihre Technik.* Berlin: Julius Springer.

Steward, Jill. 2002. "The Culture of the Water Cure in Nineteenth-Century Austria, 1800–1914." In *Water, Leisure and Culture: European Historical Perspectives*, edited by Susan C. Anderson and Bruce H. Tabb, 23–35. Oxford: Berg.

Struve, Friedrich Adolph August. 1824. *Über die Nachbildung der natürlichen Heilquellen.* Dresden: Arnoldische Buchhandlung.

Taiani, Rodolfo. 1991. "L'acqua e la sua anima: il contributo della scienza chimica alla sfruttamento delle fonti di acqua minerale nella prima metà del XIX secolo." *Nuncius* 6: 84–107.

Teuteberg, Hans Jürgen. 2004. "Vom 'Gesundbrunnen' in Kurbädern zur modernen Mineralwasserproduktion." In *Geschichte des Konsums. Erträge der 20. Arbeitstagung der Gesellschaft für Sozial- und Wirtschaftsgeschichte 23–26. April 2003 in Greifswald*, edited by Rolf Walter, 123–57. Stuttgart: Steiner.

Wanktin, Lucie. 2006. *Have You Bottled It? How Drinking Tap Water Can Help Save You and the Planet.* London: Sustain.

Chapter 3

Environmental anxieties in 1980s Athens

Mediatization and politics

Panagiotis Zestanakis

Introduction

> Visitors turn away their eyes from the marbles' holy beauty looking at
> the sea of cement that besieges Acropolis. [...] The smog is choking the
> capital, engulfing the Parthenon [...] Big, dark ditches nest [sic] where
> air doesn't blow enough: they look like sources pouring pus [...]. The
> Karyatides[1] have been taken out of the Erectheion. In their place stand
> copies. They are uncovered and nobody admires them. When smog [...]
> has destroyed even the top of the temple's Dorian capitals and Phidias'
> happy frieze what will attract this many people to the sacred rock?[2]

The article is by Italian journalist Enzo Siciliano; it was published in
the Italian newspaper *Corriere della Sera* and republished in the Greek
Kathimerini in September 1981. Describing his visit to Athens, Siciliano
focused on air pollution or *nefos*, a problem that troubled the city throughout
the 1980s. This chapter explores how *nefos*, in combination with a number of
other environmental issues provoked anxieties about air quality (and, more
generally, life quality) highlighting how these anxieties were mediatized. It
associates this mediatization with developments in local and global politics
and with transnational environmental anxieties such as the consequences of
nuclear energy. In Athens, these issues were intertwined as anxiety about *nefos*
intensified in 1986–1987, combined with the aftermath of the Chernobyl
nuclear accident in April 1986 and the July 1987 heatwave. The Chernobyl
accident took place in Ukraine, more than 2,000 km from Athens, but since
the wind blew towards Greece, high levels of radioactivity were detected
in the country's atmosphere. The July 1987 heatwave resulted in about 1,300
deaths and was associated with *nefos* as a consequence of Attica's urbanization since the 1950s. Environmental anxieties went hand-in-hand with the
development of the interest in ecology. Engaging with then-current discourses
on Europeanization (Greece joined the European Economic Community in
1981 and relevant debates flourished throughout the decade) the concept
of the "ecologist" emerged as a modern "European" political identity. This

significantly weakened around 1990 showing that enthusiasm for ecology was ephemeral and failed to influence Greek politics in the long-term.

The chapter highlights the articulation of emotions of anxiety. Historians of emotions perceive them as de-essentialized cultural processes approachable by way of access to historical sources from letters to media texts.[3] Barbara Rosenwein argues that subjects form emotional communities with shared norms, through communication.[4] The formulation of such a community organized around environmental anxieties in 1980s Athens is examined here. "Anxiety" is a useful term because it is distinguished from fear. Fear is related to traumatic events and differs from the emotions that individuals usually develop when they face ecological threats. Problems such as air pollution are not sudden events (unlike nuclear accidents which violently affect everyday habits e.g. inflaming nutritional panic) and usually provoke weaker emotions than fear. Hine and Gifford assert that the 1980s antipollution messages resulted in verbal commitment or financial donations raising environmental concerns.[5] I feel that the term "concern" is moderate for 1980s Athens, where environmental issues permeated the public sphere, with various results such as suburbanization. Hence, in line with historian Johanna Bourke I approach fear as different to the lesser term anxiety, an emotion expressing permanence about unpleasant but not extremely threatening situations.[6]

This chapter has three parts. The first explores how anxieties around air pollution emerged. The second illustrates how these anxieties intersected with apprehensions stimulated by the events of 1986–1987 to inspire new political subjects, particularly the emergence of the Oikologoi Enallaktikoi (Ecologists-Alternatives, henceforth EA) party, which experienced noticeable success in conditions of political polarization in the late 1980s . The last part analyses why anxieties lessened around 1990 failing to lead to a powerful ecological movement. The chapter draws on textual, visual and oral sources including articles, posters, advertisements and oral testimonies.[7] It sees media discourses as expressing interactions between producers and audiences, deconstructing the media frames within which ecological anxieties were articulated.[8] Such interactions unfolded at a juncture where enthusiasm for international media trends was remarkable. As we will see, a number of new media, mainly magazines, invested ecology with connotations of post-materialist alternativity promoting ecology-friendly trends as new and attractive.

Anxieties

Athens had almost 1.4 million inhabitants in the 1950s. By the early 1980s, its population had increased to about three million largely due to domestic migration.[9] Post-war development started from a low base as Greece emerged from the devastation of the Civil War (1945–1949) but economic progress was fast from the 1950s.[10] This was reflected in the popularization of consumer durables, as post-war cinema characteristically shows. To use cars as an indicator (a commodity associated with pollution) if, in the 1950s, car ownership was limited to affluent consumers, by the 1960s, upper-middle-class consumers could afford them.[11] In the 1970s there were 358,111 private cars, 33,376 motorcycles and 1,841 public buses in Athens in 1977. This number rose to 552,263 cars, 62,449 motorcycles and 2,008 buses in 1983 and 930,942 cars, 134,108 motorcycles and 2,965 buses in 1991.[12] Around 1980, discussions about pollution from car and industrial emissions were common. Athens then hosted about 55 per cent of Greek industrial activity.[13] The city had poor rail transport links (one line connected Piraeus with northern Athens via the green line of Athens' modern metro network) and public transport was mostly comprised of old buses.[14] Central neighbourhoods suffered from traffic jams and parking problems were common.[15]

The first environmental anxieties appeared in the dictatorship years (1967–1974). The state started measuring air pollution in 1972, but complaints that control points were insufficient and that specialists could hardly intervene in policymaking remained.[16] In 1973, about 12,000 inhabitants of Megara, a town close to Athens, protested against the establishment of refineries in their area.[17]

Valavanidis argues that the term *nefos* appeared in 1977.[18] However, newspapers continued to put the word into quotation marks, suggesting that the term remained only moderately recognizable until the early 1980s.[19] These years saw environmentalist agitation: in central neighbourhoods protest groups appeared, and organized small demonstrations. These initiatives engaged with the then influential left-wing politicization.[20] According to political scientist Iosif Botetzagias, ecologists originated from nuclei of environmentalists formed in the 1970s; people who had engaged with the anti-dictatorship struggle but felt disappointed with 1980s politics and looked for alternatives, and people from a loose network of left-wingers and anarchists organized around the concept of impeachment (including a general opposition to the establishment and to existing political parties, entrenched left-wing powers such as the Communist Party of Greece (KKE)).[21]

Uncommitted ecologists found the conservatism of established political powers (entrenched left-wing parties included) unattractive as these parties were not perceived as being interested in then novel post-materialist demands that intrigued ecologists such as environmental issues, anti-racism or minority rights. Such issues mobilized incongruous groups looking for an alternative radical political agenda. Established parties and older politicians tried to engage with this trend. In the 1978 municipal elections, Dimitris Mpeis nominee of the Panhellenic Socialist Movement (PASOK) in the election for the Municipality of Athens included ecological messages in his campaign. He circulated a poster entitled "I vote for Mpeis because I love Athens" where one letter of the word Athens was replaced by a plant. An envelope being posted into a ballot box sealed with a stamp with a plant was also included in the synthesis. Further, as a woman who won such a distinction remembers, Mpeis during his service period as mayor (1978–1986) occasionally rewarded Athenians with well-planted balconies, which added to the city's amenities and to the health of its inhabitants.[22] Given that debates on pollution in Athens remained vibrant when Mpeis lost the 1986 elections after eight years in office, his environmental achievements are debatable. However, he was a pioneer in communicating ecology.

Mpeis' communication agenda engaged with wider developments. Continuing a trend of the dictatorship years, when publishers launched books by radical international intellectuals to encourage critical thinking, the late 1970s and the early 1980s saw the translation into Greek of books by acknowledged ecologists such as Murray Bookhin and Pierre Samuel.[23] *Nefos* also preoccupied media products such as "Edo Lilipoupolis" [Lilipoupolis speaking] a politicized radio programme broadcast by Greek National Radio from 1976 to 1980 or by scientific debates in the press.[24] The problem became increasingly recognizable in the early 1980s, since a growing number of Athenians sought medical help especially when *nefos* was intense, such as on public transport strike days.[25] *Nefos* was also mentioned as damaging the city's image, putting tourism (an important economic sector for Athens) at risk.[26] Around 1980, reservations in city centre hotels decreased; travel agents preferred hotels in seaside suburbs with cleaner air, such as Glyfada.[27]

The issue influenced debate before the national election in October 1981 which PASOK won. PASOK and the Left (especially the Greek Communist Party (KKE)) argued that industry was responsible for *nefos* and accused New Democracy, the party in office between 1974 and 1981, of supporting such these owners at the expense of public health. This argument was not baseless: in 1977, New Democracy voted for three environmental laws concerning the prohibition of mazut (a viscous liquid residue from the distillation of petroleum that was used as a heavy low-quality fuel oil) for central heating, the control of car emissions and the institutionalization of measures to protect industrial employees' health. This last measure remained inactive until 1981 as it entailed significant cost for industry owners.[28]

Communists interpreted *nefos* as a form of class struggle between the affluent residents of less-affected suburbs and working-class people who often lived close to industry sites.[29] Indicatively, the Public Power Cooperation factory in the working-class district of Keratsini consumed 700,000 tones of petrol annually producing 35 per cent of the sulphur dioxide in Athens; further, many oil tanks were concentrated in this area.[30] Using a rhetorical comparison with one of the most fatal pandemics in human history, the Communist Party described *nefos* as a "black death" brought to Athens by the politics of the Right.[31] This image was invoked in photos where Athens' grey buildings disappeared into a dark sky giving the impression of a damned place.[32] Communist rhetoric saw *nefos*, along with drugs and pornography, as the outcomes of capitalism and the influence of America.[33] Anxieties about *nefos* were highly spatialized. Affluent Athenians lived in or could move to cleaner districts: more simply, money could buy a healthier lifestyle. Scientific institutions such as PAKOE (the Panhellenic Centre for Environmental Studies) noticed that *nefos* was more intense in working-class districts.[34] Contrarily, New Democracy highlighted the levels of pollution created by cars, seeing *nefos* as the inevitable cost of post-war economic progress.[35]

It is hard to estimate to exactly what degree *nefos* was created by cars and industry. Measurements in the 1970s showed that industry produced 80–85 per cent of sulphur dioxide, while cars produced 95, 85 and 50–60 per cent of carbon monoxide, hydrocarbons and lead respectively.[36] As traffic jams could be dramatically visualized, newspapers often highlighted levels of traffic; public transport was of poor quality and Athenians used their cars extensively. Complaints about public transport were common and preoccupied the media.[37] Further, as cars were overtaxed and expensive in comparison with Western Europe, many Athenians used old vehicles sometimes even those constructed in the 1960s or old imported cars: according to a 1987 estimate, such vehicles accounted for 30 per cent of car sales (about 25,000);[38] the percentage of cars withdrawn was only 0.5 per cent per year.[39]

Oral interviews show that although *nefos* preoccupied casual discussions such as gatherings of family or friends, perceptions of the problem were highly variable. KZ, an upper-middle-class female left-wing student, argued that ecology and pollution often preoccupied progressive youngsters and that some went on camping holidays seeking closer contact with nature.[40] TV, a high-school student from northern Athens, occasionally discussed *nefos* with friends but never felt anxious.[41] MA had a similar approach. Born in the late 1960s and raised in a lower-middle class suburb close to the city centre, she had an adventurous youth amongst a social group who moved around the city on motorcycles, pursued nightlife, and adopted a liberal attitude to sex. For her, *nefos* was a topic created by the media.

> I remember nefos mostly photographically [...] in the public space. [...] I was not interested because I had a nice time. I loved Athens. [...] I was wandering around and never believed that I was living in an ugly city. Athens was a beautiful, very friendly, adventurous city.[42]

A female high-school student from the lower-middle-class district of Vyronas provides a more nuanced explanation. For her, Athenians discussed *nefos* because they were anxious about its health consequences, though this anxiety did not reflect a selfless interest in ecology.[43] This resonates with articles and surveys, which showed that Athenians were mildly interested in issues such as lack of green spaces in the city: 5.5 per cent thought the lack of parks and playgrounds were an important issue.[44] A male interviewee from the central lower-middle-class suburb of Kallithea argued that ecological anxieties disrupted pleasant activities such as swimming during the summer.[45]

Athenians spent time on nearby beaches in summertime. Beach bars and discothèques flourished, attracting youngsters, not least because proximity to the sea provided a fresher environment. Bonds between sea, leisure and a liberated attitude to sex are corroborated by representations of the beach in 1980s cinema (early 1980s school comedies are characteristic) and summed up by a party on Vouliagmeni beach, which attracted around 50,000 participants in 1983.

Such anxieties resonated with nervousness about Athens' tourist image, which revolved around beach vacations, as many hotels, especially in prestigious suburbs such as Vouliagmeni and Glyfada, were on the seafront.[46] This anxiety among children and youngsters is further corroborated by the campaign of the Hellenic Marine Environment Protection Association (HELMEPA), an organization aimed at protecting marine life, established in 1982. The campaign's symbol was a playful seagull; its slogans "Keep our seas clean" and "No garbage, no plastic in seas and coasts" remain recognizable even nowadays. The choice of an illustrative cartoon drew on the popularity of comics in post-war Greece and showed that HELMEPA sought to approach youngsters and kids recognizing them as a group that had to be sensitized to environmental issues.[47]

Of course, environmental anxieties were not limited to the youth. A middle-aged mother of two teenagers who lived in the central district of Victoria remembered that she often discussed *nefos* and pollution and that these issues influenced her family's decision to relocate to the northern suburb of Maroussi in 1988. She associated pollution with health anxieties and everyday problems. As her house was close to the busy crossroads between Patission Street and Alexandras Avenue, she regularly had to wash her curtains due to dirt produced by fumes. This, combined with noise pollution and the scarcity of air-conditioning at that time (balcony doors were usually open in summertime) created unpleasant conditions.[48] The decision of her family to move to the suburbs for a healthier life resonated with a wider trend. In the 1980s, the centre lost population to the suburbs and other non-urban areas for the first time.[49] Hence, more flats were available in central areas (e.g. Patissia and Kypseli) because of suburbanization.[50] Anxieties about *nefos* concerned residents in central districts more than those living in the suburbs (with the exception of those close to industry). These residents saw the centre as a polluted zone to be avoided. A teenager growing up in a northern suburb remembers that some parents discouraged their children from visiting the centre frequently because they considered it to be polluted.[51] Similarly, GP, a then middle-aged civil engineer was spending a lot of time in Lagonissi, a seaside resort about 30 kilometres south of Athens. He remembers his anxious feelings when entering Athens by car.

Entering Athens I was seeing [...] a yellow thing covering the city. It was distant and at once I was feeling that I was entering it. It was palpable.

Everybody was anxious because they could feel the consequences. Those who were more sensitive were feeling it in their lungs, in their nose. [...] It's palpable, it's not theory.[52]

Interviews mention the main factors influencing anxieties around *nefos*. First, the elderly were more anxious about health consequences as *nefos* was particularly dangerous for those with cardiovascular and respiratory problems, especially bronchitis and asthma. Obviously, such problems were less common among the young. The danger was higher on days of temperature inversion (15–20 every year in Athens) when air at higher altitudes became hotter than at ground level so the *nefos* stayed about 100–150 metres above the city irritating eyes and throats and provoking respiratory difficulties in its inhabitants.[53] The second distinction concerned residence. Those living in the cleaner, non-industrial, suburbs tended to perceive *nefos* as a problem of the centre; similarly, those living in the centre saw relocation to the suburbs as a solution provided that they had the economic means.

The 1986–1987 Conjuncture and its outcomes: Culmination of environmental anxieties and growing politicization of ecology

The Chernobyl accident in 1986 almost coincided with the 1987 heatwave and boosted existing environmental anxieties. Although the accident happened far from Athens, winds blew the radioactivity towards Greece, creating alarming in the country. Everyday routines changed; authorities advised Athenians to stay home and avoid foods that could be affected by radioactivity, such as fresh vegetables. This was a frequent topic of discussion for Athenians and (as Greece had no tradition of nuclear energy) they attempted to learn the new scientific vocabulary regularly used by the media. Children stopped playing in playgrounds and parks, to avoid exposure to rainfall (rain water carried radioactivity) and could not eat popular Greek summer foods such as ice-cream and strawberries.[54] The accident routinized discussions on how human activity could damage the environment and even inspired the cultural industry, eloquently shown by as the video movie, *O Anthropos apo to Chernobyl* [The Man from Chernobyl] in which a man affected by radioactivity loses his hair and grows a tail.[55] The mass circulation of this video was a clue that anxieties about radioactivity were widespread.[56] It is hard to evaluate who was more anxious, but there is some evidence that the elderly were particularly affected.[57]

According to ecologists at the time, Chernobyl motivated an unprecedented interest in environmentalism[58] and posters featuring ecological messages flourished in Athens for the first time.[59] For some, Chernobyl represented a sort of fateful moment, when subjects were confronted by an event that shockingly affected their everyday lives.[60] Coinciding with the 1987 heatwave,

Chernobyl reorganized the conceptualization of risk for Athenians. In his classic book on risk society, whose first edition discussed the aftermath of the Chernobyl shock, sociologist Ulrich Beck (1986) sees late 1980s society as living with anxiety about future risk more than any other in the past. In Athens, Chernobyl intensified the lower-level anxieties generated by *nefos*.[61] Chernobyl led to shocking images – dead firemen or employees hospitalized with radiation sickness (ARS) – illustrating how lethal environmental disasters could be.[62]

The 1987 heatwave offered further shocking experiences. Athenian summers are hot and dry. In the 1980s, the average temperature in June, July and August was 25, 28 and 27 degrees Celsius respectively, while temperatures between 35 and 40 degrees were not uncommon.[63] On 10 July 1977, Athens experienced a temperature of 48 degrees in a heatwave which killed three inhabitants.[64] The July 1987 heatwave saw unprecedented high temperatures and humidity. Temperatures began to rise on 20 July; on 23 July, Athens saw 40 degrees and 60 per cent humidity. By the next day, 95 people had died; overconsumption meant that in some areas there were water shortages. The combination of heat and lack of water provoked panic. As air-conditioning was rare, Athenians sought cooler air by sleeping on the beaches, in the open air, in nearby mountains or even by diving into fountains.[65] On 26 July, the thermometer climbed to 46 degrees. On 30 July, the temperature returned to normal levels, leaving more than 1,000 victims (the authorities never provided a final number and some reporters argued that there were around 1,300) mainly in Athens. Mortuaries were full and corpses were kept in hospital yards.[66] Missing elders were found dead in apartments after days, questioning Greek family solidarity. The heatwave further trivialized discussions about climate change as some media approached it the outcome of the disorderly reconstruction of Athens in the 1950s–1970s.[67] In this period, lower houses were replaced by higher (often four- to six-floor) buildings with small and medium-sized flats to shelter domestic immigrants.[68] This effect was underlined because about 90 per cent of victims were in Athens. Most victims were in central neighbourhoods rebuilt in the early post-war years (e.g. Pangkrati) and in working-class districts (e.g. Aigaleo).[69]

Ecologists took further action. The most noticeable development was the formation of Ecologists-Alternatives (EA). Discussions intensified in 1988–1989 leading to the establishment of a fresh, radical party.[70] The advertisement used before the November 1989 elections argued that a new policy had been born.[71] Despite the basic graphic design because of its limited funding, it still effectively conveyed global ecological anxieties such as those about nuclear energy associating them with local problems, mainly *nefos*. It recalled the clichés used by PASOK and New Democracy about environmental issues throughout the 1980s and employed shocking images (e.g. from the Chernobyl accident) before concluding that EA would fight for a greener and healthier future. The spot used electronic music, unusual in political advertisements of the time, which focused on the supposed charisma of political leaders and blamed political opponents through negative advertising (this trend weakened after the mid-1990s). EA had no recognizable leader, which influenced this choice. It is not easy to ascertain its effectiveness, but the spot certainly carried novel characteristics and is the only 1980s material on the party's YouTube channel today.[72] Combining fast-moving graphics with electronic music it engaged with topical music trends and highlighted the party's fresh character, capitalizing on issues such as endangered animals and pro-cycling messages, which appealed to educated audiences. Emphasis on endangered animals shows that EA followed trends in juvenile cultures: Panini Hellas and World Wildlife Forum circulated stickers at that time picturing endangered animals.[73] EA received 0.58 per cent and 0.77 per cent of votes in the November 1989 and April 1990 general elections performing better in Athens centre (A Athens) than in the suburbs (see Table 3.1). EA also used pro-feminist rhetoric with some success: in the November 1989 elections, female candidates performed much better than males, unique for a Greek political party at that time.[74] EA's performance shows that a number of Athenians looked for alternative political expression highlighting environmental issues even in polarized times.[75] The results also demonstrated that residents in the suburbs were less anxious about environmental issues.

EA enjoyed media coverage disproportional to its electoral performance. The party earned one seat in the November 1989 elections; this was crucial as, due its system of proportional representation, Greece had three elections between June 1989 and April 1990 before New Democracy achieved a slim majority. Marina Dizi, EA's parliament member between November 1989 and April 1990, attracted significant media attention. Dizi had studied marketing and advertising and had been arrested by the military regime. She had participated in the Marxist-Leninist Epanastatiko Kommounistiko Kinima Elladas (Revolutionary and Communist Movement of Greece) until 1976 when she resigned, remaining an independent left-winger until she joined the EA in the late 1980s. She was a thirty-something woman in a male-dominated parliament, which attracted media attention. Further, her communication style challenged parliament's communication customs. Dizi shared flowers before taking her oath in November 1989 and, while in a meeting in March 1990, opened a placard writing "Enough with the theater with nefos" while other EA members who attended the meeting in the parliament's public gallery shouted slogans in support. Eight of them were sentenced for violating parliament's rules. Conservative MPs castigated her "for allegedly transferring the behaviour of the anarchist district of Exarchia into the parliament". One of them, actress Anna Synodinou, resigned condemning the reaction of her party (New Democracy) as inexcusably lenient.[76] EA's radical aura had an impact among left-wing voters (e.g. N.P., then a male student in the University of Athens, voted for EA seeing them as fresher than traditional left-wing parties).[77] Similarly, (a male born in the early 1960s) who previously

Table 3.1 Performances of "Ecologists – Alternatives" in the November 1989 and April 1990 general elections.

Electoral prefecture	Votes (November 1989)	Percentage % (November 1989)	Votes (April 1990)	Percentage % (April 1990)
A Athens	5,949	1.33%	7,052	1.60%
B Athens	8,855	1.12%	10,643	1.36%
A Piraeus	1,346	0.79%	1,658	0.98%
B Piraeus	1,382	0.75%	1,940	1.06%
Rest of Attica	960	0.53%	1,310	0.73%

Source: Selected data compiled by the author: *Apotelesmata ton vouleytikon eklogon tis 5is Noemvriou* 1989, 37–42; *Apotelesmata ton vouleytikon eklogon tis 8is Apriliou* 1991, 40–47.

had abstained from voting joined the EA recognizing in them a dynamism that left-wing parties lacked.[78]

Contextualizing, EA profited from ecology's popularity in European and Greek politics.[79] In Germany and the Netherlands, Green parties influenced politics from the late 1970s. The German Green Party received 1.0 per cent of the vote in the 1980 elections. In the 1984 European Parliament elections, the Greens won twenty out of 434 sets. As already stated, in Greece, most political parties started to claim that they had an eco-friendly identity at that time. The Left promoted the activities of Athenian ecologists, such as small demonstrations, in its media;[80] PASOK developed an eco-friendly rhetoric highlighting the anti-*nefos* measures it had taken in 1982, particularly the provisional elimination of cars in a ring around the center of the city according to the last digit of their registration numbers.[81]

Some right-wing politicians also claimed an eco-friendly identity. Miltiadis Evert was Mayor of Athens between 1986 and 1989. Evert won the 1986 election supported by New Democracy. His rhetoric combined an interest in ecology with enthusiasm for infrastructure facilitating the use of cars in the city's saturated centre such as multi-level underground parking, which irritated a number of residents.[82] He was also an animal lover, owning various pets, including a monkey. Adopting a left-wing idiom of protest, in November 1987 Evert called for a cycle rally asking the government to create infrastructures for cyclists as cycling was a nature-friendly means of transport which could help reduce *nefos*. The race was successful in attracting Athenians of various ages.[83] Discussions on cycling as an alternative means of transport had started in the early 1980s, with the appearance of Greek translations of books by physical activity specialists such as German cycling expert Franz Wöllenzmüller.[84] It is questionable whether Evert ever intended to promote cycling. PAKOE had conducted preliminary studies on the creation of a network of cycle lanes in the early 1980s.[85] It is hard to estimate what results such an initiative would have had. At the time, there were few cyclists as hot weather, pollution, lack of infrastructure and the city's hilly landscape rendered it very difficult.[86] However, in Athens and other Greek cities, there were small collectivities of cyclists promoting cycling under tough conditions.[87] Evert did not capitalize on this expertise but developed a rhetoric targeting nature-friendly lifestyle enthusiasts. Such attempts established Evert as a pioneer of political communication.[88] Not coincidentally, he was selected to give an interview to the first talk show on commercial television "Psila ta Cheria" ("Hands Up") on 25 November 1989. An emphasis on ecology seemed to be an effective strategy and was adopted by the winner of the next municipal elections, Antonis Tritsis (1990).[89]

Evert's agenda was not irrational. He targeted groups of voters that had appeared in various western European countries in the 1980s. Franklin and Rüdig, have examined the 1980s Green vote: Well-educated youngsters and middle-class voters were those usually touched by ecology rhetoric. Women voted green more often than men. The association between an interest in ecology and left-wing positioning differed among countries: in Germany and the Netherlands this link was strong, while in France and the United Kingdom, the Greens attracted voters from various backgrounds.[90] Evert capitalized on the disassociation of radicalism from left-wing politics attempting to attract voters interested using post-materialist claims. In Greece, late-1980s youngsters increasingly saw the left-wing politicization, which had dominated earlier juvenile culture, as a new form of establishment and looked for new radical referents in consumer and other cultural trends.[91] In 1988, university students voted Right for the first time after the 1974 political changeover.[92] Such youngsters were often interested in lifestyle media which succeeded (especially among urban audiences) in contrasting the promotion of unhealthy habits such as drinking alcohol with an enthusiasm for fitness.[93] Interest in ecology was included in this narrative. *Cosmopolitan* magazine asked its readers "how Green they are" while *Elle* advertised pricey clothing alongside eco-friendly designs by Greenpeace.[94] They also published articles on phenomena such as climate change, Green politics or deforestation.[95] As the extract below shows, ecologists were positioned as activists fighting for post-materialist issues, different from those by established political subjects such as trade-unionists and as representing a respectful lifestyle carrying connotations of hope for a healthier world. The publisher of lifestyle magazine *Status* (a title popular among affluent young urban residents) criticized the limited participation in an anti-*nefos* demonstration.

> The country's future is not undermined only by the hazardous sensitivities of [...] absurd minorities. It is equally if not more threatened by the 'don't give a damn attitude'. [...] A demonstration [...] against *nefos* attracted only a few hundreds of protesters. The event passed unnoticed. The same people who run kilometers holding plastic flags of political parties remained untouched. They preferred not to sacrifice their afternoon even

if in recent years they have forgotten what color the famous Athenian sky was.[96]

The ebb of the early 1990s

Dramatic mediatization of *nefos* fizzled out around 1990. According to a survey, those seeing the environment as a major source of anxiety reduced from 55.4 per cent in 1987 to 23.4 per cent in 1990.[97] From 1988, journalists argued that the situation had improved due to measures such as the "ring", restricting motorists' access to central Athens according to the tear their car was registered.[98]

Further, Athens saw a new environmental threat: drought. In 1989, the Company of Water Supply and Drains (EYDAP) announced that Athens had water reserves of only a few weeks and calling on Athenians to use water frugally.[99] Drought was not seen as directly resulting from human intervention in the environment and could not be impressively visualized (at least not compared to *nefos*) as it did not entail palpable health symptoms. In media terms, drought rendered environmental discourses less visible and appealing. Further, as drought could not provoke political mobilization, the ecologists lost ground. Early 1990s pop culture ridiculed ecology and nature-friendly lifestyles such as vegetarianism.[100] In an episode of the popular TV series *Oi Apadarektoi* [The Unconvential] screened in 1992, Nikos (performed by Nikos Alexiou), an ex left-winger, ecologist and vegetarian appears as an obsessive and grotesque character.[101]

In 1990, the Minister of the Environment, Stefanos Manos, assumed that Athenians discussed *nefos* less because they had become more used to living with it.[102] As we have seen, various new issues preoccupied the media but one factor, namely migration, influenced the process. As historian Ivan Berendt argues, migration was the most crucial cause of population growth in late-twentieth-century Europe.[103] After 1990, Greece attracted immigrants mostly from Albania and Eastern Europe: immigrants constituted 2 per cent of Athens' population in 1991 but this had risen to 13 per cent by 2001.[104]

Contrary to the international trend whereby segregation marks such urban transformations, in Athens immigrants co-existed quite harmoniously with established residents.[105] Their arrival affected the real estate market. The 1960s and 1970s saw the mass construction of apartments based on *antiparochi*, a pattern where a plot of land was exchanged for flats usually constructed by small companies. Small companies and landowners participated in a mutually beneficial deal offering affordable housing in the form of small or medium-sized apartments. Many of these apartments were vacant due to suburbanization in the 1980s and immigrants found affordable dwellings left available by their owners.[106] Most immigrants settled in an imaginary line connecting the Port of Piraeus and its industrial districts with western Athens via the centre and in rural areas in Attica working in agriculture.[107] Immigrants settled in

ecologically impoverished areas had few possibilities to mediatize environmental anxieties or to participate in politics due to limited (or no) knowledge
of Greek, lack of political rights and issues such as residence status. This is
only one of the ways in which interactions between migration and suburbanization transformed Athens after 1990: this affected everyday life in multiple
ways and deserves more scholarly attention.

Epilogue: The anxiety that marked a decade

In the late 1990s, I was a teenager growing up in the central Athenian district
of Pangkrati. I remember *nefos* less as a current concern and more as something from the past. In the meantime, the economic and political climate had
changed. Greece saw a period of development and adjustment to European
legislation largely based on a consensus towards Europeanization.[108]
Regarding the environment, growing prosperity and political mobilization
contributed to the replacement of older cars. A programme subsidizing
the purchase of new cars with catalytic convertors increased sales of those
types of vehicles from about 350 in 1988 to about 205,000 in 1992.[109] New
infrastructures improved everyday life: the gradual replacement of old buses
and the construction of two new metro lines, a suburban rail network and
peripheral highways contributed to the reduction of pollution.[110] The city
never again experienced a heatwave as severe as that of July 1987; shorter
heatwaves remained common, but not fatal. Athenians equipped their homes
with air-conditioning. According to an early 1990s estimate, 7.7 per cent of
Greek households owned air-conditioning, a percentage probably higher
in Athens, one of the country's warmer cities.[111] A late-1990s study argued
that half of households then owned air-conditioning without specifying its
source.[112] From my experience, middle-class households usually had air conditioning from around 2000, while cafés or restaurants were almost always
air-conditioned. Individual acquisition intervened where the state failed.

Interest in ecology foundered. The Ecologists-Alternatives were disbanded.
The party failed to solve disputes among its groups, which emerged due to
new topics such as the Macedonian Question, the dispute between Greece
and North Macedonia about how the latter would be named after the dissol-
ution of Yugoslavia in the early 1990s.[113] The party's members did not agree
a common position on this issue.[114] Some ecologists supported the left-wing
Synaspismos tis Aristeras kai tis Proodou [Coalition of the Left and Progress]
in the 1993 elections: the latter earned 2.94 per cent of the vote, but no par-
liamentary seats as the electoral law had changed. Other members comprised
the party Politiki Oikologia [Political Ecology], which earned 17,017 votes
(0.26 per cent) in the 1994 European Parliament elections, ironically less than
half of the 41,157 votes won by a party that was fighting for hunters' rights.
Almost five years after its peak in the 1986–1990 moment, enthusiasm for
ecology already seemed to belong to history.

Notes

1 Karyatis was an epithet of ancient Greek goodness Artemis whose priestesses were named Karyatides. Six Karyatides in marble supported the temple of Erechteion in the Acropolis of Athens.
2 Siciliano 1981.
3 Bourke 2011; Scheer 2012.
4 Rosenwein 2010.
5 Hine and Gifford 1991.
6 Bourke 2011, 268–72.
7 Except for one recent interview, the oral testimonies were collected for my PhD research project and originate from wider interviews where Athenians implicated in 1980s modern lifestyles narrated their lives, "sensitive" issues (e.g. sexuality) included. Protecting their privacy, I use initials instead of full names, except for one interview (with MA Kessariani, 9 August 2012) where I use the false initials, as requested by the interviewee. As interest in novel lifestyles such as ecology usually required relevant economic security, most interviewees were middle or upper-middle class. Hence, lower-class Athenians are underrepresented in the oral sources employed here.
8 For frame theory see Reese 2007; and Entman 1993.
9 For Athens' expansion, see Leontidou 1990, especially 127–71, and Maloutas 2018.
10 For a classical account of this post-war development see McNeil 1978.
11 See indicatively the movies Tzavellas, *I Kalpiki Lira* (1955) and Sakellarios, *I Soferina* (1964).
12 Tsakirides 2004, 524.
13 Valavanidis 1981.
14 Tsakiris 1984. For this network in detail see *Odorama*, 1983, 212–14.
15 "I afthaireti" 1981.
16 Theochari 2010; Valavanidis 1981.
17 "En aganaktisei" 1973.
18 Valavanidis 1981.
19 "Kykloforiako chaos" 1982.
20 For this politicization until the early 1980s (especially in the urban context), see Papadogiannis 2015.
21 Botetzagias 2003, 77–78.
22 VP (interview).
23 Kornetis 2013, 161; Bookhin 1977; Samuel 1981.
24 Charzidakis and Kipourgos 2010. For scientific debates see Tsarouchas 1982 and Valavanidis 1981.
25 "Nefos aithalomichlis" 1979; "Kykloforiako chaos" 1982.
26 For the development of tourism in post-war Athens, see Nikolakakis 2015.
27 "Akriveia" 1981.
28 Valavanidis 1981.
29 Filikos 1980. For the development of such a working-class district in Piraeus (that of Drapetsona), see Kyramargiou 2019.
30 Valavanidis 1981.
31 Filikos 1981.
32 For example, "O vrachnas tou nefous" 1981.

33 "Oi dimoi, oi koinotites" 1978.
34 "I aithalomichli" 1981.
35 Verykaki 1981; "Thalamos aerion" 1988.
36 Valavanidis 1981.
37 Stavropoulos 1987.
38 "Akrivynan kata 631%" 1987.
39 Stamou 1987.
40 KZ (interview).
41 TV (interview).
42 MA (interview).
43 GZ (interview).
44 Papachristos 1988.
45 GT (interview).
46 In the late 1970s, the coastal suburbs of Varkiza, Voula and Vouliagmeni had 69 hotels in total (26 of them classified as of four and five stars). In comparison, central Athens had 187 hotels (30 of them classified as of four and five stars respectively). See *Ellas Touristikos Odigos* 1976, 137–40.
47 For the popularity of comics, see Gerakopoulou 2018.
48 IZ (interview).
49 Kyriazi-Alisson 1998, 283–84.
50 Grigoriou 1984.
51 GS (interview).
52 GP (interview).
53 Valavanidis 1981.
54 Zestanakis 2017,320.
55 "Amok gia treis" 1986; Psara 2010; Efstratiadis 1986.
56 Kassaveti 2014, 174–76.
57 Zestanakis 2017, 320.
58 PV (interview).
59 Psychas in Botetzagias 2003, 84.
60 Giddens 1991, 113.
61 Beck 1986.
62 ARS: bodily symptoms appear in the first hours of exposure to high ionizing radiation. Symptoms depend on the amount of radiation exposure; large doses result in neurological effects, including seizures, tremors, lethargy and rapid death.
63 Brucher et al. 1986, 217.
64 "Pyraktomeno diimero" 1977.
65 Zestanakis 2017, 315.
66 Markatas 2010.
67 Papadopoulos 1987.
68 Kandylis et al. 2012, 283. See also Maloutas 2007 and Maloutas 2018.
69 Antonopoulos and Karpathiou 1987.
70 See "Koini symfonia" 1988; Deltio, "Deltio ekdiloseon" 1989; and Giannakopoulou 1989. EA published a journal under various names. Changes expressed fluid hierarchies in a party comprised of many minor groups (See also: Botetzagias 2003). The journal was initially named *Deltio ton Synergazomenon Oikologikon Enallaktikon Kiniseon kai Omadon* [Bulletin of collaborating ecological alternative movements and groups] and from 1989 *Deltio: Oikologoi Enallaktikoi kai*

Synergazomenes Oikologikes kai Enallaktikes Ekdoseis (Bulletin: Ecologists-Alternatives and Collaborating Ecological and Alternative Editions). For brevity in references, I use the term *Deltio* for all these editions.

71 "Oikologoi Enallaktikoi" (TV Spot).
72 Oikologoi Enallaktikoi 1989.
73 *Zoa pros diasosi* 1989.
74 Kampylis 1989.
75 In 1989–1990 Greece experienced a political crisis. It started when members of PASOK governments appeared implicated in economic scandals and continued due to a highly proportional electoral law, which hardened the creation of government between June 1989 and April 1990. The country experienced three elections in this period. For details see Voulgaris 2002, 346–59.
76 For details on this incident see Kampylis 1990 and Papazoglou 1990.
77 NP (interview).
78 VP (interview).
79 For the overview, see Müller-Rommel and Poguntke 2002.
80 For example, Zalaoras 1981.
81 "Entos dietias" 1982.
82 Papachristos 1987; "I epistoli tou k. Evert" 1987; Livieratos 1988.
83 "Protos podilatikos gyros Athinas" 1987.
84 Wöllenzmüller 1984.
85 *34 Chronia gia to Perivallon* 2013, 22.
86 AC (interview).
87 Stavropoulou 1987.
88 "To image tou kyriou Evert" 1987.
89 Tritsis 1990.
90 Franklin and Rüdig 1992.
91 Sakellaropoulos 2001, 472–74.
92 For this turn, see also Lakopoulos 1988.
93 Zestanakis 2017, 97–101.
94 Alexiou 1990; "Sto sfygmo tis fysis" 1989.
95 Krauer 1989; Iliopoulos 1989; Kochaimidou 1988; "Podilato: to ochima tou mellontos" 1989.
96 Lyberis 1988.
97 Varouxi and Fragkiskou 2004, 679.
98 Zalaoras et el. 1988.
99 "Prosechoume gia na echoume" 1990; "Nero" 1990.
100 E.g. *To Retire* 1992.
101 "Oi Aparadektoi" 1992.
102 Konstantinea 1990.
103 Berendt 2010, 231.
104 Kandylis et al. 2012, 269.
105 Maloutas 2007.
106 To provide an example, Aghios Panteleimonas, a central district much affected by *nefos*, had 44,798 and 43,730 residents in 1991 and 2001 respectively. 42,984 of them were Greeks in 1991 and 31,312 in 2001. For details, see Arapoglou et al. 2009.
107 Kandylis et al. 2012, 271.
108 Pagoulatos 2003, 128.

109 Bitsika 1998.
110 OECD 2009, 206–07.
111 Panellinia erevna 1991.
112 Hassid et al. 2000.
113 I employ the term North Macedonia as established by the Prespa Agreement
     on 12 June 2018. In the 1990s, Greeks usually referred to North Macedonia as
     Skopje, while North Macedonians were self-defined Macedonians.
114 Botetzagias 2003, 102–04.

References

Interviews

AC Ilioupoli, Athens. 15 March 2012.
GT Kallithea, Athens. 25 May 2012.
GP Pangkrati, Athens. 16 February 2012.
GZ Pangkrati, Athens. 23 March 2012.
IZ Marousi, Athens. 8 July 2012.
KZ Filothei, Athens. 28 June 2012.
MA Kessariani, Athens. 8 August 2012.
NP Rethymno. 14 July 2012.
PV Kifissia, Athens. 1 April 2019.
TV Melissia, Athens. 11 May 2012.
VP Patissia, Athens. 6 January 2012.

Published sources

"Akrivynan kata 631% ta IX se deka chronia." 1987. *Kathimerini*, 3 October 1987.
Alexiou, Lena. 1990. "Poso prasini eiste." *Cosmopolitan*, July 1990.
"Amok gia treis." 1986. *Eleftheros Typos tis Kyriakis*, 10–11 May 1986.
Antonopoulos, L. and A. Karpathiou 1987. "Ta synora tou thanatou." *Ta Nea*, 31
    July 1987.
*Apotelesmata ton vouleytikon eklogon tis 5is Noemvriou 1989. Tomos protos:
    sygkentrotika apotelesmata*. 1991. Athens: Ethniko Typografeio.
*Apotelesmata ton vouleytikon eklogon tis 8is Apriliou 1990. Tomos protos: sygkentrotika
    apotelesmata*. 1991. Athens: Ethniko Typografeio.
Arapoglou, Vassilis, Karolos Iosif Kavoulakos, Yorgos Kandylis, and Thomas
    Maloutas. 2009. "I Nea Koinoniki Geografia tis Athinas. Metanastefsi, Poikilotita
    kai Sygkrousi." *Sygchrona Themata* 107: 57–67.
"Akriveia – molynsi diochnoun tous tourists." 1981. *Avgi*, 26 April 1981.
Beck, Ulrich. 1986. *Risikogesellschaft. Auf dem Weg in eine andere Modern*. Frankfurt
    am Main: Suhrkamp.
Berendt, Ivan T. 2010. *Europe since 1980*. Cambridge: Cambridge University Press.
Bitsika, Panagiota. 1998. "Ti tha ginei me toys katalytes." *To Vima tis Kyriakis*, 12
    April 1998. www.tovima.gr/2008/11/24/archive/ti-tha-ginei-me-toys-katalytes/
    (accessed 25 August 2020).
Bookhin, Murray. 1977. *I Oikologia kai I Epanastatiki Skepsi*. Athens: Eleftheros
    Typos.

Bourke, Joanna. 2011. *Fovos. Stigmiotypa apo ton politismo tou 19ou kai tou 20ou aiona*. Athens: Savallas.

Botetzagias, Iosif. 2003. "I omospondia oikologon enallaktikon. To elliniko prasino peirama." *Elliniki Epitheorisi Politikis Epistimis* 22: 69–105.

Brucher, Ambos, Peter Gobel, Wolfgang Gogol, Ronald Hahn, Udo Moll, Jörg Nunnenmocher, Gutner Putz, Dieter Richter, and Werner Storkebaum. 1986. *Yfilios. To Panorama ton Kraton tis Gis*. Athens: Giovanis.

Chadjidakis, Manos and Nikos Kipourgos. 2010. "To nefos." In *Edo Lilipoupoli*, CD 6, director Manos Chadjidakis. Athens.

"Deltio ekdiloseon EKEA sto theatro kalon technon." 1989. *Deltio,* 7 August 1989.

Efstratiadis, Omiros. 1986. *O Anthropos apo to Chernobyl*. Athens: Hi-Tech.

Ektheseis perivallontikon epidoseon: Ellada. 2009. Athens: Ypourgeio Perivallontos, Energeias kai Klimatikis Allagis.

Ellas Touristikos Odigos. 1976. Athens: ELPA (Elliniki Leschi Periigiseon kai Aytokinitou).

Entman, M. Robert. 1993. "Framing. Towards Clarification of a Fractured Paradigm." *Communication* 43 (4): 51–58.

"En aganaktisei oi katoikoi tis periochis Megaron synekrotisan megalin sygkentrosin dia tin mataiosin tis idryseos diilistirion." 1973. *Makedonia*, 16 October 1973.

"Entos dietias evelpistei i kyvernisi na dioksei to nefos apo tin Attiki." 1982. *Kathimerini*, 16 January 1982.

Filikos, Nikos. "Sos, to nefos." 1980. *Rizospastis*, 17 December 1980.

Filikos, Nikos. "To Nefos." 1981. *Rizospastis*, 7 February 1981.

Franklin, Mark N. and Wolfgang Rüdig. 1992. "The Green Voter in the 1989 European Elections". *Environmental Politics* 1 (4): 129–59.

Gerakopoulou, Patricia. 2018. "Amfisvitisi kai amerikaniko fandom sti metapolemiki Ellada: protoleia pagkosmiopoiimenis cheirafetisis meso tis systimatikis katanalosis amerikanikon comics kai tileoptikon serials." In *Oi apeitharchoi. Keimena gia tin istoria tis neanikis anaideias ti metapolemiki periodo*, edited by Kostas Katsapis, 21–37. Athens: Okto.

Giannakopoulou, Smaro. 1989. "O Megalos oikologikos tromos diamorfonei ena neo politiko kai koinoniko topio." *Deltio*, September 1989.

Giddens, Anthony. 1991. *Modernity and Self-Identity. Self and Society in the Late Modern Age*. Stanford, CA: Stanford University Press.

Grigoriou, Avra. 1984. "Poleitai I Athina. Sto sfyri 40,000 diamerismata." *Eleftheros Typos tis Kyriakis*, 18–19 August 1984.

Hassid S. et al. 2000. "The Effect of the Athens Heat Island in Air Conditioning Load." *Energy and Buildings* 32 (2): 131–41.

Hine, Donald W., and Robert Gifford. 1991. "Fear Appeals, Individual Differences and Environmental Concern." *The Journal of Environmental Education* 23 (1): 36–41.

"I aftheraiti stathmefsi sinechizetai stous dromous tis Athinas." 1981. *Kathimerini*, 6 November 1981.

"I aithalomichli stin Athina dimiourgei kai pali anapnefstika provlimata." 1981. *Makedonia*, 3 February 1981.

"I epistoli tou k. Evert pros ton kyrio Papandreou." 1987. *Vima tis Kyriakis*, 8 March 1987.

Iliopoulos, Yorgos. 1989. "Thermokipio i Gi." *Status*, August 1989, 59–65.

Kampylis, Takis. 1989. "Proigountai oi kyries." *Ta Nea*, 7 November 1989.

Kandylis, George, Thomas Maloutas, and John Sayas. 2012. "Immigration, Inequality and Diversity: Socio-ethnic Hierarchy and Spatial Organization in Athens, Greece". *European Urban and Regional Studies* 19 (3): 267–86.

Kassaveti, Orsalia-Eleni. 2014. *I elliniki videotainia (1985–1990). Eidologikes, koinonikes kai politismikes diastaseis*. Athens: Asini.

Kochaimidou, Eleni. 1988. "Deka chronia prasinoi sti Dytiki Germania. O realismos mias outopias." *Playboy*, April 1988.

"Koini symfonia ton synergazomenon oikologikon omadon." 1988. *Deltio*, November 1988.

"Koinonikoi kai politikoi thesmoi." 1989. *Deltio*, February–March 1989.

Konstantinea, Marita. 1990. "I epistrofi tou Stefanou Manou." *Ena*, 30 May 1990.

Kornetis, Kostis. 2013. *Children of the Dictatorship. Student Resistance, Cultural Politics and the "Long 1960s" in Greece*. Oxford: Berghahn.

Krauer, Sebastian. 1989. "Ta dentra pethainoun orthia." *Status*, May 1989.

"Kykloforiako chaos, 'nefos', apergies sta trolei kai leoforeia talaiporisan xthes tous Athinaious." 1982. *Kathimerini*, 6 November 1982.

Kyramargiou, Eleni. 2019. *Drapetsona, 1922–1967. Enas kosmos stin akri tou kosmou*. Athens: Ethniko Idryma Erevnon.

Kyriazi-Alisson, Elissavet. 1998. "Esoteriki metanastefsi stin Ellada: taseis – provlimatismoi – prooptikes." *Elliniki Epitheorisi Koinonikon Erevnon*, no. 96–97: 279–309.

Lakopoulos, Yorgos. 1988. "Giati oi foitites psifisan deksia." *To Vima tis Kyriakis*, 20 March 1988.

Leontidou, Lila. 1990. *The Mediterranean City in Transition. Social Change and Urban Development*. Cambridge: Cambridge University Press.

Livieratos, Yannis. "Garage kai provlimata." *To Vima tis Kyriakis*, 20 November 1988.

Lyberis, Antonis. 1988. "Editorial." *Status*, April 1988.

Maloutas, Thomas. 2007. "Segregation, Social Polarization and Immigration in Athens during the 1990s: Theoretical Expectations, and Contextual Difference." *International Journal of Urban and Regional Research* 31 (4): 733–58.

Maloutas, Thomas. 2018. *I koinoniki geografia tis Athinas. Koinonikes omades kai domimeno perivallon se mia notioevropaiki mitropoli*. Athens: Alexandreia.

Markatas, Yorgos. 2010. "Kafsonas: to anthropistiko drama, i yperpolitikopoisi kai i lithi." In *I Ellada sti Dekaetia tou 1980. Koinoniko, Politiko kai Politismiko Lexiko*, edited by Vassilis Vamvakas and Panayis Panagiotopoulos, 258–60. Athens: To Perasma.

McNeil, William. 1978. *The Metamorphosis of Greece Since World War II*. Chicago: University of Chicago Press.

Melissinos, Yorgos, Dimitris Pagadakis, and Stathis Papoulias. 1990. "Gaia, i athanati." *Click*, May 1990.

Müller-Rommel, Ferdinand, and Thomas Poguntke, eds. 2002. *Green Parties in National Governments*. London: Frank Cass.

"Nefos aithalomichlis skepase pali Athina kai Peiraia." 1979. *Makedonia*, 18 October 1979.

"Nero. Giati prepei oloi na synechisoume." 1990. *Avgi tis Kyriakis*, 4 November 1990.

Nikolakakis, Michalis. 2015. "Athens. The Tourist Capital of Post-War Greece." *Pharos* 21 (1): 21–36.

Odorama. Enchromos Odigos Lekanopediou Protevousis. 1983. Athens: Tri-color.

"Oi Aparadektoi." 1992. Episode 30 of "Oi Aparadektoi" titled "Leventes oikologoi". Broadcast by Mega Channel, 13 May 1992.

"Oi dimoi, oi koinotites kai ta propyrgia gia ti dimokratia". 1978. *Rizospastis*, 22 October 1978.

"Oikologoi Enallaktikoi." 1989. TV Spot. www.youtube.com/watch?v=gZzN_JfkdLM (accessed 29 July 2020).

"O Vrachnas tou nefous emfanistike kai pali." 1981. *Rizospastis*, 19 July 1981.

OECD, *Ektheseis Perivallontikon Epidoseon: Ellada.* Athens: Ypourgeio Perivallontos, Energeias kai Klimatikis Allagis.

Pagoulatos, George. 2003. *Greece's New Political Economy. State, Finance and Growth from Postwar to EMU.* Houndmills: Palgrave.

"Panellinia erevna Bari tis Focus." 1991. In *Odigos Dimosiotitas.* Athens: Infopublica, 198–200.

Papachristos, Yorgos. 1987. "Chreiazontai exypnes lyseis. Oi protaseis tou neou dimarchou Miltiadi Evert." *To Vima tis Kyriakis*, 8 March 1987.

Papachristos, Yorgos. 1988. "To perivallon kaiei tous Athinaious." *To Vima tis Kyriakis,* 11 December 1988.

Papadogiannis, Nikolaos. 2015. *Militant around the Clock? Left-wing Youth Politics, Leisure and Sexuality in Post-dictatorship Greece, 1974–1981.* Oxford: Berghahn.

Papadopoulos, Thanos. 1987. "Den einai o kafsonas, alla i poli pou skotonei." *Avgi tis Kyriakis*, 26 June 1987.

Papazoglou, Minas. 1990. "Ena pano, mia paraitisi kai okto syllipseis." *Ta Nea*, 5 March 1990.

"Podilato: to ochima tou mellontos." 1989. *Klik*, September 1989.

"Prosechoume gia na echoume." 1990. *Avgi tis Kyriakis*, 8 July 1990.

"Protos podilatikos gyros Athinas. Ekanan sta aytokinita ti zoi podilato." 1987. *Ta Nea*, 2 November 1987.

Psara, Maria. 2010. "Chernobyl: I Ellada ton rem kai ton bekerel, tou diatrofikou panikou kai tis oikologikis agonias". In *I Ellada sti dekaetia tou 1980. Koinoniko, Politiko kai Politismiko Lexiko*, edited by Vassilis Vamvakas and Panayis Panagiotopoulos, 597–600. Athens: To Perasma.

"Pyraktomeno diimero se olokliri tin Ellada." 1977. *Rizospastis*, 12 July 1977.

Reese, Stephan. 2007. "The Framing Project: A Bridging Model for Media Research Revisited." *Journal of Communication* 57 (1): 148–54.

Rosenwein, Barbara. 2010. "Problems and Methods in the History of Emotions. Passions in Context." *Passions in Context: International Journal for the History and Theory of Emotions* 1. www.passionsincontext.de

Sakellarios, Alekos. 1964. *I Soferina.* Greece: Damaskinos Michailidis.

Sakellaropoulos, Spyros. 2001. *I Ellada sti metapolitefsi. Politikes kai koinonikes exelixeis, 1974–1988.* Athens: Livanis.

Samuel, Pierre. 1981. *Oikologiko manifesto. Ti einai kai ti thelei i oikologia.* Athens: Andromeda.

Scheer, Monique. 2012. "Are Emotions a Kind of Practice (And Is That What Makes Them Have a History)? A Bourdieuian Approach to Understanding Emotion." *History and Theory* 51 (2): 193–220.

Siciliano, Enzo. 1981. "Athina. Oneiro gia touristes poliorkimeno apo to nefos." *Kathimerini*, 23 September 1981.

Stamou, Dimitris. 1987. "Sto eleos tou chronou kai tou kratous to I. X." *Kathimerini*, 25–26 October 1987.

Stavropoulos, M. 1987. "Leoforeion o pothos." *4 Trochoi*, April 1987.

Stavropoulou, L. 1987. "Oi kryfes chares ton dyo trochon." *Avgi tis Kyriakis*, 22 November 1987.

"Sto sfygmo tis fysis." 1989. *Elle*, December 1989.

"Thalamos Aerion." 1988. *Eleftheros Typos tis Kyriakis*, 7–8 May 1988.

Theochari, Christina. 2010. "Nefos: i syneiditopoiisi tis perivallontikis rypansis stin protevousa." In *I Ellada sti Dekaetia tou 1980. Koinoniko, Politiko kai Politismiko Lexiko*, edited by Vassilis Vamvakas and Panayis Panagiotopoulos, 365–67. Athens: To Perasma.

"To image tou kyriou Evert." 1987. *Klik*, July 1987.

To Retire, episode 10. 1992. Broadcast by Mega Channel, 21 November 1992.

Tritsis, Antonis. 1990. *I Athina Chreiazetai Programma Tritsi. Me Tolmi, Gnosi, Ergo.* Pre-electoral programme. Athens.

Tsakirides, Olga. 2004. "Daily Mobility." In *Recent Social Trends in Greece, 1960–2000*, edited by Dimitris Charalambis, Laura Maratou-Alipranti and Andromachi Hadjiyanni, 515–24. Montreal: McGill–Queen's University Press.

Tsakiris, Yorgos. 1984. "Leoforeia: aytes einai oi allages." *Eleftherotypia*, 8 January 1984.

Tsarouchas, Kostas. 1982. "Poso fountonei to nefos to kykloforiako." *Kyriakatiki Eleftherotypia*, 16 May 1982.

Tzavellas, Giorgos. 1955. *I Kalpiki Lira*. Greece: Anzervos.

Valavanidis, Thanasis. 1981. "To mavro nefos kai oi aities gia tin atmosfairiki piesi stin periochi tis Athinas." *Synchrona Themata* 11: 3–4.

Varouxi, Christina and Amalia Frangkiskou. 2004. "Perception of Social Problems." In *Recent Social Trends in Greece, 1960–2000*, edited by Dimitris Haralambis, Laura Maratou Alipranti and Andromachi Hadjiyanni, 676–81. Montreal: McGill–Queen's University Press.

Verykaki, Eleni. 1981. "Nefos kai agchos adeiazoun tin Athina." *Avgi tis Kyriakis*, 26 April 1981.

Voulgaris, Yannis. 2002. *I Ellada tis Metapolitsfsis 1974–1990, Statheri dimokratia simademeni apo ti metapolemiki istoria.* Athens: Themelio.

Wöllenzmüller, Franz. 1984. *Afti einai i podilasia. Apo ti theoria stin praksi.* Athens: Alkyon.

Zalaoras, Nikos. 1981. "I oikologia katakta ti zoi mas." *Avgi tis Kyriakis*, 5 July 1981.

Zalaoras, Nikos et al. 1988. "Diplo prosopeio edosan ta imimetra stin Athina." *Avgi tis Kyriakis*, 19 January 1988.

Zestanakis, Panagiotis. 2017. *Style Zois, Emfyles Scheseis kai Neoi Koinonikoi Choroi Stin Athina tis Dekaetias tou 1980.* PhD dissertation. Rethymnon: University of Crete.

Zoa pros diasosi. 1989. Athens: Panini and WWF.

34 Chronia gia to perivallon kai ton katanaloti gia poiotita zois. 2013. Athens: PAKOE.

Chapter 4

The woodland cure

Tuberculosis sanatorium patients' perceptions of the healing power of nature

Heini Hakosalo

Introduction

Tuberculosis is a disease with protean manifestations and a notoriously unpredictable and often chronic course. Even prior to the introduction of effective medication, not everyone who was infected fell ill (only 5–10% did) and not everyone who fell ill died. It was impossible to predict with any certainty if and when a latent infection turned into a manifest disease, and if and when the disease took a fatal course. These features made tuberculosis a particularly tough nut for medical science to crack, and they also crucially influenced the patient experience. Given the nature of tuberculosis, it was particularly difficult to judge the relative weight of the many factors that might have an influence on the course of the disease. Prior to the discovery of the tuberculosis bacterium (1882) – and also after it, as the presence of bacteria alone clearly does not suffice to explain why one person falls ill while another does not – relevant pathogenic and etiological factors were sought far and wide: in heredity and constitution, in individual lifestyle choices and behaviours, and in the social, material and natural environment. For centuries, the quality of the natural environment played a significant role both in explaining the disease and especially in the search for cure.

This chapter looks at the notion of the therapeutic environment in the context of mid-twentieth century Finland, primarily from the point of view of the sanatorium patient. Since Roy Porter issued his famous call for "medicine from below" (1985),[1] patients have indeed become more visible in the historiography of tuberculosis. Patients' experiences are present, in various ways, in for instance Linda Bryder's *Below the Magic Mountain* (1988); W.B. Smith's *The Retreat of Tuberculosis* (1988); Katherine Ott's *Fevered Lives* (1996) and Sheila Rothman's *Living in the Shadow of Death* (1994). Anne Shaw and Carole Reeves's *The Children of Craig-y-nos* (2009) and Stacie Burke's *Building Resistance* (2018) focus on the experiences of child patients.[2] None of these studies has been specifically concerned with the patients' perception of the role of the natural environment. In general, historians of tuberculosis have been more interested in patients' emotions than in their beliefs. It may also be the case that researchers have not paid attention to patients' environmental experiences because they have assumed that the belief in the healing power of nature had already vanished by the beginning of the antibiotic age. As we will see, this is not exactly true.

The chapter relies on a major collection of illness narratives, mainly written by former sanatorium patients. The "Collection Competition for Sanatorium Tradition" (henceforth *ST*) was organized in 1971 by the Finnish Literature Society and the Chest Patients' Union, on the occasion of the latter's thirtieth anniversary.[3] The material – over 9,000 pages of text and over 1,000 photographs – is held by the Finnish Literature Society.[4] The collection is both large and heterogeneous. Around 350 people[5] sent in written contributions, whose length varied from half a page to over 1,000 pages. The youngest participants were under twenty and the oldest over eighty. The genders are represented in roughly equal proportion, while the Swedish-speaking minority and the highest social classes are clearly underrepresented, even if we take into account the socially selective nature of the disease. The writing call was accompanied with a list of 21 "writing topics" which, as the call stressed, were in no way binding.[6] Some participants addressed one or more of these topics, while others paid scant attention to them. As the list included no questions about the natural environment, we may assume that those who wrote about it did so because they felt it was an important part of their overall sanatorium experience.[7] I will ask how patients perceived and made use of the natural environment and whether they attributed any therapeutic value to it. I distinguish three different forms of interaction with the environment – aesthetic, pragmatic or instrumental and therapeutic – and will, after a short introduction on sanatorium history, discuss them in turn.

A healing spot

Since antiquity, a cure for *phthisis* (the closest equivalent to pulmonary tuberculosis) has been sought in the natural environment. It was commonly assumed that there were places where various natural elements (e.g. climate, air, water, soil, vegetation) aligned in a way that allowed them to exert a healing influence on a consumptive. However, opinions varied as to where such therapeutic sites were to be found and how they could be recognized. For instance, in nineteenth-century New England, doctors first urged consumptives to sail towards the South in search of a temperate climate; they then recommended the northern borderlands, and then, as the colonization of the West advanced, started to refer them to its mountains and deserts.[8] In Europe, traditional bath resorts attracted and catered for many consumptives, at least until the bacterial origin and thus the infectiousness of the disease was established in the 1880s.

During the last third of the nineteenth century, it seemed as if the consumptives' Shangri-La might have been found at last. Dr Hermann Brehmer (1826–1889) opened what is commonly considered as the first modern, specialized tuberculosis sanatorium in the hills of Görbersdorf (Sokołowsko), Silesia, in 1859. According to him, the region was "immune" to consumption: it was not only naturally free of tuberculosis but also able to exert a curative influence on those who were already sick. Brehmer also formulated a theory of the pathogenesis of tuberculosis, a theory that lent credibility to his environmental claim. In addition to the healing natural environment, Görbersdorf offered institutional care that combined a mixture of discipline, comfort and paternal medical authority which many patients found appealing and many doctors thought was worth imitating.[9]

Brehmer's sanatorium concept was adopted and elaborated on by many medical entrepreneurs, first in the German-speaking countries and then elsewhere. By the end of the century, sanatorium treatment was considered best practice in pulmonary medicine. As the number of sanatoria grew, they were often established in places that bore little resemblance to the pioneering high-altitude sanatoria. The strong environmental claim – that it was the place itself, its unique combination of natural qualities and traits which accounted for the eventual improvement – was replaced by weaker, less site-specific claims, where fresh air, sunlight and the presence of coniferous trees were sufficient qualifications for a salubrious sanatorium site. A central task of sanatorium architecture was to allow these elements to work on the patient. As the twentieth century advanced, architectural choices were more likely to be grounded on the needs of specific medical procedures and the cost-effective circulation of people and goods within the institution rather than on the needs of environmental therapies. The sanatorium gradually shed its idiosyncratic architectural features and regimen, eventually losing its *raison d'être*.[10]

The first sanatorium on what was then Finnish soil was the Halila Sanatorium on Karelian Isthmus, close to St Petersburg.[11] It was established in 1889 by Dr W.G. Dittman, a private practitioner from the Russian capital. High-altitude sanatoria were the order of the day, and Dittman was painfully aware that the fate of his "air sanatorium" crucially depended on whether he was able to convince his potential clientele – mostly middle-class consumptives from St Petersburg – that the Karelian Isthmus, a region which was anything but mountainous, could be just as therapeutic as central European mountain areas. Newspapers offered him a helping hand. One of them wrote that "Finland, this land of granite, coniferous woods and lakes, can, thanks to its meteorological and geographical and other conditions, be regarded as relatively immune with regard to consumption and tuberculosis."[12] Dittman was apparently unable to convince his potential patients of the curative power of the Karelian environment, as he was forced to sell the sanatorium a few years later. That the new proprietor happened to be the Russian Imperial house allowed Halila to grow into a major institution without having to worry about making a profit. The medical staff of the Imperial Halila Sanatorium nevertheless eagerly continued to search for links between the successful treatment of tuberculosis and the local "meteorological and geographical" conditions. The sanatorium had a meteorological station, and the research activities of the medical staff were heavily focused on studying the relationship between the local natural conditions and tuberculosis.[13]

In 1889, while Dittman was busy getting his sanatorium started, Richard Sievers (1852–1931), Finland's leading tuberculosis expert, gave a presentation at the biannual general meeting of the national medical society. The topic was the sanatorium treatment of tuberculosis, and the key question was whether this form of treatment could possibly have any future in a country with no proper mountains. Sievers asserted that while Finland had no absolutely "immune places" à la Görbersdorf, it did have plenty of forested gravel ridges that could be considered as "relatively immune" and could therefore serve as sites for sanatoria.[14] The site described by Sievers would indeed become the standard sanatorium landscape in Finland.

With a few exceptions, Finnish tuberculosis sanatoria came into being between 1900 and 1939. The total number of sanatoria operational over the course of the twentieth century was around 100. They were a heterogeneous lot, with major differences in size and facilities and minor differences in treatment regimens. But regardless of the size and form of the sanatorium, the natural environment was considered important. This deep-seated environmentalism was already indicated in basic planning choices. First, the healthiness of the prospective site was carefully inspected by tuberculosis experts before the building plan was accepted. It was considered essential that the building site was dry, elevated and surrounded by coniferous woods. Pines signalled that the soil was dry, and were also considered health-inducing in themselves. The presence of swamp or marshland was a clear counterindication, while the presence of a deep, clear-water pond, lake or river was considered a bonus.[15] The preference for the presence of water lacks a clear medical grounding, and is therefore due to aesthetic reasons, perhaps also to the age-old associations between water and healing.[16] Second, many of the characteristic features of sanatorium architecture were designed to allow the natural environment to exert a beneficial influence on the patient: the orientation of the building, the narrow patient wards, the efficient natural ventilation, as well as the large windows, balconies and terraces. The result was an idiosyncratic building that Thomas Mann famously characterized in *Zauberberg* as "pierced and porous as a sponge."[17] Third, a well-tended park and extensive wooded grounds were considered important. Even urban sanatoria had parks or easy access to woodland paths.[18]

Beautiful nature

In writing about their sanatorium stay, former patients frequently, almost routinely, described the surroundings as "beautiful." Those who provided

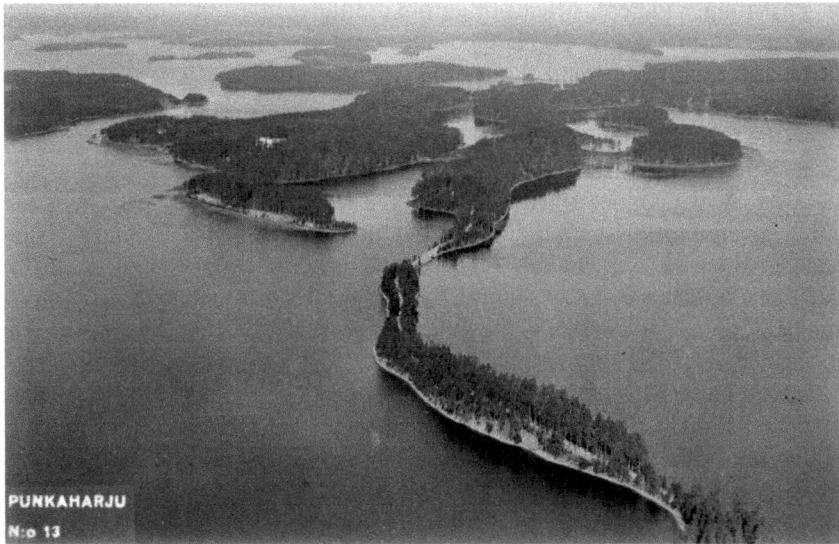

Figure 4.1 Aerial photograph of the surroundings of Takaharju Sanatorium in Punkaharju. The sanatorium building is the white blotch on the large island on the left. (The Archive of the Finnish Lung Health Association (FILHA), Helsinki.)

details usually singled out the same features as tuberculosis experts: high sandy ridges, tall pine trees, and a clear lake or a river glimmering between the trees.[19] The image of the sanatorium as a white castle set against the backdrop of a dark forest is evoked in several illness narratives. For instance, a visitor characterized the Satalinna Sanatorium as "large and castle-like. Seen from the Harjavalta bridge it resembles an old Medieval castle on the banks of the Rhein. The banks of Kokemäki River are high and forested, and the tall tower of the sanatorium rises above the tree-tops."[20] The institution which attracted the highest praise for the beauty of its natural surroundings was Takaharju Sanatorium, located in the lake district of southwestern Finland (Figure 4.1). In contrast, patients very seldom characterized the sanatorium building, or any part of it, as beautiful. Architecturally famous buildings such as the Paimio Sanatorium are no exception.[21] Sanatoria took pride in their surroundings and made full use of them in their promotional material. It would be difficult, and perhaps futile, to sharply separate therapeutic promise from aesthetic appeal. The "sanatorium landscape" closely coincided with "the national landscape" that had been canonized as quintessentially Finnish in and by the paintings of the so-called "golden age" of Finnish art (at the turn of the twentieth century).

Some patients also expressed their admiration for the well-tended sanatorium park with its rare, even exotic, plants. Sanatoria indeed took pride in and invested in their gardens: the larger ones employed at least one full-time gardener, and many matrons and physicians-in-chief took a special interest in gardening.[22] Patients often came from a different part of the country, and their sanatorium stay brought them into contact with landscapes that were novel and exciting to them. Thus a patient from a flat western province was impressed by the varied landscapes of eastern Finland, while a young woman from the north of the country described the leafy south-eastern spring as "a huge experience."[23] The highest praise for the rural landscape came from city-dwellers. A woman described in great detail the overwhelming beauty of the snow-covered forest surrounding the inland sanatorium where she had been treated when she was young: "Oh what a wonderful experience it was for a genuine city-dweller like myself, the forest that glimmered in the reflection of the hall lights in a winter's night. I had never before been in the countryside in the winter."[24]

Patients often wrote poetry, which they published in sanatorium magazines and occasionally included in their retrospective narratives. Their poems abounded with nature metaphors. In the hundreds of poems published in Paimio Sanatorium's magazine, for instance, spring was the single most common theme, standing as it did for hope and rejuvenation. Another popular theme was a wild bird caught in a cage. A poem called "The Flame" is representative of this thematic: "Like a bird, imprisoned in a room, / I fly against the glass and fall / Again and again I sigh / crying in pain."[25] Several poems contrasted "the house" and the outside world, associating the former with confinement, sickness and death, and the latter with health and freedom. The window of the patient's room, awash with rain or rattling in the wind, figured as the transparent, but unbreachable, boundary that separated the two worlds from each other.[26]

Useful nature

Patients associated the natural environment with increasing freedom of movement and improving health not only metaphorically but also concretely. Large sanatoria divided their patient population into three categories: "bed patients," "up-patients" and "walk-patients." Patients of the first kind usually had fever and were supposed to stay in bed at all times, even if they felt subjectively well enough to move about. Those in the second category had their meals in the joint dining room and took part in the regular rest hours on the communal balconies, but were not allowed to leave the building. Patients in the third group "had the walks," i.e. were considered well enough to stroll in the garden or walk along the winding footpaths in the surrounding forest. Bed rest was associated with the acute, debilitating phase of the disease, and walks in the park and around the grounds offered the hope of convalescence. Becoming a "walk-patient" was a sign of improvement and could be an exhilarating experience, especially when preceded by prolonged confinement.[27]

The natural surroundings were an important source of diversion for patients. Those confined indoors derived pleasure from observing birds and squirrels, the changing shapes of clouds or the colours of the forest.[28] Sometimes "nature" came to the bed-ridden patient through an open window. A man described in his diary how tits escaped the cold winter weather coming into the patients' rooms and the communal balcony (known as "the hall"): "They hop along our bodies, sit on the edges of our milk cups, pecking their cream-covered edges. We can often catch them when we lay on our beds in the hall."[29] Another man recalled watching from his bed, unable to move, how birds flew in and pecked on his newly excised ribs. He had just undergone a thoracoplasty and a nurse had placed his ribs, which he had requested as a memento, on a table in front of an open window.[30] Birdsong could be a prominent part of the sanatorium soundscape, especially in the spring. The daily diary entries of a woman treated in Paimio Sanatorium in 1940 typically opened by making a note of the lovely early morning birdsong. Birdsong restored her faith in life after yet another sleepless night listening to her very sick and delirious roommate cough and mumble.[31] Birdsong emerges in this narrative in a therapeutic light, as an antidote to the toxic soundscape of the patient room. Unsurprisingly, not all patients responded to natural sounds the same way. One patient wanted to see all the crows in the vicinity of the sanatorium killed, while others were disquieted by the eery nighttime owl calls.[32]

The natural environment also emerges in the patient narratives as a resource to be exploited, albeit on a very modest scale. Fishing and crabbing seem to have been relatively common in some remote wilderness sanatoria. One man even trapped small game, catching four rabbits and an ermine. Patients picked berries and mushrooms, sometimes for fun, sometimes as a form of "work therapy."[33] Such activities were gendered much the same way as they were outside the institution: men fished and crabbed, women cleaned up and cooked the prey, and both picked berries. Sanatoria certainly did not starve their patients, but such activities provided variety to their diet and offered an escape from the rigid daily routine. These activities were fondly remembered, partly, no doubt, because they allowed patients to engage in activities that had been part of their normal, everyday life before it had been disrupted by disease.

Patients also wrote about using the natural environment as a source of medication. This may seem surprising, given that sanatoria were very much part of regular medicine, with nothing "alternative" about them. One explanation for the relative prominence of this theme may be that many *ST* participants were highly aware that they were participating in a folklore collection and allowed the assumed wishes of the organizers to steer their choice of topic. However, there is no doubt that folk remedies were widely used in rural Finland well into the twentieth century. Patient narratives referred to many remedial substances derived from local nature and supposedly effective against (the symptoms of) tuberculosis: juniper bark, bird cherry and creeping willow; lichen; bog-rosemary; resin; juniper branches and berries; black salsify; common comfrey; Labrador tea; ant urine; and lye (made of birch tree ash). These ingredients were infused and drunk by the spoon- or cupful or used in ointments and medicinal baths. By far the most frequently mentioned nature-based remedial substance was tar, which was applied externally and internally, symptomatically and with the hope of actually curing tuberculosis. Patients' expressed trust in natural remedies sometimes caused friction with their doctors.[34]

The sanatorium grounds were also the primary location for *lumpustus*, known in American sanatorium slang as "cousining."[35] The word, which does not exist in Finnish outside the sanatorium context, referred to male-female relationships. *Lumpustus* is one of most extensively discussed themes in *ST*, both because the organizers encouraged the participants to write about it and because it really was an important part of sanatorium life until the end of the 1950s. This is hardly surprising. The average age of patients in pre-chemotherapeutic sanatoria was low and their average stay was long. Many patients had little contact with the outside world during that time, and they could be in a relatively good health. While the word *lumpustus* could be applied to basically any female-male interaction, it typically took the form of walks in the woods. During such walks, the strict gender segregation that prevailed inside the sanatorium was temporarily relaxed. Naming practices highlight the role of the natural environment as a scene of romance. Sanatoria were surrounded by "Love Ponds," "Love Paths," or "Kissing Alleys."[36] One winding footpath started out as "Path of Love," continued as "Path of Sin" and ended in "Bridge of Sighs."[37]

Lumpustus shows how thin the line between appropriate and inappropriate behaviour could be. While walking, talking and holding hands was fully acceptable and even encouraged by many physicians-in-chief, patients in folk sanatoria were sternly warned against "going too far." It is impossible to say how common intimate relationships were. Some informants deny any knowledge of such goings-on, others assert that veritable "orgies" were taking place in the woods. When it comes to writing about sex, the narratives are blatantly gendered. Women never described themselves as active parties in clearly sexual acts, while men sometimes did. Class also played a role; explicit first-hand descriptions of sexual acts were exclusively produced by working-class men.[38] Other clandestine activities taking place in the woods – smoking, drinking and playing cards – also emerge as distinctively male activities (Figure 4.2).[39] The risks involved in such activities (drinking, in particular, could result in immediate discharge) was part of their attraction, making them more exciting and thus more effective as a distraction. Retelling such incidents also allowed the authors to show that they had, in a small way, stood up to the authorities – a feature that the oral historian Alessandro Portelli has identified as a regular component of hospital narratives.[40]

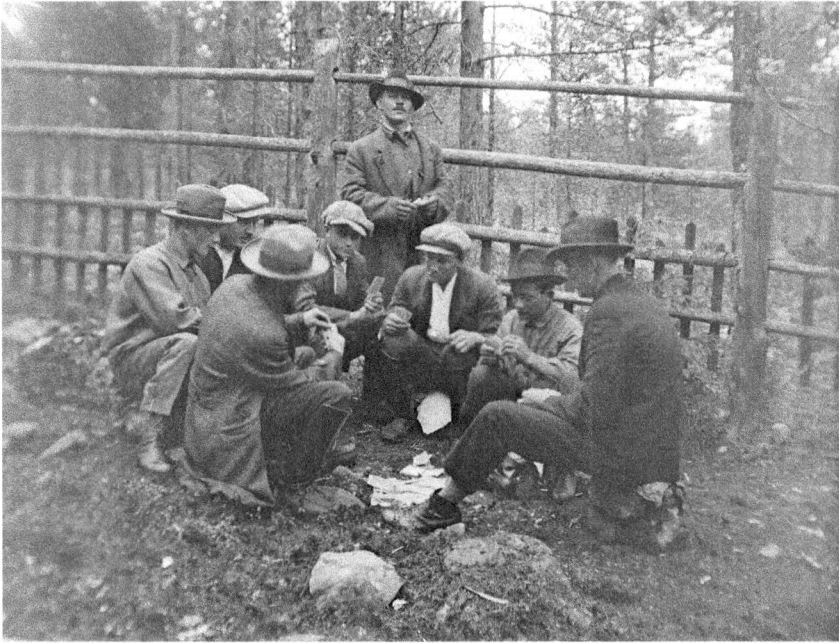

Figure 4.2 Men playing cards on the grounds of Muurola Sanatorium, Rovaniemi. (Photograph by: Matti Körkkö. The Archive of Rovaniemen Totto, Provincial Museum of Lapland.)

Therapeutic nature

Patients recognized that the natural environment contributed to their wellbeing and that the sanatorium landscape was not only beautiful but also salubrious.[41] However, they were seldom specific about what it was in the environment that supposedly enhanced their wellbeing. If and when a particular natural element was singled out, it was almost always the air.[42] Fresh air, together with rich food and rest, was the basic component of the so called "general treatment," aimed at making the body strong enough to fend off the disease. All three categories of patients were put into contact with fresh air – bed patients by means of open windows and ventilation, up-patients during the "hall hours," and "walk-patients" during their outings. The patient room window was to be kept open at all times, and feeling cold was a widely shared and frequently described physical experience. Some patients commented wryly that if cold were an effective cure for pulmonary tuberculosis, the disease would not exist in Finland, while others accepted the chill as a useful, if unpleasant, way to build up resistance.[43]

The principle of the fresh-air cure is epitomized by *halli*, the rest hall (derived from the German word *Liegehalle*). The same word was used to

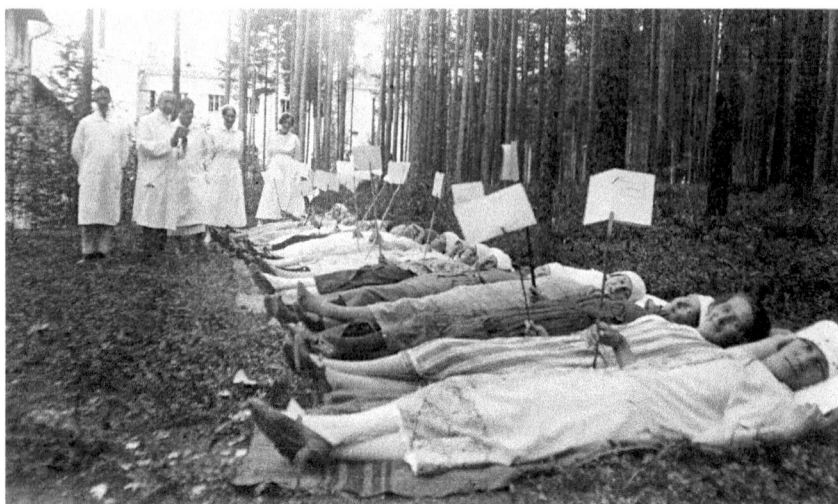

Figure 4.3 Patients taking their fresh-air rest in a "forest hall" in the grounds of Takaharju Sanatorium. (Unknown photographer. Helsinki University Museum.)

refer both to an architectural structure (the communal balcony or terrace), a social unit (the group of patients using the same hall) and the curative practice of resting in the hall. Halls were the single most distinctive feature of sanatorium architecture. Whereas individual balconies were the rule in continental Europe, they were an exception in Finnish sanatoria, where the fresh-air cure usually took place on large communal balconies located at the ends of the patient wings and disconnected from the patient rooms.[44] Bed-ridden patients did not visit the hall; it was used only by patients with no fever and well enough to walk and to carry their own sleeping bags and blankets. The women's and men's halls were usually separate. In older, smaller sanatoria, the hall could also be a free-standing construction, disconnected from the main building. In the summer, sanatoria might place patients in open "forest halls," where they rested on wooden platforms or lay directly on the ground (Figure 4.3).

Patients prescribed outdoor rest lay on their reclining chairs one to three times a day, for one to two hours at a time. The noon rest hour was called "the silent hall," and patients were not supposed talk, do needlework or read during it. "The doctors said that the silent hall was the pillar of the treatment of consumption," recalled a patient.[45] Patients were allowed to stay indoors if the weather was colder than -15 or -20 C°. The recumbent patients had their winter clothes, blankets, fur coats and perhaps also fur-lined sleeping bags to keep them warm, but many still remembered feeling cold in the hall.[46] The emotional valence of recollections relating to the rest hours, like patient experiences in general, varied a great deal. Thus, a patient might recall that it had been downright torture to lie quiet in the hall, doing nothing, like a mummy.[47] Others remembered the silent hall as "absolutely lovely" or "sweet" and the pine-smelling air as "so clean and so easy to breathe."[48]

Prior to the introduction of effective medication, patients seldom left the sanatorium fully recovered. Many continued with sanatorium-style outdoor rest hours at home, where basically any well-ventilated place such as a porch, an attic, a shed, a hammock or a plank bed might serve as a "hall."[49] A women noted in her diary during her convalescence: "My folks take good care of me. I have a fine private hall on the porch. [...] Treatment continues much the same as in the sanatorium: hall rest, walks in fresh air, and plenty of milk and good food. The only medications are Aspirin and brandy [mixed] with egg and milk. [...] I put the expectorations in a paper bag which I get to burn in the oven."[50] The popularity of such domestic arrangements show, first, that patients and doctors had faith in the therapeutic value of outdoor rest and, second, that they no longer believed that the curative effects were related to a particular geographical site.

Whereas fresh air was regarded as a *sine qua non* in the treatment of pulmonary tuberculosis, the benefit of sunbathing was a moot point. Sunlight had been firmly associated with health since the beginning of the twentieth century, when its germicidal qualities had been established. The flood of health education literature produced by the anti-tuberculosis associations during the first decades of the century instructed women to expose both their homes and their children to sunlight in order to prevent disease. Sunlight was considered important not only in tuberculosis control but also in combating rickets, a common health problem at the time.[51] Hospital and school architecture favoured large windows and a south-eastern orientation in order to increase the solar exposure of surfaces and people.[52] Interwar Europe also had several social and youth movements which promoted outdoor life and linked a tan to health and moral uprightness.[53]

However, sunbathing was not prescribed to patients with pulmonary tuberculosis and, by the 1950s, it was squarely counterindicated.[54] Evidence had been accumulating since the beginning of the century that direct solar exposure could aggravate pulmonary tuberculosis, increase body temperature and, most dangerously, trigger haemoptysis. Some *ST* patients had first-hand experience of the risks involved. One man described a haemoptysis he had suffered during his treatment at the Halila Sanatorium in his youth. On a midsummer night's eve, he had been left in the sanatorium with a handful of other patients and a night nurse while the others had gone down to the lake to see the midsummer bonfire. The day had been warm, and the balcony on which the patients rested was stifling hot.

Of course temperature and blood pressure rose. The older patient coped with the heat. We two younger ones suffered haemoptyses. The other one, an 18-year-old refugee from Eastern Karelia, died the next day. Circa two litres of blood spurted out of me that midsummer night's eve. I was close to suffocation. I was the night nurse's first 'blood patient' [...]. This business turned both our noses white, to the extent that they could be made out from the blood.[55]

Paediatric sanatoria for extrapulmonary tuberculosis differed from adult sanatoria in many respects, including the way they construed and made use of the natural environment for therapeutic purposes. The average treatment times in children's sanatoria were even longer than in adult sanatoria. Prior to the introduction of efficient medication, a person could spent the whole of his or her childhood in a sanatorium. Those suffering from bone tuberculosis spent much or all of this time immobilized in their beds, which precluded all spontaneous contact with the natural environment. At the same time, exposing children to the elements was considered an essential part of the treatment. Heliotherapy (natural sunlight) and phototherapy (artificial light) were routinely administered in paediatric sanatoria; seaside paediatric sanatoria also relied on sea bathing. For instance, in the summer, the children treated at the Högsand Seaside Sanatorium (founded 1901), located on the southern coast of Finland, spent practically all their waking hours, and sometimes their nights as well, outdoors. They bathed in the sea and lay in the sun. Weight gain and a deepening tan were considered signs of improvement[56] (see Figure 4.4).

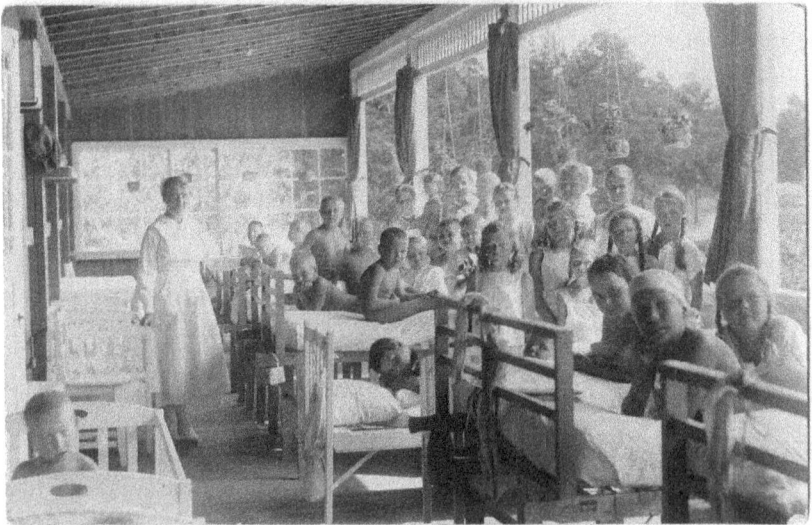

Figure 4.4 Children on the terrace of Kalevanniemi Paediatric Sanatorium in the early 1920s. (Unknown photographer. The Image Collection of the Åbo Akademi University.)

While sea bathing was not part of the regimen in inland paediatric sanatoria, fresh air and sunbathing were. Child patients would be rolled onto the terrace in their beds and left there for hours. On summer days, they sunbathed naked, with only their heads covered, and ate and napped on the terrace.[57] A female narrator recounts that "Our beds were put on the balcony side by side the first thing in the morning, right after morning porridge. [...] Some oil was applied on our skin and Doctor often measured our tan with a piece of equipment." During her years in the institution, she developed an intense dislike for both sunbathing and superalimentation. "I started to hate food. I hated it. I used to say that when I get out I will eat hardly anything, not until I'm really hungry. And I hated the summer sun. You 'fatface', I used to repeat when it burned my skin with full force."[58]

Experts were divided as to the relative merits of the coastal and inland climate and environment in treating paediatric tuberculosis. The authoritative committee of the Swedish Anti-Tuberculosis Association stated in its 1929 report that the seashore offered no discernible benefit in the treatment of children with extrapulmonary tuberculosis, at least not in the Swedish climate. The report was carefully studied in Finland as well. A.J. Palmén, a doctor at Salpausselkä Paediatric Sanatorium, believed that "it would be important to carry out a comparative study" on the treatment results of inland and coastal sanatoria. He was probably contemplating undertaking such a study himself, as he had equipped his sanatorium with meteorological equipment.[59] At this time, adult sanatoria were no longer concerned with climatological or meteorological studies. Indeed, the link between the healing environment and tuberculosis seems to have persisted longer in the context of paediatric than adult sanatoria. This can be explained by the nature of extrapulmonary tuberculosis, but it also resonated with deep-seated notions about children's special relationship with nature. Swedish historians Karin Aronson and Bengt Sandin have noted that in many cultures, including early twentieth-century Western culture, children were regarded as being closer to nature than adults and were talked about using plant metaphors, as growing organisms reaching for the sun.[60]

Effective anti-tuberculosis drugs were introduced at the beginning of the 1950s, but it took some time before they were effectively and routinely used, and the whole decade should be regarded as a transitory period. As one patient put it, writing about the early 1950s: "we were, so to speak, at the turning point between old and new ways of treatment." The sanatorium regimen still included compulsory hall rest, woodland walks, and overeating, but treatment also relied heavily on surgical operations and the new drugs.[61] Effective medication became universally available only at the beginning of the 1960s, when it was made free to the patient. In the course of the 1960s, traditional sanatorium practices such as hall rest and gradated woodland walks first became voluntary and then increasingly rare, and halls were either demolished or converted into indoor space. The sanatorium building closed upon itself, as it were, and the long history of environmental therapy for tuberculosis came to an end.

Conclusion

Patients taking part in the *Collection Competition for Sanatorium Tradition* did not subscribe to the notion of immune places, i.e. to the idea that there are specific geographical locations that – thanks to a fortuitous combination of natural qualities – could contain or even cure tuberculosis. This is hardly surprising, given that most of them wrote down their recollections in 1971, when the notion had long since vanished from mainstream medical thinking. The connection between healing nature and lung health had not been completely severed, however. Patients still associated some features of the natural environment, for instance pines and the smell of resin, with lung health. They did this on a fairly general level, and sometimes distanced themselves from such beliefs by their choice of words, writing, for instance, that the air around pines "was considered to be" or "was supposedly" healthy.[62]

That is not to say that they did not value the natural environment. Despite the often severe physical restrictions caused by their disease, sanatorium patients found many ways of enjoying and making use of the natural environment. It emerges in their narratives as a source of diversion, food and remedies, as well as granting them some privacy and freedom. On the grounds, patients were temporarily able to free themselves from the strict social control which prevailed inside the sanatorium and to regain a degree of agency and individuality. While they appreciated the beauty of the natural environment, they were more likely to describe it in pragmatic than romantic or aesthetic terms. Patients' matter-of-fact attitude towards the natural environment is no doubt related to the fact that the majority of them originated in the countryside, in the small farms that were the distinctive feature of the rural landscape and economy until the end of the 1960s. Activities such as fishing or berry-picking were very much part of their normal lives.

The notion that tuberculosis was a product of modern urban life and should be counteracted by "immersion in nature" has been identified as being central to the development of sanatorium treatment in the European context. This conception found very little resonance with the patients represented in *ST*. The absence of the theme reflects both the distribution of tuberculosis in Finland and the social outlook of the patient population. In contradistinction to many other European countries, tuberculosis was more common in the countryside than in the cities. Finland was still an agrarian country, and many people worked in primary production, i.e. farming and forestry. By Central and Western European standards, the degree of urbanization and industrialization remained low until the early 1970s. The average farm was small; all family members, including children, were involved in farming work.[63] The majority of the patients participating in *ST* came from this kind of background. They had been "immersed in nature" most of their lives, also when they fell ill. It is little wonder that the idea of immersion in nature as restorative in itself found little resonance among them.

When patients describe their contacts with nature, they make little distinction between emotional and physical wellbeing. One patient wrote: "April ushered in spring, snow melted on the slopes, and it was nice, during the walking hours, to wander around in the woods and sit in the sun. Life felt downright enjoyable."[64] Another patient exclaimed: "Oh you wonderful OZONE that quicken my imagination and stimulate my reason. PINE has always been an object of my admiration. How straight and brave it raises its top towards the skies. Oh if only one could become as straight, brave and life-enhancing."[65] The latter quotation may be untypically florid, but it is entirely typical in representing nature as a source of mental as well as physical wellbeing and in drawing parallels between plants (or animals) and humans. Patients firmly believed that emotional states impacted the course of the disease. In their intrinsically psychosomatic interpretative framework, the therapeutic value of any aspect of sanatorium life – including the natural environment – was predicated upon its capacity to keep the spirits up despite the constant presence of disease and death.

Notes

1 Porter 1985.
2 Bryder 1988; Smith 1988; Ott 1996; Rothman 1994; Shaw and Reeves 2009; Burke 2018. In addition, Boon (2010) discusses lay narratives of tuberculosis in the context of health education and Condrau (2001) has used a hall diary to investigate patients' self-organization and experience.
3 There is a strong tradition of collecting such testimonies in the Nordic and Baltic counties. In Finland, several cultural organizations, most importantly the Finnish Literature Society, have been actively involved in collecting written narratives on a wide variety of topics. These collections have often been framed as "competitions", although the prizes were too modest to account for their popularity. Data collected this way has been used above all by folklore scholars and oral historians. On thematic writing calls and collections, see e.g. Heimo 2016 and "The folklore activities" 2009.
4 "Parantolaperinnettä 9000 sivua" 1972, 7.
5 Although the majority of the people who answered the writing call were former sanatorium patients writing about their own experiences, the contributions also include second-hand accounts and entries written by staff and people who had not been treated in sanatoria but nevertheless felt that they had something to say about the issue. While the texts were mainly written in 1971 as an answer to the call, people also sent in "remnants" such as (excerpts from) diaries, letters and patient magazines.
6 "Parantolaperinnekilpailun kutsu" 1971, 8.

7   The folklore scholar Aili Nenola has written a book on patients' sanatorium culture and self-organization (Nenola 1986), using *ST* as her material, and parts of the collection have been used as source material in unpublished MA theses (Uurtamo 2010; Taskila-Åbrandt 2000).
8   Teller 1988, 6, 11; Rothman 1994, 19, 132, 134.
9   Rothman 1994, 195; Ott 1996, 147–48; Bynum 2012, 129–30; Châtelet 2006; Châtelet 2014, 107–08; Burke 2018, 281.
10 On the architectural history of the tuberculosis sanatorium, see, e.g. Cremnitzer 2005; Adams, Schwarzman and Theodore 2008; Heikinheimo 2016; Kisacky 2017, 178–81, 253; Willis, Goad and Logan 2019, 8, 163–64. The latter two books are also useful in relating the history of sanatorium architecture to broader development of environmentalism in hospital architecture in the late nineteenth and twentieth centuries.
11 From 1809 to 1917, Finland was part of the Russian Empire as an autonomous Grand Duchy. Karelian Isthmus was part of Finland until 1940.
12 "Halila Sanatorium" 1999.
13 Blomqvist 1986.
14 Sievers 1890.
15 Sievers 1890; Hirvensalo 1931, 6; Proceedings of the Relief Association for Consumptives of Little Means 23 May 1913 § 4 (The Archive of the Finnish Lung Health Association, Helsinki); Hannes Ryömä and Severi Savonen to the Sanatorium Committee of South-Western Finland, 27 June 1928. Proceedings of the Building Committee of Sanatorium of South-Western Finland 1928–1934 (Ca:1) (The Archive of the Paimio Hospital, Paimio).
16 On these beliefs, see Foley 2010.
17 *Zauberberg* (1916), cited in Châtelet 2014, 111.
18 Harju 32–38, Poijärvi 14 (*ST*). In the following, the source material deriving from *Sanatorium Tradition* is referred to by the surname of the author of the contribution, followed by the abbreviation of the collection (= *ST*).
19 Rantanen 15–16, Tolsa 1, Arola 5–7, Holopainen 2, Kivilahti 22, Koponen 11, Kuhlberg 4, Kylmäaho 1, Pehkonen 11, Yli-Jyrä 2, Forss 3–4, Kaario 32, Kiander 4–5, Kleemola 2, Korhonen-Jolma 1–3, Leino 2–3, Stadius 2–3, Tiainen 8, Pönkkö 9, Kapiainen 11 (*ST*); Raunio-Hietanen in Hoffren et al. 2006, 123–25.
20 Soini 23 (*ST*). Th original diary entry is from September 7, 1928.
21 Paimio Sanatorium was designed by the office of Alvar Aalto and opened in 1933. It is among the most well-known buildings of the early modern movement.
22 Lindqvist 8, Aro-Heinilä 5, Lohi 26, Kapiainen 11 (*ST*); Hakosalo 2015a, 151; Hakosalo 2015b, 150.
23 Tavasti 1, Lohi 25, 26, Pönkkö 9 (*ST*).
24 Kaario 21, 45 (*ST*).
25 *Pasuna* 1949, quoted in Aitamäki 364 (*ST*).
26 Kanervisto 27, Saarikoski 2, Piikamäki 2 (*ST*).
27 Hannula 10, Meilo 6 (*ST*).
28 Mäki-Petäjä 27, Aitamäki 932, Kivimäki 12–13 (*ST*).
29 Aimo-Koivisto 9 (the original diary entry is from December 12, 1907). See also Bogdanoff 27–28 (*ST*).
30 Ijäs 8 (*ST*).
31 Karke 4–5, 8, 15 (the original diary entries are from May 1940) (*ST*).

32 Aitamäki 827 (*ST*); Hoffren et al. 2006, 73–4.
33 Lohi 28, Hiiro 2, Jaatinen 16, Jaskari 3, Jääskeläinen 11–12, 18, Rantanen 15–16, Yli-Jyrä 10, Mäki-Petäjä 27, Pönkkö 9, Heikkilä 17–18, Jokinen 3, Mäki-Petäjä 27 (*ST*).
34 Leskinen 344, Korhonen 26, Heikkinen 2–3, 8–9, 18–25, Kivilahti 18–19, Eerola 4, Suoniemi 17, Kasurinen 3–4, Torvinen 6, Huotari 1–2, Järvinen 3, Kuisma 3, Savolainen 1–2, Aitamäki 22–23, Rontu 3–4, 5–6, 8–9, Soini 4–5, Karke 18 (*ST*).
35 Rothman 1994, 236–37.
36 Liukko 4, Koskell 7, Korkeakoski 5, Anttonen 3–4, Hannula 15, Viljanen 25–26, Yli-Jyrä 10, Jääskeläinen 18, Kivilahti 5, Jaskari 3 (*ST*).
37 Koponen 11 (*ST*).
38 Nevalainen 29–30, Harju 32–38, Kivilahti 5–6, 35, Tuominen 35–36, Tuberkuloosi- ja keuhkovammaliiton aineisto 233, Aitamäki 174 (*ST*).
39 Kautto 81–85, Kivelä 3–4, Koskelin 7, Aitamäki 145, Leskelä 5, Ijäs 30 (*ST*).
40 Portelli 1997, 7–8.
41 Korja 1 (*ST*).
42 On beliefs and practices concerning the purity of air and tuberculosis in more industrialized parts of Europe, see Worboys 1992, 50.
43 Huvinen 15, Lahti 9–10, Salmu 25, Salo 2 (*ST*).
44 Cremnitzer 2014, 116–17.
45 Kuusisto 8 (*ST*).
46 Kanervisto 20, Aarnio 7–8, Heikkilä 11–13, Reiman 8, 15–16, Wessman 9, Aitamäki 932–33, Aimo-Koivisto 4–5 (*ST*).
47 Viiliäinen 13 (*ST*).
48 Saarinen 11, Tomppo 9, Kapiainen 8, Forss 5 (*ST*).
49 Heikkilä 4, Karke 28, Korhonen 5, Torvinen 7–8, Aro-Heinilä 7, Finnilä 18–19, Tuberkuloosi- ja keuhkovammaisten liiton aineisto 188, Aitamäki 20 (*ST*).
50 Soini 17 (*ST*).
51 The disease was related empirically to lack of sunlight before the connection between UV light and vitamin D synthesis on the skin was discovered in the 1950s.
52 On hospital design and sunshine exposure, see Kisacky 2017, 149.
53 Carter 2011, 95–97.
54 *Instructions for the Patients of Paimio Sanatorium* (1971), quoted in Aitamäki 261, *Totovaaran Joiku* 1956, quoted in Arvola 35 (*ST*).
55 Piikamäki 4. Another example can be found in Tuberkuloosi- ja Keuhkovammaliiton aineisto 169 (*ST*).
56 *Journal of the History of Childhood and Youth* published a special issue on paediatric seaside sanatoria in 2009, edited by Janet Golden.
57 Kivimäki 12–13, Sivula 31–32, Tynkkynen 1 (*ST*).
58 Peltoniemi 9–10, 14–15 (*ST*).
59 Alho and Palmén 1930, 4–6; Proceedings of the Relief Association for Consumptives with Little Means 11 March 1925 § 9 (The Archive of the Finnish Lung Health Association, Helsinki). Sweden had several seaside sanatoria, established at the beginning of the twentieth century. On Swedish seaside sanatoria, see Nelson and Förhammer 2009.
60 Aronsson and Sandin 1996, 190, 194–96, 199.
61 Naskali 4–5 (*ST*).
62 Harju 114–15, Nevalainen 29 (*ST*).

63 Koponen and Saaritsa 2019.
64 Mäki-Petäjä 29 (*ST*).
65 Pajunen-Kivekäs 39 (*ST*). Capitals in the original.

References

Unpublished sources

Proceedings of the Relief Association for Consumptives of Little Means (Vähävaraisten keuhkotautisten avustamisyhdistys). The Archives of the Finnish Lung Health Association (FILHA), Helsinki.
The Proceedings of the Building Committee of the Tuberculosis Sanatorium of South-Western Finland 1928–1934. The Archives of the Hospital District of South-Western Finland, Paimio and Turku.

Published source

Adams, Annemarie, Kevin Schwatrzman, and David Theodore. 2008. "Collapse and Expand: Architecture and Tuberculosis Therapy in Montreal, 1909, 1933, 1954." *Technology and Culture* 49: 908–42.
Adams, Jane M. 2015. *Healing with Water: English Spas and the Water Cure, 1840–1960*. Manchester: Manchester University Press.
Alho, Ensio and A.J. Palmén. 1930. "Tuberkuloositaistelun vastaiset suuntaviivat Ruotsissa." *Tuberkuloosilehti* 6 (1): 1–8.
Aronson, Karin and Bengt Sandin. 1996. "The Sun Match Boy and Plant Metaphors: A Swedish Image of a 20th-century Childhood." In *Images of Childhood*, edited by C. Philip Hwang, Michael E. Lamb, and Irving E. Sigel, 185–202. New York & London: Psychology Press.
Blomqvist, Tore. 1986. "Ryska tuberkulossanatorien på Karelska näset från slutet av 1800-talet till Ryska revolutionen år 1917." *Hippokrates*, no. 3: 124–49.
Boon, Timothy. 2010. "Lay Disease Narratives, Tuberculosis, and Health Education Films." In *Tuberculosis Then and Now: Perspectives on the History of an Infectious Disease*, edited by Flurin Condrau and Michael Worboys, 24–48. Montreal & Kingston: McGill-Queens University Press.
Bryder, Linda. 1988. *Below the Magic Mountain: A Social History of Tuberculosis in Twentieth-Century Britain*. Oxford: Clarendon Press.
Burke, Stacie. 2018. *Building Resistance: Children, Tuberculosis and the Toronto Sanatorium*. Montreal and Kingston: McGill-Queen's University Press.
Bynum, Helen. 2012. *Spitting Blood: The History of Tuberculosis*. Oxford: Oxford University Press.
Carter, Simon. 2011. "Leagues of Sunshine: Sunlight, Health and the Environment." In *Environment, Health and History*, edited by Martin Gorsky and Virginia Berridge, 94–112. Basingstoke: Palgrave Macmillan.
Châtelet, Anne-Marie. 2006. "La naissance du sanatorium en Europe et aux États-Unis (1860–1902)." In *Les Quinze glorieuses de l'architecture sanatoriale*, 16–20. Assy: Centre de Recherche et d'étude sur l'Histoire de'Assy.
Châtelet, Anne-Marie. 2014. "Early Days of the Sanatorium (1860–1902)." In *Alvar Aalto Architect: Paimio Sanatorium 1929–1933*, edited by Mia Hipeli and Esa Laaksonen, 106–11. Helsinki: Alvar Aalto Foundation and Rakennustieto.

Condrau, Flurin. 2001. "Who is the Captain of All These Men of Death? The Social Structure of Tuberculosis Sanatorium Patients in Postwar Germany." *Journal of Interdisciplinary History* 32 (2): 243–62.

Cremnitzer, Jean-Bernard. 2014. "The Sanatorium in Europe in the 1920s and 1930s." In *Alvar Aalto Architect: Paimio Sanatorium 1929–1933,* edited by Mia Hipeli and Esa Laaksonen, 113–17. Helsinki: Alvar Aalto Foundation and Rakennustieto.

Cremnitzer, Jean-Bernard. 2005. *Architecture et santé. Le temps du sanatorium en France et en Europe.* Paris: Editions A&J Picard Paperback.

Foley, Ronan. *Healing Landscapes: Therapeutic Landscapes in Historical and Contemporary Ireland.* Farnham: Ashgate, 2010.

"The folklore activities of the Finnish Literature Society". 2009. The web pages of the Finnish Literature Society. www.folklorefellows.fi/the-folklore-activities-of-the-finnish-literature-society/

Golden, Janet. 2009. "Editor's Introduction" (To a Special Issue on Children's Seaside Sanatoria). *Journal of the History of Childhood and Youth* 2 (2): 217–19.

Hakosalo, Heini. 2015a. "'En vacker kvinnogärning': Rita Gripenberg ja Muurolan parantola." In *Lisää tällaista! Marianne Junilan juhlakirja,* edited by Heini Hakosalo, Seija Jalagin, and Tiina Kinnunen, 145–60. Oulu: Oulun historiaseura.

Hakosalo, Heini. 2015b. "Elin och Ille. Syskon, kön och medicinsk karriär i det tidiga 1900-talets Finland", *Historisk Tidskrift för Finland* 100 (2): 125–60.

"Halila Sanatorium." 1899. *Finland,* June 17, 1899.

Härö, Sakari. 1992. *Vuosisata tuberkuloosityötä Suomessa: Suomen tuberkuloosin vastustamisyhdistyksen historia.* [Helsinki]: Suomen tuberkuloosin vastustamis-yhdistys.

Heikinheimo, Marianna. 2016. *Architecture and Technology: Alvar Aalto's Paimio Sanatorium.* Helsinki: Aalto University.

Heimo, Anne. 2016. "Nordic-Baltic Oral History on the Move." *The Journal of Oral History Society* 44 (2): 37–46.

Hirvensalo, V[äinö]. 1931. *Selostus Tarinaharjun parantolan eli Pohjois-Savon kansanparantolan alkuvaiheista ja rakentamisesta. Parantolan vihkimistilaisuuteen joulukuun 27 p:nä 1931.* Kuopio: Pohjois-Savon Kansanparantolan rakennus-toimikunta.

Hoffren, Raimo et al. 2006. *Elämää Tarinanmäellä. Tarinanharjun parantolan perinnettä sanoin ja kuvin.* Kuopio: KYS sairaalamuseo.

Jauho, Mikko. 2007. *Kansanterveysongelman synty. Tuberkuloosi ja terveyden hallinta Suomessa ennen toista maailmansotaa.* Helsinki: Tutkijaliitto.

Kisacky, Jeanne. 2017. *Rise of the Modern Hospital: An Architectural History of Health and Healing, 1870–1940.* University of Pittsburgh Press.

Koponen, Juhani and Sakari Saaritsa, eds. 2019. *Nälkämaasta hyvinvointivaltioksi. Suomi kehityksen kiinniottajana.* Helsinki: Gaudeamus.

Mansén, Elisabeth. 2001. *Ett paradis på jorden. Om den svenska kurortskulturen 1680–1880.* Stockholm: Atlantis.

Nelson, Marie C. and Staffan Förhammar. 2009. "Swedish Seaside Sanatoria in the Beginning of the Twentieth Century." *Journal of the History of Childhood and Youth* 2 (2): 249–66.

Nenola, Aili. 1986. *Parantolaelämää – tuberkuloosipotilaat muistelevat.* Helsinki: Keuhkovammaliitto.

Ott, Katherine. 1996. *Fevered Lives: Tuberculosis in American Culture since 1870.* Cambridge, MA: Harvard University Press.

"Parantolaperinnekilpailun kutsu." 1971. *Silmu. Tuberkuloosi- ja keuhkovammaisten liiton jäsenlehti*, no. 1: 6–8.

"Parantolaperinnettä 9000 sivua." 1972. *Jousi. Tuberkuloosi- ja keuhkovammaisten liiton lehti* 27 (1): 6–8.

Portelli, Alessandro. 1997. *The Battle of Valle Giulia: Oral History and the Art of Dialogue*. Madison: University of Wisconsin Press.

Porter, Roy. 1985. "The Patient's View: Doing Medical History from Below." *Theory and Society* 14: 175–98.

Rothman, Sheila M. 1994. *Living in the Shadow of Death: Tuberculosis and the Social Experience of Illness in American History*. Baltimore and London: The Johns Hopkins University Press.

Shaw, Anne and Carole Reeves. 2009. *The Children of Craig-y-nos: Life in a Welsh Tuberculosis Sanatorium, 1922–1959*. Milton Keynes: Wellcome Trust Centre.

Sievers, Richard. 1890. "Är inrättandet af ett sanatorium för lungsiktige i Finland ändamålsenligt och önskligt? Om så är fallet hvar bör ett sådant lämpligast förläggas?" *Förhandlingar vid Finska Läkaresällskapets tolfte allmänna möte i Helsingfors den 19, 20 och 21 september 1889*, 50–77. Helsingfors: J.C. Frenckell & Son.

Smith, F.B. 1988. *The Retreat of Tuberculosis, 1850–1950*. London: Croom Helm.

Taskila-Åbrandt, Taina. 2000. *"Elämää ihmispelkona". Tuberkuloosipotilaan leimautuminen parantola-ajan Suomessa*. An unpublished MA thesis. University of Helsinki.

Teller, Michael E. 1988. *The Tuberculosis Movement: A Public Health Campaign in the Progressive Era*. New York: Greenwood Press, 1988.

Tiitta, Allan. 2009. *Collegium medicum. Lääkintöhallitus 1878–1991*. Helsinki: Lääkintöhallitus.

Uurtamo, Teija. 2010. *"Siitähän paranee, ellei kuole!" Keuhkotaudin kokeminen nuoren naisen päiväkirjoissa 1938–1941*. An unpublished MA thesis. University of Turku.

Willis, Julie, Philip Goad, and Cameron Logan. 2019. *Architecture and the Modern Hospital: Nosokomeion to Hygeia*. Abington & New York: Routledge.

Worboys, Michael. 1992. "The Sanatorium Treatment for Consumption in Britain, 1890–1914." In *Medical Innovations in Historical Perspective*, edited by John V. Pickstone, 47–71. New York: Palgrave MacMillan.

Part II

Colonial environments and health

Chapter 5

From the "wooden world" to "London in miniature"
Charlotte Bristowe Browne's diary, nursing, and the French and Indian Wars

Marcel Hartwig

Introduction

In 1924, the Library of Congress acquired a photographic copy of the diary of a Madame Browne from the collection of an S.A. Courtauld in London. The document details the events of her travels in the North American colonial space between November 1754 and January 1757, the first year after the Seven Years' War was officially declared. The diary was made available as a full scan by the New York Historical Society, via digital long-term archiving, so anyone can now read about Browne's daily routine as an appointed Matron first in General Braddock's and later Lord Loudoun's military hospitals during the war. This version of the diary was originally presented to the New York Historical Society by Samuel V. Hoffmann on 12 April 1932.[1] So far, the diary has been edited in excerpts for two scholarly contributions and proved to be an insightful addition to captivity narratives, colonial travelogues, and the historical study of the French and Indian Wars (1754–1763).[2] The diary was written in an era that is marked by utilitarian and enlightenment rationale: "The eighteenth century was an era of 'useful' knowledge. The utilitarian dynamic of empire, travel and intercultural encounter fostered practices of collection and codification, and a model of 'improvement' which focused on intervention."[3] Browne's diary rather stands for the aspect of collection, as she wrote up her experiences not solely for herself, but, as will be shown, for an intended audience. Her writing coincides with the popularity of travelogues in England: "[T]ravel writing proliferated in the eighteenth century, gaining a prestige and popularity which it maintained until well into the nineteenth century."[4]

Incidentally, Browne's diary provides insight into the North American colonial space by offering brief notes on daily life in the colonies and the organization of medical services. Being also "the doctor's country woman,"[5] Madame Browne's sporadic notes may give readers an insight into the application of medical knowledge from the metropolitan institutions in distant peripheries. Charlotte Browne's diary is here discussed as a primary reading to understand what it was like to be an English gentlewoman in the North

American theatres of the Seven Years' War. From this angle, then, her diary serves as an intriguing study of the New World as a transnational contact zone and allows insights into military medical practice and a woman's role in maintaining the health of soldiers. As will be shown in the following pages, Browne's diary particularly accentuates the community-driven aspects of medical knowledge production in the New World. Since the diary's author witnesses her experiences through a marked English lens, it is necessary to also consider the influence of a cultural filter on the assessment of a truth value in colonial medical practice.

This chapter studies Browne's diary with regard to the specific medical work and application of cures in order to explore which modes of knowledge production informed British military nurses and their experiences in the North American colonies during the French and Indian Wars of 1754–1763.[6] The following pages will be devoted to Browne's diary in order to discuss (1) how Browne particularly accentuates the community-driven aspects of medical knowledge production in the New World; (2) in what ways Browne's distinct English point of view influences a cultural filter on the assessment of colonial medical practice; and (3) what it meant to be a female nurse in the Seven Years' War.

As a member of General Braddock's wagon train, Browne travelled with the British Forces across the Atlantic aboard the ship *London*, which she repeatedly refers to as a "wooden world," to provide care for the sick. Browne was a civilian officer of the medical unit and the ship was "laden with stores for the hospital"[7] which was to be set up at Fort Cumberland.[8] The voyage across the Atlantic took little more than three months before the ship "cast anchor in Hampton Road"[9] in Chesapeake, Virginia. The medical staff of the Braddock regiments were to remain aboard the ships for an additional month. Browne's entries in her diary on 26 March 1754 imply some confusion regarding the provision of lodgings for her fellow comrades: "5 of the Doctors being at a Loss where to go, came to board with us staid 3 Weeks and then were order'd to Will's Creek" – an access point to the Potomac River at Cumberland.[10]

After Browne and the remaining staff were allowed to leave the *London*, she reports a short stay in Chesapeake, which seemed to be a "very agreeable place."[11] Browne soon had to move to Bellhaven,[12] a small town so densely populated with soldiers waiting for their orders that she barely managed to find a place to stay. Her comments on these first stations identify Browne's narrative voice as that of a gentlewoman. Whereas Hampton Road is a "very agreeable place" to her, Belhaven is merely "as agreeable a place as could be expected, it being inhabited but 4 years."[13] Here, the Matron is commenting on the progress of the civilizing effects of colonialism and appears to be very much in favour of the latter. These imperial notions frequent the diary in a plethora of episodes, for example when Browne writes about the many well-esteemed families she is invited to visit, the dances she attends, and the teatimes she is asked to join. Browne hails these occasions as a generally positive civilizing progress in the colonies. As a frequent guest in colonial genteel circles, Browne's diary invites readings on the "webs of exchange between Britain and its colonies" that, according to Sarah Fatherly, are "a critical factor in shaping colonial gender, as well as class, [and] norms."[14]

For example, when Browne attended a meeting with the commanding colonel, Hubert Marshall, at Fort Albany in New York, she reports an unpleasant encounter with some Dutch guests: "Went to the Fort to deliver a Letter from Dr. Bard at New York to Col' Marshall and was receiv'd with great politeness but the Dutch had a very bad Opinion of me saying I could not be good to come so far without a Husband."[15] With comments like these, the heteronormative and patriarchal perspectives of the elite local circles become evident. However, Browne distinguishes between the politeness of the English colonel and the rudeness of the Dutch locals and thus foregrounds the preferable manners of the English in the colonies. Such an assessment speaks volumes about the reputation of independent women medical workers during the French and Indian Wars. Indeed, on several occasions, Madame Browne had to defend her status as a widowed civilian officer on her journeys in the North American colonies. Either she reports on "money disputes" with her friend, the surgeon John Cherrington, who was put under General Braddock's command in 1755 and did not share with Madame Browne "the same opinion as to [her] sex,"[16] or she is in need of her dear friend to have her status explained when trying to obtain lodgings, or rather a room of her own,[17] while marching from fort to fort.

On another occasion, Browne even reports that another gentlewomen had to vouch for her because the Dutch mistook her for the Miss of General Braddock after which she "had convinced them, that I [Charlotte B. Browne] was not for that her Father had known me Maid, Wife and Widow and that nobody could say any thing (sic!) bad of me."[18] While Browne was stressing the active role of women in accommodating her or protecting her reputation, "she was indeed responding to something familiar: women's instrumental activity in creating a stable, defined elite" in the British colonies in North America.[19] Browne's perspective is thus informed by a specific cultural filter which very much informs the narrative point of view in her diary.

Upon the regiment's arrival in Bellhaven, the civilian officer of General Braddock's units was soon to receive the order to join a wagon train to Will's Creek "with one Officer, my Brother, self and Servant, 2 Nurses, 2 Cooks, and 40 men to guard us, 12 Waggons with the sick, Lame, and Blind, my Waggon in the Rear."[20] This exhausting journey, along what is today's Braddock Road, led Browne through "heavy forests, every mile of which would have to be widened and graded."[21] "The Roads are so bad that I am almost disjointed," reads one of her comments on this long march.[22] Two weeks later she was to arrive – sick and exhausted – at Fort Cumberland at Wills Creek on the Potomac River to take up her quarters. Soon both her brother and her maid are "taken ill with a Fever and Flux and Fits"[23] – a condition her brother will not survive.

After receiving news of the disaster on the Monongahela, a battle that cost the lives of many men including General Braddock himself, Browne is in the fort, waiting for new marching orders. In the meantime, a scalped boy appears, announcing the approaching enemy. Luckily, she manages to escape to Frederick's Town, where she waits for the sick to be brought from Fort Cumberland. Her new marching orders take her first to Philadelphia, a city she describes as "London in miniature,"[24] then New York, and finally to Albany, where she is stationed at the military hospital of Fort Frederick. The narrative ends abruptly in August 1757 right after she reports that 700 French soldiers are closing in. Browne, however, used a part of her diary as a daybook,[25] a form of record-keeping concerning bills, costs and income. These last pages of her diary reveal both Browne's return to England and her payment scheme. The date of the last fiscal entry is 19 July 1765.

Historically, the Braddock expedition is mostly of interest because of its disastrous failure and the early disadvantage it caused British troops during the French and Indian Wars.[26] Browne's diary not only documents the stages and direct impact of the losses during the campaign, but also its medical aspects. In addition, she shared a personal tragedy with her fellow soldiers due to an infection that befell many of them at Will's Creek en route to Fort Cumberland: a "bloody flux."[27] In Browne's episode, the "flux" would eventually end the life of her brother, the apothecary Robert Bristowe. Out of 2,041 men overall, only "705 regulars [were] fit for duty, 127 sick, 250 wounded" by the end of the campaign.[28]

The colonial medical context of Browne's Diary

In the following, this episode of Browne's personal ailment will be of interest. At first, it is necessary to elaborate on some of the historical contexts before taking a closer look at Browne's few days in Fort Cumberland. Two developments which had arisen briefly before and during the French and Indian Wars – one in medicine and one in the organization of military hospitals – furthered the tendency towards new theories of a disease's nature and subsequent treatments. Browne's diary is to be read against the backdrop of colonial medicine and the particulars of its geographical environment. In colonial medicine the established practice from the Old World concurs with the existence of local fairs and native folk medicine of the respective colonial context. Surgeons and apothecaries, such as Browne's brother who is accompanying her on her journey, "were part of a new discipline regime that aimed to protect their employers' human capital and improve its productivity."[29] During the long eighteenth century, it was common practice that British surgeons, physicians, and apothecaries who, due to the Empire's colonial endeavours, accompanied British troops, began to establish their own networks to share the information they had gathered and which had proved useful for keeping the British troops fit for service. In addition, the *Philosophical Transactions of the Royal Society* had come to be an established resource for practicing physicians across the Empire. Since the second half of the seventeenth century, the journal had been inviting peer-reviewed publications by practicing medical "professionals"[30] and, in return, circulated their findings to doctors who were employed both in the "mother country" and in the colonies.

Three observations appear to be of particular importance in such a setting: (1) The medical staff accompanying British troops in the colonies had to deal with unknown plagues and diseases (e.g. viral diseases such as yellow fever) that very often had long-lasting consequences for the Europeans stationed in these environments. (2) Due to the colonizer's rule and the said medical states of emergency, the dissection of dead bodies was less regulated in the colonies than in the "mother country"[31] (the number of accessible dead bodies for dissection peaked during times of colonial warfare). (3) The geographical particulars of a colony's location gave rise to an interest in the climate conditions (e.g. precipitation, temperatures, natural disasters) in the context of newly studied diseases.

Taken together, the findings gathered in the colonies challenged accepted concepts about the human body. Due to new concepts such as "miasma theory" or the notion of "the torrid zone,"[32] traditional diagnostic routines concerning the origins of an affliction such as, for example, the wrong diet, poor sanitary conditions, or unethical behaviour became disputable. Body concepts, such as those based on Newton's classical mechanics, regarded the inner workings of the patient as a pneumatic environment that was directly influenced by external conditions. In Charlotte Browne's diary, which is, but primarily has not yet been read as, a medical notebook, we encounter the contagious and lethal effects of dysentery, we learn about the Matron's access to see the dead and dying, and repeatedly read about the weather conditions and, in one particular case, how the extremely hot temperatures and heavy rains had an immediate effect on the health of the soldiers Browne was accompanying.

These encounters are testimony to a more general view of the affliction of disease. Two theories – Herman Boerhaave's physiological approach to disease and Thomas Sydenham's miasma theory – reiterate a more mechanical body concept that is very much taken for granted in Browne's irregular diary entries. Indeed, such conceptions of the human body were sound views to colonial surgeons and physicians, who witnessed a direct connection between tropical fevers and tropical climates.[33]

Boerhaave's theories also inform a book that, according to Sarah Fatherly,[34] was widely read by military staff throughout the Seven Years' War – John Pringle's *Observations on the Diseases of the Army* (1752). The author, himself a former student at Leiden University, closely followed Boerhaave in believing that fever is a body's lifesaving defence mechanism and that both circulation and digestion follow mechanical principles. His account was aimed at "classing the diseases common to a military life"[35] and advocates improvements for military hospitals. A particular focus is on "the bilious, and malignant fevers, and the dysentery, as they are distempers less frequent in this country [England]."[36] Pringle also served the household of the Duke of Cumberland, who chose General Edward Braddock "to assume the supreme command in North America"[37] during the French and Indian Wars. Sarah Fatherly[38] underlines that Pringle's book must have had an impact on both Braddock's command and the Duke of Cumberland's orders on the design of military hospitals. Following Pringle's *Observations,* Braddock received orders to establish a hospital that was to abandon the hitherto dual model of military hospitals, consisting of both a flying and a general hospital, in favour of "an enhanced version of the general hospital."[39] This integrative model was supposed to have both a mobile unit and a permanent physical location and followed Pringle's idea "that hospitals [...] should be considered as sanctuaries for the sick."[40] Thus, rather than having sick soldiers removed from the military camps, they were now to be treated and restored within it. Such a plan suggests the "centrality of economical considerations to military medical reform" and thus the direct influence of utilitarian thinking with regard to general medical treatment common in "nearly all the military and naval medical works of the eighteenth century."[41]

In some entries, Browne's diary hints at the use of such a mobile hospital. During the two-week trip from Will's Creek to Fort Cumberland, Browne was at the end of a bigger wagon train that counted 12 wagons full "with the sick, Lame, and Blind."[42] This implies that it was the matron's duty to organize the care for the sick en route and in wagons that were furnished as mobile medical units. Koppermann[43] stresses:

> A list of necessaries for the hospital prepared in late 1754 suggests [an ample supply for Braddock's medical facilities]. Heading the list were eight hundred flock beds and bolsters, each bed six by three feet, along with one pair each blankets and sheets, eight marquees, eight troopers' tents, and several associated items. Since eight hundred beds for an army consisting primarily of two regiments was a rather generous allotment, the number may suggest that planners were anticipating an extended struggle, with consequent buildup of forces. The inclusion of marquees and tents indicates that the hospital was expected to be mobile.

Such a generous planning, however, did not bank on Maryland's bad roads and poor weather conditions. Charlotte Browne takes note of these and tends to use hyperboles to point out the immediate impact the weather had on the progress of the wagon train. At one point, there was such "[a] great Gust of Thunder and Lightning and Rain so that we were allmost [sic!] drown'd."[44] On another occasion, Browne's "[w]aggon and every thing (sic!) in it Wet and all the Sick allmost drown'd."[45] On the one hand, these conditions slowed the progress of the wagon train, while, on the other hand, it shows that there were not enough staff and they were not well enough prepared for the journey. The weather took its toll on the troops: some of them suffered from a "bloody flux" upon their arrival at Fort Cumberland. A greater part of the soldiers marched on towards Fort Duquesne after their arrival in Fort Cumberland. There they were met by enemy troops in early July. The British units were defeated: two-thirds of the officers died or were wounded, and only a little more than 450 soldiers were left unharmed.[46] This put an early end to the campaign, and Braddock's regiments began their long withdrawal to Philadelphia.

Dysentery in Browne's diary

Both the developments in colonial medicine and the environmental conditions frame Browne's diary. As the author mainly uses a plain style[47] when jotting down her observations, her diary also leaves room for conjecture. For example, Browne never reports about the detailed plans for the mobile hospital, as discussed above, but waiting times, remarks on the weather, and its observed consequences paints a bigger picture of the infrastructure of Braddock's regiments, the hardships the military and non-military staff had to endure, and the immediate impact this had on their health.

This merits a closer look at an episode from Browne's march from Will's Creek to Fort Cumberland, which eventually led to her being sick for more than six weeks. In addition to the abovementioned heavy gusts of rain, her entries leading up to the arrival at the Fort repeatedly underline "extremely hot" temperatures, cold nights and exhaustion due to lack of sleep.[48] These focused and brief meteorological remarks point to an understanding that highlights the nexus between climate and physical health. On 14 June 1755, the first day after her arrival at Fort Cumberland, she writes: "I was taken ill with a Fever and other Disorders which continued 10 days and was not able to get out of my Bed." The next entry of 1 July, written more than two weeks later and reporting on both her sick brother and her maid, marks her statement as indicative of her inability to write. However, the tempus of the 14 June entry and the stress on the duration of her indispensability show that this note was written in retrospect. This is not the only occasion the diary tests the reliability of Charlotte Browne's narrated reports. In earlier entries, the Matron repeatedly mixes up dates (e.g. she mistakes both the Mondays of 3 February 1755 and 10 February 1755 for Sundays). Thus, Browne tends not to make notes in her diary on the same day as the events she is reporting on took place. Interestingly, then, all the entries from 1–17 July report in minute detail on the condition of her brother until his death. The form of the entry of 14 June 1755 as well as Browne's occasional errors in correctly dating her entries, challenge the function of her diary. Together with further moments of poetic decorum, such as situational irony and the use of metaphor (e.g. the use of "wooden world" to describe her ship in her entry of 23 March 1755), the whole diary appears to be written for an audience to whom Browne is attempting to present a cohesive narrative. It was meant to be read by others. This would also clarify her need to explain herself for the abrupt ending of her diary on 4 August 1757, when she writes: "I here End My Journal having so much Business on my Hands that I cannot spare Time to write it." For this, yet unspecified, audience, Browne, among other observations, in her notes of July and September 1755 documents symptoms, progress and remedies of dysentery.

"My Brother was taken ill with a Fever and Flux and Fits," writes Browne on 1 July 1755. This follows her longer descriptions on the experiences she made on the trail leading up to Fort Cumberland, including the abovementioned reports on the changing weather conditions. In the following, Browne's readers are to learn that her brother Robert is blistered (7 July) and given "2 drafts" (13 July). Bloodletting and blistering are mentioned in Herman Boerhaave's *Aphorisms* as having a positive effect on "facilitat[ing] the Discharge" of undesired liquids from the lungs and thus restoring a hydraulic balance in the body of the diseased.[49] On 13 July, Robert Browne, a layman and apothecary, gives in and seeks assistance of what Browne describes as trained medical staff: "I am in great Distress my Brother told me if he was not better he could not live but a few Days he submitted to have Mr Tuton, one of the Dr. to attend him." The direct discourse of this entry merges the voices of Robert and Charlotte Browne and emphasizes the strong bond that exists between them. Also it renders the decision to call out for one of the doctors a mutual one. The siblings thus acknowledge the need for someone who represents an established medical practice from the learned traditions of Europe. For a moment, this help had a positive effect: "he [Dr. Tuton] gave Him [Robert] 2 Drafts which had a supprizing (sic!) effect and I hope that he is better."[50]

The Matron then stays with her brother and jots down every change in his condition in her diary. Only a night later, she is to find Robert "so convuls'd I thought he was dying."[51] He would live for three more days. The note on convulsions, together with the repeated blistering and bloodletting, indicate this "bloody flux" as a case of dysentery. Upon her brother's demise, Browne resorts to apostrophe to lament Robert's death in her diary: "Oh! how shall I express my Distraction this unhappy Day at 2 in the After Noon (sic!) deprived me of my dear Brother in whom I have lost my kind Guardian and Protector and am now left a friendless Exile from all that is dear to me."[52] Such an assessment sounds harsh and quite reductive as to the role and function Browne's brother held for her, but at the same time it indicates the narrative performance of affect, as the death of Browne's brother is introduced as a "distraction" from her duties at the Fort. While she was taking care of her brother, Browne herself still suffered from the affliction she had contracted during the trail to Fort Cumberland. This would last until a few weeks after her brother's death. Because her servant has deserted the camp to be with her husband,[53] she orders a nurse to look after her, but she appears "to be a very bad one."[54]

In Fort Cumberland, she remained afflicted by the loss of her brother and her condition. The fact that beef provided the only nutrition had a devastating effect on her regimen and Browne seemed to be malnourished for several days.[55] On 16 August, the director of the fort gave orders to leave for Frederick's Town, today Frederick, MD. This is a trip of about 75 miles that Charlotte Browne, in her condition, made on horseback. Upon her eventual arrival at Frederick's Town, she "was very ill with a Fever and Flux."[56] Shortly before her arrival, her conditioned worsened and she asked to see the accompanying doctor of the wagon train. He gave her "a Draft to take every 2 hours."[57] This suggests that Browne was treating herself by bloodletting. This time the remedy appeared to be working against her flux and her fever. After her arrival in Frederick's Town, she reported that she was getting better every day until her health was once more fully restored. On 15 September 1755, the affliction no longer occupied her mind and she stopped reporting about her health.

Conclusion

In conclusion, the notes on the climate, sleep deprivation, blistering and bloodletting of the above episode suggest a model of the human body according to which fevers are contracted through external, environmental factors. Bloodletting and blistering, in particular, appear to be measures to hydraulically restore the volume of the body. Here, Browne indirectly integrates Boerhaave's theories into New World contexts and witnesses both their applicability and their failure. Browne's work, as both a Matron and a nurse, results from a mutually constitutive process of her seeking knowledge and surgeons who rely on knowledgeable women.

In addition, being written in the context of the new and more economic model of the military hospital, Browne's diary also highlights the community-driven aspect of medical discourse. In her role as Matron she is to supervise 'volunteer'-medical workers, she is to decide when to hire and to fire her staff, and when to take up the services of individual nurses as maids. The staff, however, is part of the regiment, motivation to work for the hospital is given by the need to stay with either the families, brothers or husbands these women were accompanying.[58] In this manner, then, a continuous care is set in place which, despite the economic dictum of the new hospital model, is contrary to only episodic encounters with patients. As the example of Browne's care for her brother has shown, she is accompanying the progress of his disease until the end. It is in particular moments like these that Browne gains meaning and power in her own nursing identity. Her insights, translated into the concise notes of her diary, convey a certain notion of professionalism that evidently results from medicine as a social experience rather than from utilitarian or economic reasons.

The example of Browne's diary suggests that prescriptions, recipes and printed theories on the nature of maladies applied in the field work of medical practitioners in the British-American colonies of the late seventeenth and early eighteenth century are to be read as transnational translations of the findings of European contemporaries such as Boerhaave or Sydenham. Visions and versions of American medicine then need to be thought of in light of the existing access to and the various ways medical writings were circulated. It is vital to any understanding of the discursive construction of American medical knowledge to be able to connect American medicine to both the specific experience of emissaries such as Browne in the British-American colonies, including their established socioeconomic contact zones, and, by the same token, to established knowledge networks.

While underlining a nurse's mobility in a highly literary sense, the diary also points out the conditions of Browne's movements via written maps, routes, vehicles, authorizations that allow her mobility and the cost of her travels. In the sense of Stephen Greenblatt's "Mobility Studies Manifesto," Browne can be read as a "mobilizer"[59] whose travels allow for contact zones between healers of the Old and the New World and "shed light on hidden as well as conspicuous movements of peoples, objects, images, texts, and ideas."[60] Hence, the connectivity between English and North American adaptations and reconsiderations of medical writings as a result of transatlantic contact during the French and Indian Wars makes visible the tropes and selective transformations of orally transmitted medical therapies, experiences, and experiments into medical diaries that are conceived for the general public such as that of Charlotte Bristowe Browne.

Notes

1 The New York Historical Society indicates that their "Diary is probably a fair copy made by Mrs. Browne from her original notes" (Browne, Charlotte Bristowe, *Diary*, n.p.).
2 For excerpted and edited versions of the diary see Calder 1967, 169–98 and Harrison 1924.
3 Easterby-Smith and Senior 2013, 471.
4 Thompson 2011, 45.
5 Diary entry of 3 June 1755.
6 Moreover, it serves as a document that, on the one hand, confirms a popularization of then new perspectives on health and the human body and, on the other hand, it reports on the then contemporary circumstances of a woman's geographic mobility and economic independence.
7 Diary entry of 7 November 1754.

8 According to Fatherly, "six women were typically allowed to accompany each army company. This meant that hundreds of women served in the British forces during this war" (Fatherly 2005, 26). However, Browne remains the only woman to be included in the eventual *Army List* (see Koppermann 2004, 265).

9 Diary entry of 10 March 1755.

10 See Calder 1967176, footnote 19: "Wills Creek flows south into the Potomac River at Cumberland."

11 Diary entry of 11 March 1755.

12 Even though this settlement had, at this point in time, already been named Alexandria, both names were commonly used for this area in Fairfax County (see Calder 1967, 175).

13 Diary entry of 22 March 1755.

14 Fatherly 2008, 14.

15 Diary entry of 16 April 1756.

16 Diary entry of 16 October 1755.

17 Diary entry of 18 October 1755.

18 Diary entry of 26 April 1756.

19 Fatherly 2008, 14.

20 Diary entry of 1 June 1755.

21 Anderson 2001, 90.

22 Diary entry of 2 June 1755.

23 Diary entry of 16 June 1755.

24 Diary entry of 18 October 1755.

25 "In eighteenth century New England, farmers, craftsmen, shopkeepers, ship's captains, and perhaps a very few housewives kept daybooks, running accounts of receipts and expenditures, sometimes combining economic entries with short notes on important family events and comments on work begun or completed" (Ulrich 1990, 8).

26 For a comprehensive study of the Braddock Campaign see Anderson 2001.

27 "'Bloody flux' [was] used interchangeably with dysentery, although it is possible that some were victimized by some other disease that caused violent, repeated purgation, such as acute severe gastroenteritis, then commonly called 'cholera morbus' or even a severe case of diarrhea" (Koppermann 2004, 266).

28 Koppermann 2004, 261.

29 Harrison 2010, 5.

30 The category of "professional" has to be put in doubt as the semiotic dimensions of such a term imply a distinction between useful knowledge and useful value. In this context, it remains particularly unclear how value is assessed. Nevertheless, it has to be stressed that the category of usefulness results from the creation of tightly-knit, state-regulated and utilitarian institutions. It is remarkable, however, that such concepts seem to emerge unbound to specific nations. Knowledge and value referencing the notion of the "professional" rather desire to be expressive language substitutes for a notion of something universal assuming the consensus that they are of use. This begs the question for whom they are of use or for what, and also if this can be assumed as universally right and the ways this is to be regarded as right to whom. Admittedly the term "professional" is an anachronism at this point as it can only be applied retrospectively in a figurative sense. It would not have been used by individual actors of this paper.

31 See Harrison 2010, 4.

32 "The torrid zone" became a term that was highly popularized in the travelogues of the seventeenth and eighteenth centuries, mostly in reference to regions in the Americas, Asia, Africa and the Middle East. As Felicity Nussbaum has shown, the term not only references climate conditions found in these regions, but also served to produce hetero-stereotypes about the cultural character of the people living there. Nussbaum was particularly interested in the representation of women in the travelogues of the said period. She found that they were often rendered as promiscuous, feisty and slothful. Such representations, however, had a regulating effect on the self-image of the British readers: "The representation of polygamous, torrid, and savage woman made visible through British imperial designs enabled the consolidation of the cult of domesticity in England itself" (Nussbaum 1995, 97). According to Anne McClintock, the term "torrid zone" needs to be rethought as a concept that encompasses both the geographic and rhetorical dimensions of the European view. She suggests to label it "porno-tropics", as "Renaissance travelers found an eager and lascivious audience for their spicy tales, so that, long before the era of high Victorian imperialism, Africa and the Americas had become what can be called a porno-tropics for the European imagination – a fantastic magic lantern of the mind onto which Europe projected its forbidden sexual desires and fears" (McClintock 1995, 22). Even though Browne never uses the term 'torrid zone' itself, she makes a particular endeavour to highlight the extreme weather conditions in the North American East. As a result, the setting of her travelogue is not only to be connected to the personal health of the Matron and her company, but also to the many references to Native American savagery (i.e. scalping, abduction, and attacks) (see Diary entries of 24 October 1755, 8 November 1755, or 16 December 1755).

33 For example, Georgius Cleghorn's *Observations on the Epidemical Diseases of Minorca from the Year 1744 to 1749* (1750) or William Hillary's *Observations on the Changes of the Air and the Concomitant Epidemical Diseases in the Island of Barbados* (1759) maintained a strong relationship between fevers and climate. Sydenham's miasma theory, popularized in the third edition of his *Observationes Medicae* (1676), will eventually pave the way for the so-called "sanitary revolution" in the nineteenth century.

34 Fatherly 2012, 568.

35 Pringle 1812, 273.

36 Ibid., 273.

37 Anderson 2001, 86.

38 Fatherly 2012, 583.

39 Ibid., 567.

40 Pringle 1812, 274.

41 Harrison 2010, 17.

42 Diary entry of 1 June 1755.

43 See Koppermann 2004, 265–66.

44 Diary entry of 6 June 1755.

45 Diary entry of 7 June 1755.

46 See Koppermann 2004, 260.

47 Plain style describes a more straightforward way of writing that uses simple words and syntax. It does not attempt to create poetic decorum by the extensive use

of tropes and schemes. In the context of American Literature, Browne's diary could be linked to the established tradition of introspection in Puritan culture. While studying Puritan literature as a cultural imaginary, Larzer Ziff debunked the notion of plain style as the sole characteristic in Puritan writing. He came across several examples for passionate expressions and the use of rhetorical figures: "plain style and passionate allegorizing are related elements of Puritanism" (Ziff 1974, 40). Thus, Browne's diary still can be taken as a typical diary of its time, written mostly in plain style, even though it sometimes deviates from neutral reports and occasionally uses rhetorical figures.

48 See Diary Entries of 21 May, 30 May and 10 June 1755.
49 Boerhaave 1752, 232.
50 Diary entry of 13 July 1755.
51 Diary entry of 14 July 1755.
52 Diary entry of 17 July 1755.
53 Diary entry of 25 July 1755.
54 Diary entry of 1 August 1755.
55 On 15 August 1755, Browne notes: "A little better but can get nothing that I can eat for here is nothing to be had but beef."
56 Diary entry of 30 August 1755.
57 Diary entry of 29 August 1755 (NB: "Draft" was wrongly transcribed as "bottle" in Calder 1967,186, a draft would indicate bloodletting in this case.)
58 See, e.g., the Diary entry of 25 July 1755, when Browne's nurse leaves her for her husband.
59 Greenblatt 2009, 251.
60 Ibid., 250.

Bibliography

Anderson, Fred. 2001. *Crucible of War: The Seven Years' War and the Fate of Empire in British North America, 1754–1766*. New York: Vintage.

Boerhaave, Herman. 1752 [1728]. *Boerhaave's Aphorisms: Concerning the Knowledge and Cure of Diseases*. Reprinted in English Translation with Preface in London: Printed for W. Innys, at the West End of St. Paul's, and C. Hitch, in Pater Noster Row.

Browne, Charlotte Bristowe. *Charlotte Browne Diary, 1754–1757, 1763–1766*. New York Historical Society, American Manuscripts Collection (dataset). https://cdm16694.contentdm.oclc.org/digital/collection/p16124coll1/id/9830/rec/1. Accessed 31 August 2019.

Calder, Isabel, ed. 1967 [1935]. *Colonial Captivities, Marches and Journeys*. Port Washington, NY: Kennikat P.

Easterby-Smith, Sarah and Emily Senior. 2013. "The Cultural Production of Natural Knowledge: Contexts, Terms, Themes." *Journal for Eighteenth-Century Studies* 36 (4): 71–6.

Fatherly, Sarah. 2005. "Daughters of Empire: Women and the Seven Years' War in Philadelphia." *Pennsylvania Legacies* 5 (1): 26.

Fatherly, Sarah. 2008. *Gentlewomen and Learned Ladies: Women and Elite Formation in Eighteenth-Century Philadelphia*. Bethlehem, PA: Lehigh UP.

Fatherly, Sarah. 2012. "Tending the Army: Women and the British General Hospital in North America, 1754–1763." *Early American Studies: An Interdisciplinary Journal* 10 (3): 566–99.

Greenblatt, Stephen. 2009. "A Mobility Studies Manifesto." In *Cultural Mobility: A Manifesto*, edited by Stephen Greenblatt, 250–53. Cambridge: Cambridge University Press, 2009.

Harrison, Fairfax. 1924. "With Braddocks Army: Mrs. Browne's Diary in Virginia and Maryland." *The Virginia Magazine of History and Biography* 32 (4): 305–20.

Harrison, Mark. 2010. *Medicine in an Age of Commerce and Empire: Britain and Its Tropical Colonies, 1660–1830*. Oxford: Oxford University Press.

Koppermann, Paul. 2004. "The Medical Aspect of the Braddock and the Forbes Expeditions." *Pennsylvania History: A Journal of Mid-Atlantic Studies* 71 (3): 257–83.

Leach, Douglas Edward. 1973. *Arms for Empire: A Military History of the British Colonies in North America, 1607–1763*. New York: Macmillan.

McClintock, Anne. 1995. *Imperial Leather: Race, Gender, and Sexuality in the Colonial Contest*. New York and London: Routledge.

Nussbaum, Felicity. 1995. *Torrid Zones: Maternity, Sexuality, and Empire in Eighteenth-Century English Narratives*. Baltimore, MD: Johns Hopkins University Press.

Pringle, John. 1812 [1752]. *Observations on the Diseases of the Army*. Reprinted with Preface and Notes by Benjamin Rush. Philadelphia, PA: Anthony Finley, Medical Bookseller, S.E. Corner of Chestnut and Fourth Street, 1812.

Thompson, Carl. 2011. *Travel Writing*. New York and London: Routledge.

Ulrich, Laurel Thatcher. 1990. *A Midwife's Tale: The Life of Martha Ballard, Based on Her Diary, 1785–1812*. New York, Vintage.

Ziff, Larzer. 1974. "Literary Consequences of Puritanism." In *American Puritan Imagination: Essays in Revaluation*, edited by Sacvan Bercovitch, 34–44. Cambridge: Cambridge University Press.

Chapter 6

The geography of Arctic food

The northern environment and Sámi health in transition, c. 1750–1950

Ritva Kylli

Introduction

According to a very well-known phrase, "you are what you eat," but there is also a less-known geographical phrase that says, "you are where you eat." When food is considered, there has always been a strong connection between nature and society. According to Peter Atkins and Ian Bowler, food has been an essential part of the political ecology, which is related to the interfaces between the environment and society.[1] Nature–society relations are also important in the *geography of food*, which focuses on food production and consumption at the local and global level. This field is also concerned with global food networks and connections, as well as the politics of justice, food security and dynamics in food accessibility related to these issues.[2]

Eating and drinking have had close links both to health and the environment. Connections have also been very evident in the Arctic. Arctic mines and hydropower plants, for example, have had a strong impact on the nutrition and health of the Sámi and other Arctic indigenous peoples. Due to hydropower plants, the rise of salmon in the northern rivers has been disturbed, which has affected the diet of the inhabitants as they have had to start buying more food from grocery stores. Similarly, the establishment of mines has changed the geography of Arctic food. Due to the mines, many new inhabitants have moved to the area and new grocery stores have been established for them. Local residents also began to use the services of these grocery stores despite the fact that store selections in the Arctic regions have often been small and the products have been expensive. Store-bought foods have not usually been as healthy as foods provided by gathering and hunting.[3] At the same time, traditional knowledge about fishing, hunting and foraging has deteriorated, which has been particularly problematic in situations where mining operations have suddenly stopped, and the grocery stores have gone out of business.[4]

This chapter examines the connection between the environment and health in Finnish Lapland from the perspective of the food history from the eighteenth century to the mid-1900s. The research focuses especially on the sub-arctic border region between Finland and Norway and especially on the area of Utsjoki (*Ohcejohka*), which is situated on the northernmost border of Finland. Utsjoki was inhabited almost completely by the Sámi population. Most of the inhabitants lived along the Teno River (*Deatnu*), which separates Finland and Norway. The Utsjoki area will be compared to the area of Inari (*Aanaar*), situated south of Utsjoki. The environment and health of the northernmost Finnish border region is also examined in the wider context of the Arctic and northern indigenous peoples. Sámi history-related sources are available in official and private archives, newspapers, memoirs and travelogues.

From healthy environments to the geography of colonialism

According to Stephen Le, cuisines of different areas are "a result of centuries of evolution, finely tuned to our biology and surroundings." Traditional combinations of food with balanced nutrients have supported health in the best possible way.[5] During the early modern period, most of the people around the world were still involved in food production, and people consumed most of their food locally. Diets were seasonally very restricted.[6] However, food has always been very transnational and it has constantly crossed borders. The traditional Sámi diet contained a lot of foods (e.g. fish and meat) from the surrounding area, but tax records from sixteenth-century Utsjoki and Inari villages show that fur buyers who came to the area sometimes paid with loaves of bread, salt and butter.[7] At this stage, both food production and consumption were still tied mostly to the local products of subarctic Lapland.

In the eighteenth and nineteenth centuries, the reindeer-herding Sámi of Utsjoki ate a lot of meat, and the Sámi who lived along the Teno River fished salmon, hunted and kept cows. In the summertime they ate wild berries and plants from the forests and marshes, so they had some sources of vitamin C, in their nearest environment.[8] They also needed to drink a lot of water because of their protein-rich diet; freshwater resources were crucial for Sámi well-being. Reindeer-herding Sámi, who followed annual migrations, preferred to erect their tent-like huts in locations where water was available nearby. As they did not spend a long time in one location, the water was not contaminated and would not cause diarrhoea. In the wintertime it was possible to melt snow to produce good quality drinking water.[9]

According to the Finnish officials of the time, the Sámi people, who had adapted to their northern living environment and had an opportunity to use their land without restrictions, were considered to be very healthy. In 1791, the minister of Utsjoki wrote that the good health of the Utsjoki Sámi was based on a cheerful outlook on life and fresh air. According to him, Utsjoki's location, where the mountains and hills alternated, caused a blast of wind that cleaned the air. Utsjoki inhabitants ate food that was difficult to digest, but they ate very moderately. At this point, there were 15 families practicing salmon fishing along the river Teno and 28 mobile reindeer herder families. The Sámi spent a lot of time outdoors, and their continuous mobility made them feel good.[10] Based on this description, health and the environment obviously had a very close connection. At the same time, while colonizing new continents, European people were also collecting knowledge of medical geography. In 1768, a Scottish doctor, James Lind, wrote that it was possible for the Europeans to manage in hot climates if the places were "located on high ground and ventilated by breezes."[11] Even though the Utsjoki Sámi had good ventilation, the cold climate could also cause some health problems. Jacob Fellman, who worked as a minister of Utsjoki in the 1820s, wrote that even if the coldness cleaned the air, hardened the body and increased the appetite, it could also cause gout and throat diseases.[12]

The Sámi, living in Finnish Lapland, were in constant contact with the northern coast of Norway, and their diet differed from the agricultural areas of southern Finland and areas that were not open to the ocean. The Sámi of Finnish Lapland ate a lot of sea fish, such as cod, and also fish oil, which contained omega-3 fatty acids. Elsewhere in Finland, cod liver oil was sometimes bought from pharmacies, but in Utsjoki it was eaten fresh and frequently – and was considered to be very healthy. Saimi Lindroth, who worked as a "health sister" in Utsjoki during the 1930s was delighted to learn how wise the people in Lapland were. She noted that when the dark, sunless winter meant that the people had spent their vitamin D supplies, they took a new healthy elixir to maintain their health, which was why they could withstand the polar night.[13] Some other foods that were staples in the Sámi diet got very positive reviews from visitors from outside the Sámi area. One such food was *Angelica archangelica* (commonly known as garden angelica, wild celery, or Norwegian angelica) which seemed to be a great antiscorbutic.[14]

The reindeer-herding Sámi of Utsjoki spent their summers in Norway on the coast of the Arctic Ocean and wintered in the interior part of what is now known as Finnish Lapland, for example the forest zone of Inari. This was easy at the time, when there were no solid borders between the kingdoms. The situation changed in 1751, when the Strömstad Treaty (between Norway and Sweden, which Finland belonged to before 1809) defined the current Norwegian–Finnish border along the river Teno. The situation did not change too much, however, because there was an addendum to this Treaty, called the *Lapp Codicil*, the aim of which was the "survival of the Sámi people."[15] Thanks to this codicil, the Sámi were able to maintain their traditional way of life and also their traditional diet. They were able to continue their traditional migratory reindeer herding across the new border and, at the same time, their fishing and hunting on the coast of the Arctic Ocean. In the treaty, the kingdoms officially confirmed that the Sámi of Norway and Sweden (as well as Finland) had the right to use the waters and lands of a neighbouring country to maintain themselves and their animals because they were known to require the territories of both kingdoms for their livelihoods. The right was also valid in wartimes. The residents of Utsjoki, who remained residents of the Swedish Empire, were also guaranteed the opportunity to trade in the same way as the Sámi of Norway.[16]

As the Strömstad Treaty proves, traditional Sámi land use and livelihoods were still being supported in the eighteenth century, but by the nineteenth century, their environment – and hence their diet and overall health – were increasingly affected by the surrounding states and their governance. The Sámi of the current Finnish Lapland could cross the border between Finland and Norway freely until the first half of the nineteenth century, but after that pressure started to grow against the *codicil* from governmental authorities and expanding agricultural interests. Fishing rights in the Arctic Ocean for the Sámi people living on the Finnish side of the border began to be restricted from the 1820s. Reindeer herding met with difficulties during the first half of the 1850s, when the border between Finland and Norway was closed. After that, Utsjoki reindeer herders had to search for summer pastures on the Finnish side of the border.[17]

The Sámi area of current Finnish Lapland had been part of the Swedish Empire during the eighteenth century but, since 1809, it had belonged to the Russian Empire in the same way as the rest of Finland. According to some writers, the Norwegians were afraid that Russia would try to take over the good ports of northern Norway, which was believed to be a threat to the security of the whole of Europe. Norway became suspicious of all the inhabitants of the Russian Empire, and the rights of the Sámi people living in the Finnish area were restricted in the Norwegian region. The Sámi suffered "because of the envy and distrust of the kingdoms."[18]

During the latter half of the nineteenth century, many indigenous communities around the world struggled to feed themselves as land use and resource management caused problems for food production. Some northern indigenous peoples were even prevented from producing foods in traditional ways,[19] while at the same time new mines, forestry working sites and urban centres were established in the Arctic. In Kirkenes, situated in Norway in the vicinity of Utsjoki and Inari, the Bjørnevatn iron mine was established in 1906.[20] The Sámi who lived in Finland were not forbidden to engage in their traditional livelihoods, but as the use of land and water areas became more restricted over the years, it inevitably affected their food culture. Environmental injustice also brought food injustice.[21] Finnish authorities tried to control Sámi livelihoods and living environments from the late 1800s by establishing reindeer herding cooperatives and changing the status of the northernmost forests of Lapland to protected forests.[22]

The ecosystems of Finnish Lapland were changing during the nineteenth century. Beaver had been hunted to extinction by the mid-1800s.[23] Wild reindeer also vanished around the same time.[24] The decline in game was used to put pressure on indigenous people to cultivate land in the northern and Arctic regions. Many indigenous people faced a situation where power relations started to impact their food production patterns. Also in Finland, the authorities tried to convert reindeer herding and fishing Sámi into agriculturalists. The Economic Society of Finland, established in 1797, gave prizes during the nineteenth century to Sámi, who were known to be hard-working, for clearing and ditching fields. Officials also admired Finnish settlers who had managed to change the swamps of Lapland into thriving hay or grain fields.[25] Such visions have been seen as the "anticipatory geography of colonialism." Taking over the territory was justified as a way to pursue the "correct" and "civilized" use of the land.[26]

Changes in biodiversity affected the availability of the food sources, and the loss of certain animal species might have affected the health and resilience of northern residents.[27] When the ecosystems became impoverished, it was all the easier to become dependent on imported foods. By the end of the nineteenth century, more and more Sámi became settlers, as this came with many benefits: it was easier to overcome disputes over meadows and fishing grounds if there was an official document of land ownership. Long tax exemptions were also of interest from the Sámi point of view.[28] The living environment changed and, during the 1920s, many Utsjoki Sámi already had small potato patches near their subarctic homes. At the same time, they started to eat more sugar and flour.[29] Infectious diseases also increased in the latter part of the nineteenth century as a non-nomadic lifestyle became more prevalent.[30]

Transnational food and widening networks

Traditional Arctic foods have sometimes been seen as a threat to food safety – for example, there are health risks from eating raw fish and meat. However, traditional foods have been seen as important for the physical, spiritual and mental health of the indigenous communities. Food gained from the immediate surroundings has connected people with the land and increased their well-being in many ways.[31] According to H.V. Kuhnlein and H.M. Chan, traditional food systems include "all of the food species that are available to a particular culture from local natural resources and the accepted patterns for their use within that culture." This term also includes the health consequences of these factors as well as the traditional knowledge connected to the use of natural environments.[32] However, underlining the term *traditional* in the context of indigenous peoples gives a very stagnant image of them and their diet. According to Coll Thrush, traditional diets "assume static ecological contexts, static networks of exchange, and static palates."[33] The food supply of the Sámi, for example, had been delocalizing at a relatively early stage. Trade brought edible consumer products beyond the local environment, as the Sámi wanted to take advantage of global commodity flows. The Utsjoki Sámi were active merchants, and they eagerly used the opportunities presented by commerce to change and expand their diets.

Where the Sámi are concerned, one can easily forget how big a change to their lifestyle and diet – and at the same time to their environment and health – the intensification period of reindeer pastoralism had been before the seventeenth century. In addition, the Sámi of Utsjoki had begun to raise cattle at a fairly early stage. From milk they had made butter, which could be sold in Norway and the proceeds could be used to purchase interesting consumer goods from the Norwegian marketplaces.[34] In the twentieth century, the Utsjoki municipality was sometimes even described as its own republic which did not need Finland for anything. Geographer Ilmari Hustich wrote: "We should also remember that the Utsjoki Sámi are not nomads, but often affluent fishermen, the wealthiest of whom have large houses with painted buildings, well-kept lawns, and cowsheds with several cows."[35] In the 1920s, exports from Utsjoki consisted of salmon, reindeer meat and hides, beef, willow grouse and butter. Flour, coffee, and sugar were essential imported products, but a lot of frozen cod was also imported during the early spring when the Utsjoki Sámi were running out of salmon.[36]

The steady supply of imported foods demanded special efforts in the Arctic. There could be a shortage of products, for example, during *rasputitsa* (the spring and autumn periods when the roads become difficult to navigate). Also, sudden price changes on the Norwegian side of the border sometimes caused concern. Residents of the Teno river valley were already accustomed to the fact that during wars and crises food could suddenly be more expensive on the Norwegian side of the border. For example, the Crimean war in the 1850s had an effect on food prices: according to the minister of Utsjoki, merchants of Norway took advantage of the war by insisting on higher prices for foodstuffs such as flour, sugar and coffee.[37]

Even when the food production and transportation faced changes during the nineteenth century,[38] there were still regional differences in food availability. In the early twentieth century, Utsjoki's food production and consumption was hampered by the lack of infrastructure. In 1939, Utsjoki was characterized as a border region municipality, with only ten kilometres of roads.[39] The Sámi were already accustomed to their imported foods but, because there were no roads leading to Utsjoki, food cargoes were transported from the Norwegian coast by reindeer, horse and boat. The distances were long and the transport costs were expensive. One important trading venue was the town of Vadsø (140 km from the centre of Utsjoki) at Varanger fjord.[40]

Through governance, it has been possible to smooth out differences between regions when trying to make food available as equally as possible.[41] Additionally, the State of Finland, which became independent in 1917, tried to ensure food sufficiency in northernmost Lapland through legislation. Northern forestry working sites required a lot of food products, and Finland's government paid special carriage fees for food transporters in the northernmost border area. In principle, food products eligible for carriage fees should have been domestic imports but, for the northernmost municipalities, the fees were also available for the transportation of goods from the Norwegian coast to satisfy local needs.[42] Before the outbreak of the Second World War, many products were the same price in Utsjoki as in the southern municipalities located right next to the railroads – thanks to the financial support from the Finnish State.[43]

In addition, on the basis of the law laid down in 1924, it was allowed to import duty-free goods for the needs of (fellow) inhabitants of the municipalities of Inari and Utsjoki. As a result, coffee and sugar were much cheaper, for example, in northernmost Lapland than in other parts of Finland.[44] The situation also affected residents on the Norwegian side, as it was cheaper for them to make food purchases in the stores in Utsjoki.[45] Officials drew attention to the fact that although the municipality of Utsjoki did not have that many inhabitants, there were many grocery stores with varied selections right next to the border.[46] Utsjoki traders had to constantly explain the sale of their products to the authorities, as well as the extent to which they sold their products to the residents of neighbouring Norway. Trader U Hagelin announced once to the rural police chief of Utsjoki that he had sold coffee, sugar, tobacco, rice groats, fruit, wheat flour, margarine, lard, petrol, canned meat and more to the residents of Norway. Hagelin had three stores in Utsjoki, and at least one of them was located within reach of Karasjok residents.[47] Karasjok was a Sámi municipality on the Norwegian side of the border.

According to Coling Sage, eating is an ecological act: "What we eat and how we eat has more impact on the Earth than almost anything else."[48] During the nineteenth century, railroads, refrigerated steamships and industrial canning started to break down the role of the environment as a principal factor that determined the geography of food. As food imports became more and more distant, the environmental impact of food production moved further away from where the food was consumed. In the late nineteenth century, fruit companies established large banana-growing areas in Central America.[49] More tropical products were also imported into the northernmost parts of Europe. The first banana ships arrived in Finland in the early years of 1900s.[50] It was not possible to buy these fruits from northernmost Lapland, as the distances were long and there was only a small postal path leading to the southern parts of the country. Instead, many kinds of products were available in Norway. During the late 1930s, a public health nurse from Utsjoki unexpectedly received an orange from a Sámi girl in the middle of the winter.[51] The orange had been bought from northernmost Norway. Based on the Norwegian newspaper advertisements, vitamin-rich oranges were already widely available in the stores at this point.[52]

The northern environment produced limited amounts of plants, and the lack of vitamin-rich foods might sometimes have negatively affected the health of people living in the Arctic.[53] Even though some of the residents of Utsjoki had tasted oranges, no fresh oranges could be found in Utsjoki cargo or customs listings from the 1930s. Oranges did not receive any customs exemptions, even though Utsjoki traders regularly attempted to apply for permission from the Finnish Ministry of Finance to import them, tax free, to Utsjoki.[54] In customs clearance reports, there are, however, mentions of other kinds of canned and dried fruit that were imported to Utsjoki: "Imported: in boats, June 16, 1937 from Karasjok: 6 cans of apricot, 6 cans of pineapple, 6 cans of peaches, 6 cans of pears. Country of origin: USA."[55] In addition to dried fruits, sources also mention fresh apples. In 1935, Sámi trader Hans Laiti would have liked to import cocoa, chocolate, and fruits for his store, but with the exception of apples, fresh fruit were not allowed to be imported free of duty.[56]

In the border regions, the selection of foods was sometimes quite exceptional compared to the rest of the country. Tea from Ceylon, biscuits from Norway and coffee sacks from Liberia could be found in the horse carts of the Sámi traders. Industrial packaged and branded goods were commonly available in Utsjoki before the outbreak of the Second World War. Trader Jouni N. Niittyvuopio had announced in July 1936 that he had imported 20 boxes of sugar cubes, mixed fruits and raisins, and two boxes of *Corned Beef* to Utsjoki from Norway by boat.[57]

The lack of transport infrastructure hampered trading in Utsjoki, but because there were not many roads, it was easier for Utsjoki Sámi to protect their own culture and livelihoods. There had been some Finnish settlers in Utsjoki during the past centuries, but not too many – largely thanks to the cold climate but also to the lack of roads. Utsjoki had remained a Sámi municipality unlike the other municipalities of Finnish Lapland. In 1925, the municipal council of Utsjoki even suggested to the Finnish Parliament that the municipality should be codified as a "Sámi area of protection" on which Finnish habitation, roads or phone network should not be established.[58] The municipality of Inari served as a warning for Utsjoki residents: since the early 1900s, roads from the south had been built in Inari and with them came a lot of new Finnish residents. The Finnish population in Inari exceeded the number of Sámi by 1915.[59]

In his newspaper writing in the late 1920s, Inari Sámi Uula Sarre told how reindeer husbandry in Inari had recently faced many problems. When the number of reindeer declined, more and more Sámi were forced to seek out a living in forestry work together with Finnish lumberjacks. This had been devastating to the Sámi culture. He noted: "In order to protect themselves in this inhospitable company from mockery, a Sámi must live, talk and dress like they do."[60] In addition, lumberjacks generally ate pork and lard, which differed from the Inari Sámi's earlier fish-based diets.[61]

The Sámi health was in a state of transition during the early twentieth century.[62] The entry of numerous new edible products had impacted on the health of the human communities in the Arctic. Some vitamin-rich foods began to be more accessible than before, but the so-called "Western diseases" (obesity, heart disease), had also became more common.[63] As a whole, the situation did not change too radically. The Sámi of Finnish Lapland still had good water resources available – and they were still able to purchase cod, cod oil and other health-promoting products on the coast of Norway. They also continued to use food products from their local living environment to their advantage, and they still knew, for example, the habitats of *Angelica archangelica* and other healthy plants.[64]

Unhealthy environments and the Second World War

According to the United Nations Food and Agriculture Organization, *food security* prevails when people have "access to sufficient, safe and nutritious food to meet their dietary needs and food preferences for an active and healthy life."[65] During the Second World War, the right to a healthy environment and food security was endangered in many parts of the world, and the Arctic indigenous peoples were no exception to this. The north Sámi area was an active front of the war because of its geostrategic position and rich natural resources.[66] The mine at Kirkenes, the Kiruna mine in Swedish Lapland and the well-situated harbours in northern Norway brought German troops to fight in the northernmost areas of Finland and Norway.[67] Political unrest also caused sudden disruptions to food availability.

The Second World War began on 1 September 1939 with the invasion of Poland by Nazi Germany. Finland's Winter War against the Soviet Union started on 30 November 1939, but the threat of a major war had begun to affect livelihoods in Finnish Lapland even before that.[68] The first concrete signs of the outbreak of the Second World War in Utsjoki were restrictions on cross-border trade. This caused difficulties for residents since they were accustomed to freely crossing the Teno River with their commodities. On 8 September 1939, Sámi merchant Isak Walle wrote about the diminished stores of local traders. Walle still had plenty of sugar, wheat flour and coffee, but stocks were already getting lower. He noted: "Due to the outbreak of war, people had an increased desire to purchase, so it was obvious that such stocks reduce very quickly."[69]

Finland fought the Continuation War against the Soviet Union in cooperation with Nazi Germany from June 1941 to September 1944. The Germans had a small air surveillance station in Utsjoki, and they soon became part of the Sámi's everyday life.[70] The Germans influenced the environment, health and diet of the Sámi inhabitants. The Sámi people had been accustomed to protecting their scarce forest resources, but the Germans took advantage of them without hesitation.[71] Especially in Inari, the Germans had large forestry working sites.[72] The Germans co-opted the former epidemic hospital in Inari for their own use, but they also helped the local residents with their health problems.[73] The Germans also influenced the region's food supply: they left canned foods, bread, and money in the households of local Sámi. In turn, the Sámi sold the Germans warm clothes and reindeer meat.[74]

The Sámi had gained a lot of knowledge over the centuries about soft ways to utilize their fragile subarctic environment.[75] During the war, indigenous knowledge (e.g. the best time for slaughtering reindeer) was useless in situations where the reindeer had to be slaughtered in large quantities for to feed the Finnish Army and civilians. Although the Sámi living in Finnish Lapland had actively imported a wide variety of new food products into their residential areas before the Second World War, reindeer herding had remained a staple which the Sámi of Utsjoki were willing to defend from the influence of Finnish culture. Reindeer herding was a livelihood which had been perfectly adapted to the northern environment and which was a guaranteed source of food and well-being in those years when other livelihoods failed or when trade connections were broken because of the *rasputitsa* or in times of crises.[76] As soon as the war in Finland broke out at the end of November 1939, reindeer herding encountered problems. One was the decline in the workforce, as many skilled herders left to fight.[77]

Food shortages in Finland escalated after 1941 and were also reflected in Lapland's reindeer herds. Under government orders, reindeer herders had to participate in the war effort by slaughtering large numbers of their reindeer every year and giving away reindeer meat by the decision from the start of the 1941–1942 winter. During the first winter, the Province of Lapland had to produce 1,600,000 kg of reindeer meat and 36,000 reindeer hides. The situation was very challenging. Despite of the slaughter requirements, reindeer herders were not sufficiently exempt from military service (despite the fact that a large part of the donated meat was going to be used by the Finnish Army) and the slaughter did not take place according to the normal timetable between October and the end of January. The lack of manpower delayed the slaughter, which meant that more reindeer had to be slaughtered than was originally expected. By mid-January – when the slaughters should already have ended – only about 12,000 reindeer had been slaughtered, which was less than a third of the required amount. In the large and sparsely populated northern reindeer herding cooperatives, slaughtering had hardly even begun. At this stage, the reindeer had already lost several kilograms per animal in weight. As the number of donations were measured in kilograms, more reindeer had to be slaughtered than had been planned.[78]

The provincial government stressed that during the same winter, 600 draught reindeer had also been donated to the Finnish Army. It was hoped that serious consideration would be given to the forthcoming slaughtering because, by continuing the first-year rate, there was a threat to the entire reindeer husbandry of Finnish Lapland. During the war, it was not possible to put an end to the compulsory slaughtering, but the obligation was reduced the following year. The slaughtering was delayed again, and the weights of the reindeer dropped. Also some very thin reindeer, which nobody would have wanted to buy in normal years, now had to be slaughtered. However, there were still enough reindeer to be donated for the general war time consumption – a new order to donate reindeer meat was given in the winter of 1943–1944.[79]

During the Lapland War in winter of 1944–1945 no mandatory slaughter was carried out, but the war disturbed reindeer herding in many other ways.[80] Military units of the northernmost Finnish Lapland were informed, on 2 September 1944, that Finland had made efforts to achieve peace or armistice: the Soviet Union had made the negotiations conditional upon the removal of German troops from Finland, and the Finnish Government had agreed. Two days later, it was announced that Finland had ended its relationship with Germany and ordered all German troops to leave the country.[81] As the Germans were expected to resist, it was considered necessary to remove the civilian population from Lapland.[82] The Sámi people from Inari and Utsjoki, were evacuated to Central Ostrobothnia in Finland: to the municipalities of Ylivieska and Alavieska. Eino Lukkari, who lived in Utsjoki, wrote later: "In the beginning of September, we became aware that we had to be evacuated. [...] The most valuable goods were packed, cows were sold to Germans, if there were any buyers, sheep were slaughtered, and meat was salted in containers. The reindeer were left without any care in the forests."[83]

Many other Sámi shared Lukkari's experience. Domestic animals were either slaughtered or transported to the gathering places, goods were packed, and some were buried in the ground or hidden otherwise.[84] Cattle could not be evacuated because of the long journeys.[85] The Sámi of Utsjoki had to slaughter or sell all their cows which had a profound effect on the diversity of livestock in the whole of Finland. Before the evacuation, cows in Utsjoki were usually the so-called "Lapland cattle breed,"[86] but after the war, as almost all the cows of Utsjoki and Inari Sámi had been slaughtered, "Lapland cows," which were very well adapted to the northern environment, were replaced by Ayrshire and other cattle breeds of western and southern Finland.[87]

During the Lapland War, some of the Sámi reindeer herders remained, but the majority of the population was evacuated. The evacuation had a great influence on Sámi health and nutrition, as there were sudden changes in diets and new diseases. Some Sámi were more fortunate than others: Sámi reindeer herders who lived in the northwestern parts of Finnish Lapland were evacuated to the residential areas of southern Sámi in Sweden.[88] Disease did not bother evacuees in Swedish Lapland to the same extent as those located in Finnish Ostrobothnia. Apart from Sweden's excellent health care system, the reason was due, apparently, to the more favourable climate for the Sámi.[89] Sweden did not participate in the Second World War, which was also reflected in the food supply of the region: people who were evacuated to Sweden had the chance to taste fruit they had longed for. According to the evacuees, the shelves of the Swedish stores were filled with plums, raisins, figs, jam, biscuits, sweets and chocolate.[90]

Utsjoki residents did not get to sample the Swedish delicacies, despite the fact that "everyone was hoping to get to Sweden." This did not happen.[91] The final location for the Utsjoki Sámi inhabitants' was Alavieska in the Province of Ostrobothnia in Finland. In Alavieska, the Utsjoki Sámi missed their reindeer meat (e.g. sautéed reindeer) and salmon meals. They were also startled by Finnish oatmeal porridge and the poor quality of the drinking water, which caused many illnesses. "Brown water" was mentioned in several sources.[92] In January 1945, a writer who wrote a newspaper article using the pseudonym Sabmelash, described how Utsjoki residents had been taken from the valley of the brave mountains and crystal-clear waters to the valley of Kalajoki (*Fish river* in English) which, in reality, had no fish at all. According to him, the former and current habitats were pretty much the opposite of each other for climatic and natural reasons, so it was no wonder that there was increasing morbidity and frequent deaths among the Sámi evacuees.[93] The district doctor of Inari and Utsjoki also wrote:

> The brown, dirty, bad smelling water of Kalajoki scared the people who had been accustomed to the clear waters of Lapland. They did not dare to wash themselves in it, neither their dishes nor their clothes. Even the water of the wells tasted very bad (...). Also the food – porridge, soup and groats, which were of course not well prepared, were not of a prime quality as the meat and fish had been in Lapland. (...) A very high percentage of the inhabitants of Inari and Utsjoki collapsed during the evacuation period. Many families broke up completely after the mother died, for example, of jaundice or diphtheria.[94]

The contrast with the Sámi home environment was great. One evacuee was annoyed by the fact that back at home there would have been a cellar full of cloudberry jam and salmon, as there had been an excellent harvest year in Utsjoki.[95] There had also been cases where the local inhabitants had given potatoes and milk to the domestic animals rather than to the Sámi evacuees.[96] Sabmelash was also concerned about their weight loss.[97]

The diet of the evacuation period affected the health of the evacuees in many ways and food was often blamed for increased levels of mortality.[98] Of the inhabitants of Inari, 15 died during the evacuation of acute inflammation of the bowels,[99] which might very well have been caused by the lack of proper food or by a sudden change in diet. Diarrhoea was a common disease among the Sámi evacuees.[100] Their changed diet (combined with unhygienic conditions) had already affected the stomachs of the evacuees during the journey,[101] and when they stayed for their first night in the church of Ylivieska, many fell ill under the new conditions. One person reported, "We had eaten, of course, strange food, and during the night started vomiting."[102] The district doctor reported later: "The church and the elementary school, (which) were full of migrants waiting for their final destinations, and the sick people were laying without treatment and helplessly on the floor, among them there were people who were giving birth and people who were dying. [...] The lack of hygiene was unbelievable."[103]

The strange environment was not favourable for the traditional Sámi cooking methods. The Sámi were used to drying meat; some Sámi had also packed dried reindeer meat before leaving Lapland.[104] The Utsjoki evacuee Hans Guttorm said later that they had not managed to dry the meat properly in the conditions at Alavieska: "We bought a heifer with Vuolab's Joosep's family. We slaughtered it, and Jooseppi was excited to put the meat to dry. He, of course, salted it properly and hung it. The days went by and we started to wonder as the meat did not seem to dry up at all but started to become slimy. Alavieska's climate was not suitable for meat drying. It was probably too moist for that purpose."[105] The Sámi placed in Alavieska were eager to go back home as soon as possible: in Utsjoki, the conditions were expected to improve immediately. At least meat and fish would have been available right away.[106]

The Second World War rapidly changed the geography of the Arctic food. The pace of change accelerated during the latter half of the twentieth century: imports of food from the Norwegian side of the border began to be controlled more strictly than before, as the Finnish Border Guard tightened its grip on Utsjoki.[107] An increase in tourism also began to have an impact on the food available in northernmost Finland. In the summer of 1947, the Finnish Border Guard unit of Utsjoki observed several foreign fishermen trying to catch salmon all along the river. These foreigners had such good quality lures and other fishing gear that they sometimes caught bigger salmon than the locals.[108] The Germans had destroyed the fishing nets when they left Lapland, and after the war there was lack of fishing lures and other kinds of fishing supplies among the local Sámi people.[109]

Crossing the state border started to be more closely controlled and connections to Norway began to break. More and more, the Inari's trade began to be directed towards Finland, due to improved road connections.[110] Roads were also built in Utsjoki during and after the Second World War.[111] New people, goods and influences came along with the new roads, but environmental and health threats also began to spread increasingly from the air. Mines and hydroelectric power plants were followed by pollution that came through the Arctic sky. The foodways of the Sámi were often colonized by spoiling their lands and at the same time their traditional food sources.[112] The period post the Second World War in the Sámi area was, in many ways, a period of contamination, which had huge environmental and health impacts.[113]

Conclusion

Food production, distribution and consumption are all related both to the environment and health. Food is associated with human rights such as the right to a healthy environment and increasing mortality rates and health issues have often been strongly connected with environmental changes.[114] The right to healthy environments has often been questionable in the Arctic. Arctic mines, hydro power plants, and pollution have impacted on the well-being and health of indigenous peoples. There were neither mines nor power plants in Utsjoki in the centuries under examination, but border closures and wars affected the environment, health and the geography of food in the Sámi area, especially since the nineteenth century. Indigenous food production was strongly connected to land rights, and there were often political decisions behind the food crises.

It is useful to study globalizing food production and consumption from a regional perspective.[115] During the past centuries, the food systems of the Arctic, its environment and health have increasingly come under a global influence. Food imported from elsewhere has contributed to a decline in the health of northern people and has changed their interaction with their living environment. The diets of the Sámi and other Arctic indigenous peoples have contained many typical elements that have remained the same throughout the centuries (reindeer and game meat, fish, berries), but the human diet, has not always correlated directly with peoples' place of residence in northern latitudes. Especially during the nineteenth and early twentieth centuries, the Sámi diet changed because of their own agency. The Utsjoki Sámi were very active in food distribution.

During the period studied, the Sámi people of northernmost Finland could usually control their own food supply. The Utsjoki Sámi faced a totally new situation during the Lapland War, when they were evacuated to the unhealthy environments –away from the Arctic environment where the means of food production were very familiar to them. After the Second World War, many indigenous Arctic people faced environmental injustice; this was reflected in food production and consumption.

Notes

1 Bell and Valentine 1997; Atkins and Bowler 2001, 253.
2 Atkins and Bowler 2001, 279; Del Casino 2015, 800–2.
3 Mead et al. 2010; Rudolph and McLachlan 2013, 1085.
4 Rudolph and McLachlan 2013, 1084–86.
5 Le 2016, 5–6.
6 Atkins and Bowler 2001, 21.
7 Kylli et al. 2019.
8 Ibid.
9 See, e.g., von Linné 1993, 63, 134–35.
10 *Åbo Tidningar* January 10 and 17, 1791.
11 Wear 2004, 321.
12 Fellman 1906, 341–42.
13 Lindroth 1970, 84.

14 Kylli 2019, 28.
15 Nahkiaisoja 2016, 20.
16 Första Bihang eller Codecill till Gränsse Tractaten. Cramér and Prawitz 1970, 108–15.
17 Fellman 1846, 113, 150–54.
18 *Kirjallinen Kuukauslehti* 1 April 1868.
19 Siddle 2012, 70–75.
20 Viken et al. 2008, 22.
21 Rudolph and McLachlan 2013, 1095.
22 *Suomen matkailu* 1 June 1939.
23 Ilvesviita 2005, 20.
24 Nahkiaisoja 2016, 198.
25 Fellman 1906, 404.
26 Thrush 2011, 5–6.
27 Morse and Zakrison 2010.
28 Nahkiaisoja 2016, 118.
29 Kylli 2019, 41.
30 Lists of deceased. Utsjoen kirkonarkisto. NA.
31 Bjerregaard et al. 2004; Pufall et al. 2011.
32 Kuhnlein and Chan 2000, 596–99.
33 Thrush 2011, 16.
34 Kylli et al. 2019.
35 Hustich 1946, 50–72.
36 Rosberg et al. 1931, 375.
37 *Oulun Wiikko-Sanomia* 26 July 1856.
38 Saunier 2016, 27–43.
39 *Maa* 1 February 1939.
40 Rosberg et al. 1931, 375.
41 Madubansi and Shackleton 2006.
42 Documents related to cargoes 1928–1941. UNA HIV:1 NA.
43 *Rajaseutu* 1 January 1943.
44 *Liiketaito* 1 June 1939.
45 *Rajaseutu* 1 January 1943.
46 Letters to the rural police chief 1938. UNA HIII:2. NA. In 1920 there were 37 Finnish and 491 Sámi speaking inhabitants in Utsjoki. Rosberg, Hildén and Mikkola 1931.
47 Letters of border trade 1927–1941. UNA HIII:2. NA.
48 Sage 2012, 1.
49 Atkins and Bowler 2001, 25, 176–79.
50 See, e.g., *Helsingin Sanomat* 21 November 1906.
51 Letters of border trade 1927–1941. UNA HIII:2. NA; Lindroth 1970.
52 See, e.g., *Nordkapp* 3 April 1933.
53 Rudolph and McLachlan 2013, 1080.
54 Letters of border trade 1927–1941. UNA HIII:2. NA.
55 J.N. Niittyvuopio's letter 25 June 1937. UNA HIII:2. NA.
56 Decision of the Ministry of Finance, 31 December 1935. UNA HIII:2. NA.
57 J.N. Niittyvuopio's letters 1936–1937. UNA HIII:2. NA.
58 Lehtola 2012, 220–21.

59 Rosberg et al. 1931, 344.
60 *Rovaniemi* 27 April 1929.
61 Suomalaista sianlihaa 1934.
62 See, e.g., Rosberg 1911, 173–78.
63 Le 2016, 1.
64 Pieski 2006, 34–35.
65 Atkins and Bowler 2001, 154.
66 McCannon 2012, 224–25.
67 Paterson 2017.
68 Governor's report 1939. LHA Hb:1. NA.
69 Isak Walle's letter to rural police chief 8 September 1939. UNA HIV:1. NA.
70 Lehtola 2019, 35–40.
71 Metsähallituksen Utsjoen hoitoalueen arkisto HX:1. NA.
72 Lehtola 2012, 368, 383.
73 Annual report 1944. ALA Db:1. NA.
74 Lehtola 2019, 35–39.
75 Lehtola 2015, 118.
76 Poro. Lapin kruunupää. *Nuorten Pellervo* 1940.
77 Governor's report 1940–1941. LHA Hb:1–2. NA.
78 Governor's report 1941–1942. LHA Hb:2. NA.
79 Ibid.
80 Governor's report 1944. LHA Hb:3. NA.
81 Taka-Lapin Isp.E:n Sotapäiväkirja No 2. 2.9.1944–4.9.1944. TIEA. NA.
82 Etto 1975, 4.
83 Evakkomatkasta matkakertomus. Eino Lukkarin arkisto Aa:1. NA.
84 Aikio 2000.
85 Kertomus siirtokarjan palautuksesta Lapin lääniin 1945. Jälleenrakennusasiakirjat (Toivo T. Kailan–Martti Ursinin kokoelma) Bc:10. NA.
86 *Rajaseutu* 1, 1943.
87 Lehtola 2012, 348; Lehtola 2019, 203.
88 *Pohjolan Sanomat* 24 November 1944.
89 Lehtola 2019, 62.
90 Etto 1977, 16.
91 Aikio 2000, 18.
92 Annual report 1944. ALA Db:1. NA; *Kansan kuvalehti* 11 October 1944.
93 *Kaleva* 25 January 1945.
94 Annual report 1944. ALA Db:1. NA.
95 Aikio 2000, 38.
96 Report 23 January 1945. Inarin siirtoväen huoltojohtajan arkisto Ca:1. NA.
97 *Kaleva* 25 January 1945.
98 Lehtola 2019, 64–71.
99 Annual report 1944. ALA Db:1. NA.
100 Aikio 2000, 95; Pohjois-Suomen päättymässä oleva evakuointi. *Pohjolan Sanomat* 1 October 1944.
101 Annual report 1944. ALA Db:1. NA; Etto 1975, 34.
102 Aikio 2000, 137.
103 Annual report 1944. ALA Db:1. NA.

104 *Etelä-Suomen Sanomat* September 22, 1944; Aikio 2000, 62.
105 Aikio 2000, 139.
106 Lehtola 2019, 132.
107 Ibid., 189–190.
108 Utsjoki patrol reports 1947. Rajajääkäripataljoona 5. 3. komppania, Lapin rajavartiosto 2. komppania Dh:5. NA.
109 Rinne 1991, 153.
110 Lehtola 2019, 191.
111 Aikio 2006, 44–45.
112 Pufall et al. 2011.
113 McCannon 2012, 236–37.
114 Hossain et al. 2018, 8–14.
115 Atkins and Bowler 2001, 34.

References

Unpublished sources

National Archives of Finland (NA):

Eino Lukkarin arkisto
Inarin ja Utsjoen aluelääkärin arkisto (ALA)
Inarin siirtoväen huoltojohtajan arkisto
Lapin lääninhallituksen arkisto (LHA)
Lapin rajavartiosto 2. komppania
Taka-Lapin Ilmasuojelupiirin Esikunnan arkisto (TIEA)
Utsjoen kirkonarkisto
Utsjoen nimismiespiirin arkisto (UNA)

Newspapers and magazines

Etelä-Suomen Sanomat
Helsingin Sanomat
Kaleva
Kansan kuvalehti
Kirjallinen Kuukauslehti
Liiketaito
Maa
Metsähallituksen Utsjoen hoitoalueen arkisto
Nordkapp
Nuorten Pellervo
Oulun Wiikko-Sanomia
Pohjolan Sanomat
Rajaseutu
Rovaniemi
Suomen matkailu

Published sources

Aikio, Niilo. 2000. *Liekkejä pakoon: Saamelaiset evakossa 1944–1945*. Helsinki: SKS.
Aikio, Niilo. 2006. "Johtolagaid ja johtinneavvuid nuppástusat." In *Dološ áiggi Muitu*, edited by Vuokko Hirvonen, 42–53. Ohcejohka: Ohcejohnjálmmi gilisearvi.
Atkins, Peter and Ian Bowler. 2001. *Food in Society: Economy, Culture, Geography*. London: Arnold.
Bell, David and Gill Valentine. 1997. *Consuming Geographies: We Are Where We Eat*. London: Routledge.
Bjerregaard, Peter, T. Kue Young, Eric Dewailly, and Sven O.E. Ebbesson. 2004. "Indigenous Health in the Arctic: An Overview of the Circumpolar Inuit Population." *Scandinavian Journal of Public Health* 32 (5): 390–95.
Cramér, Tomas and Gunnar Prawitz. 1970. *Studier i renbeteslagstiftning*. Stockholm: Norsted.
Del Casino, Vincent J. 2015. "Social Geography I: Food." *Progress in Human Geography* 39 (6): 800–08.
Etto, Jorma. 1975. *Evakkotaival: Kuvia ja muisteluksia Lapin evakosta 1944–1945*. [Rovaniemi:] Lapin Maakuntaliitto.
Etto, Jorma. 1977. *Pohjoinen taikapiiri: Lapin evakkojen maailma 1944–1945*. [Rovaniemi:] Lapin maakuntaliitto.
Fellman, Jakob. 1846. "Anmärkningar öfver 'Anteckningar om Församlingarne i Kemi Lappmark af And Joh. Sjögren' af J. Fellman." In *Suomi, Tidskrift i fosterländska ämnen*, 63–160. Helsingfors: Finska Litteratur-Sällskapets förlag.
Fellman, Jacob. 1906. *Anteckningar under min vistelse i Lappmarken 1*. Helsingfors: Finska litteratursällskapet.
Hossain, Kamrul, Dele Raheem, and Shaun Cormier. 2018. *Food Security Governance in the Arctic-Barents Region*. Cham: Springer International Publishing.
Hustich, Ilmari. 1946. *Tuhottu ja tulevaisuuden Lappi*. Helsinki: Kustannustalo.
Ilvesviita, Pirjo. 2005. *Paaluraudoista kotkansuojeluun: suomalainen metsästyspolitiikka 1865–1993*. Rovaniemi: Lapin yliopisto.
Kuhnlein, H. V. and H. M. Chan. 2000. "Environment and Contaminants in Traditional Food Systems of Northern Indigenous Peoples." *Annual Review of Nutrition* 20 (1): 595–626.
Kylli, Ritva. 2019. "Traditional Arctic Healing and Medicines of Modernisation in Finnish and Swedish Lapland." In *Healers and Empires in Global History: Healing as Hybrid and Contested Knowledge*, edited by Markku Hokkanen and Kalle Kananoja, 27–53. London: Palgrave Macmillan.
Kylli, Ritva, Anna-Kaisa Salmi, Tiina Äikäs, and Sirpa Aalto. 2019. "'Not on Bread but on Fish and by Hunting': Food Culture in Early Modern Sápmi." In *The Sound of Silence: Indigenous Perspectives on Historical Archaeology of Colonialism*, edited by Tiina Äikäs and Anna-Kaisa Salmi, 119–40. New York: Berghahn Books.
Le, Stephen. 2016. *100 Million Years of Food: What Our Ancestors Ate and Why It Matters Today*. New York: Picador, 2016.
Lehtola, Veli-Pekka. 2012. *Saamelaiset suomalaiset: Kohtaamisia 1896–1953*. Helsinki: SKS.
Lehtola, Veli-Pekka. 2015. *Saamelaiset: Historia, yhteiskunta, taide*. Aanaar – Inari: Puntsi.

Lehtola, Veli-Pekka. 2019. *Surviving the Upheaval of Arctic War*. Translated by Linna Weber Müller-Wille. Aanaar – Inari: Puntsi.

Lindroth, Saimi. 1970. *Terveyssisarena tunturipitäjässä*. Mäntsälä.

Linné, Carl von. 1993. *Lapinmatka 1732*. [Hämeenlinna:] Karisto.

Madubansi, M., and C. M. Shackleton. 2006. "Changing Energy Profiles and Consumption Patterns Following Electrification in Five Rural Villages, South Africa." *Energy Policy* 34 (18): 4081–92.

McCannon, John. 2012. *A History of the Arctic: Nature, Exploration and Exploitation*. London: Reaktion.

Mead, Erin, Joel Gittelsohn, Meredith L.V. Kratzmann, Cindy Roache, and Sangita Sharma. 2010. "Impact of the Changing Food Environment on Dietary Practices of an Inuit Population in Arctic Canada." *Journal of Human Nutrition and Dietetics* 23 (1): 18–26.

Morse, B. W. and Michelle Zakrison. 2010. "The Impact on the Inuit of Environmental Degradation to the Canadian Arctic." *Common Law World Review* 39 (1): 48–68.

Nahkiaisoja, Tarja. 2016. *Saamelaisten maat ja vedet kruunun uudistiloiksi: Asutus ja maankäyttö Inarissa ja Utsjoella vuosina 1749–1925*. Oulu: Oulun yliopisto.

Paterson, Lawrence. 2017. *Hitler's Forgotten Flotillas: Kriegsmarine Security Forces*. Barnsley: Seaforth Publishing, a division of Pen & Sword Books.

Pieski, Aslak A. 2006. "Ohcejohkalaččaid luonddu geavaheapmi = Utsjokelaisten luonnon käyttöä." In *Dološ áiggi Muitu: Eilinen Keskellämme*, edited by Vuokko Hirvonen, 32–41. Ohcejohka: Ohcejohnjálmmi gilisearvi.

Pufall, E. L., Andria Q. Jones, Scott A. Mcewen, Charlene Lyall, Andrew S. Peregrine, and Victoria L. Edge. 2011. "Perception of the Importance of Traditional Country Foods to the Physical, Mental, and Spiritual Health of Labrador Inuit." *Arctic* 64 (2): 242–50.

Rinne, Reino. 1991. *Lapin Rauha: Retkiä Lapissa kesällä 1946*. Kuusamo: Karhu-kirjat.

Rosberg, J.E. *Lappi*. 1911. Helsinki: Kansanvalistusseura.

Rosberg, J.E., K. Hildén, and E. Mikkola. 1931. *Suomenmaa: Maantieteellis-taloudellinen ja historiallinen tietokirja 9. Oulun Lääni, Pohjoisosa*. Porvoo: WSOY.

Rudolph, Karlah Rae, and Stephane M. McLachlan. 2013. "Seeking Indigenous Food Sovereignty: Origins of and Responses to the Food Crisis in Northern Manitoba, Canada." *Local Environment* 18 (9): 1079–98.

Sage, Colin. 2012. *Environment and Food*. London and New York: Routledge.

Saunier, Pierre. 2016. "Food Production: Industrial Processing Begins to Gain Ground." In *A Cultural History of Food in the Age of Empire. Volume 5*, edited by Martin Bruegel, 27–47. London: Bloomsbury.

Siddle, Richard M. 2012. *Race, Resistance and the Ainu of Japan*. London: Routledge.

Suomalaista sianlihaa metsätyömaille. 1934. Kangasala: Suomen sianjalostusyhdistys.

Thrush, Coll. 2011. "Vancouver the Cannibal: Cuisine, Encounter, and the Dilemma of Difference on the Northwest Coast, 1774–1808." *Ethnohistory* 58 (1): 1–35.

Viken, Arvid, Brynhild Granås, and Toril Nyseth. 2008. "Kirkenes: An Industrial Site Reinvented as a Border Town." *Acta Borealia* 25 (1): 22–44.

Wear, Andrew. 2004. "Medicine and Health in the Age of European Colonialism." In *The Healing Arts: Health, Disease and Society in Europe, 1500–1800*, edited by Peter Elmer, 315–43. Manchester University Press.

Chapter 7

Standardized housing concepts in the North

Sámi housing meets Western hygienic norms in twentieth-century Finland

Anu Soikkeli

Introduction

A home is a private space and domestic life is a highly individual and personal matter. However, the economic, social, and technical issues involved also make the home a public issue. This chapter discusses the tensions that existed between two cultures: the Finnish and the Sámi, over the issue of healthy housing. More specifically, the chapter investigates how Finnish ideals of good housing, health and hygiene influenced the way that Sámi housing and way of life changed during the post-Second World War period of reconstruction. This period saw the large-scale introduction of type-house planning in the regions inhabited by the Sámi people (Figure 7.1).

Normative concepts of purity influenced the way that type-planned houses were designed and (family) life in them represented and valorized. Purity is a value-laden concept with a long history. The anthropologist Mary Douglas famously emphasized that dirt is not an objectively measurable thing, but must always be interpreted in context. Filth is thus matter out of place, something that brings confusion to a well-organized world. Food on a plate represents purity, food on clothing impurity.[1] Norms, in turn, are practices of the social world in which social order is maintained. Any perception of dirtiness, including our own, stems from culture-related symbolic systems.

In late nineteenth and early twentieth-century Finland, the concept of purity was applied to a wide variety of things, ranging from material purity and hygiene to moral conduct. Finns evaluated Sámi housing and the Sámi way of life, including the latters' degree of tidiness, according to their own criteria. These criteria also increasingly became shared by the Sámi themselves. Especially after the Second World War, Finnish campaigns for health and hygiene reached both Finns and the Sámi, notably by means of schools and the health care system, especially public health nurses and midwives. Sámi housing was regarded, to an extent, as a public issue. Many Sámi also sought to be better assimilated into Finnish society as far their residence was concerned. The home, planned and implemented in a Finnish way, would then shape other aspects of the Sámi culture.

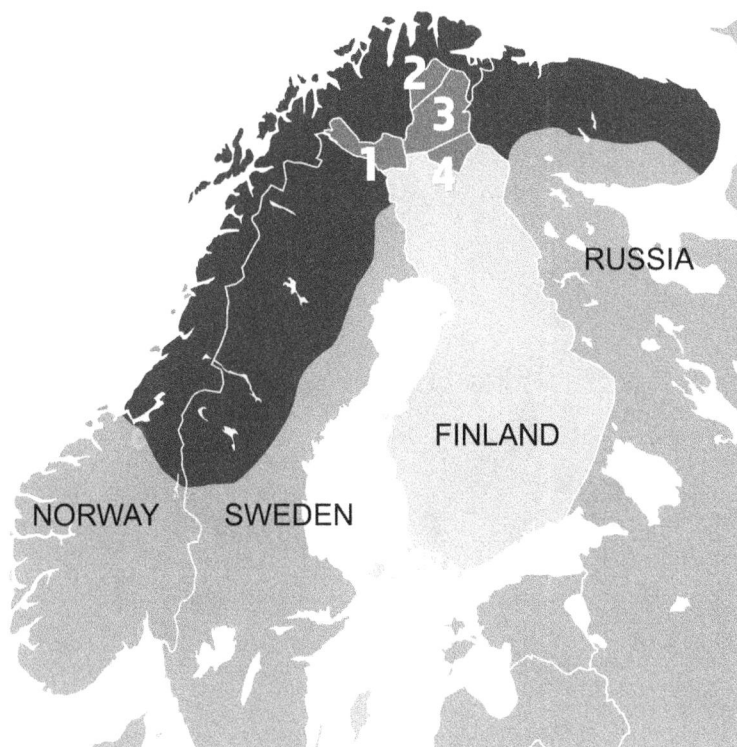

Figure 7.1 The Sámi homeland (*Sápmi*). In Finland, the Sámi homeland consists of the municipalities of (1) Enontekiö, (2) Utsjoki, (3) Inari and (4) the northern part of Sodankylä.

The general processes of the assimilation of the Sámi have been studied extensively during the last 20 years. This chapter will focus on the issue of healthy housing and exclude other dimensions of the Sámi assimilation process. The health and well-being of the Sámi has been examined by medical researchers,[2] but the influence of Finnish architecture and planning on Sámi culture has so far gone unstudied. An exception is Veli-Pekka Lehtola's thorough account of the relationship between the Sámi and the Finns during the first half of the twentieth century; Lehtola's book also includes some discussion on the new types of houses build after the Second World War.[3]

The Sámi building tradition

Traditionally, Sámi building was shaped by the available building materials, which were mainly acquired from local nature. Their nomadic or

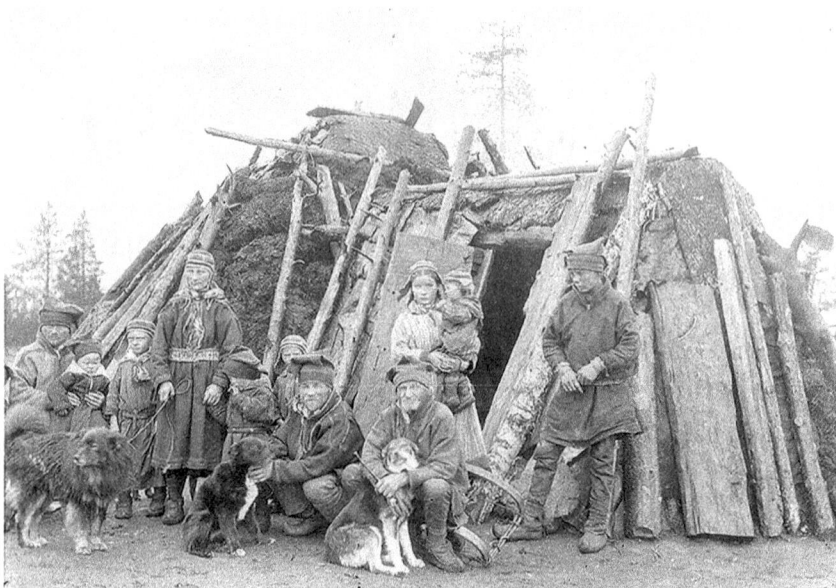

Figure 7.2 A family in front of their peat *goahti* in Vuotsotaipale, 1902. (Unknown photographer. The Image Collection of the National Board of Antiquities, Helsinki.)

semi-nomadic lifestyle favoured small-scale, movable dwellings. By the end of the nineteenth century, many Sámi families had turned from hunting and gathering to reindeer husbandry and/or fishing to farming and animal husbandry. With the gradual waning of the hunting-gathering way of life, dwellings became more permanent in nature. Log buildings became increasingly common, as wealthier Sámi hired Finnish carpenters to construct log houses for them. Larger log houses usually had two rooms and an entrance hall between them, while more modest log cottages had just one small room under the ridge.[4]

The Sámi lifestyle nevertheless maintained some nomadic features. Families lived in different places during different seasons. Winter dwellings were more permanent and more carefully built; the first log cabins would be found at winter sites. When moving between their spring, summer and autumn sites, Sámi families resorted to traditional, more easily movable buildings such as *lavvus*,[5] *goahtis*,[6] storage sheds, storage platforms and other sheltering structures (Figure 7.2). Neither did the shift from the *lavvus* and peat *goahtis* to log construction completely change the way that the dwellings were organized and used. Crafting, eating and sleeping took place indoors. Fixed furnishings were few. These might include, for instance, a side bench

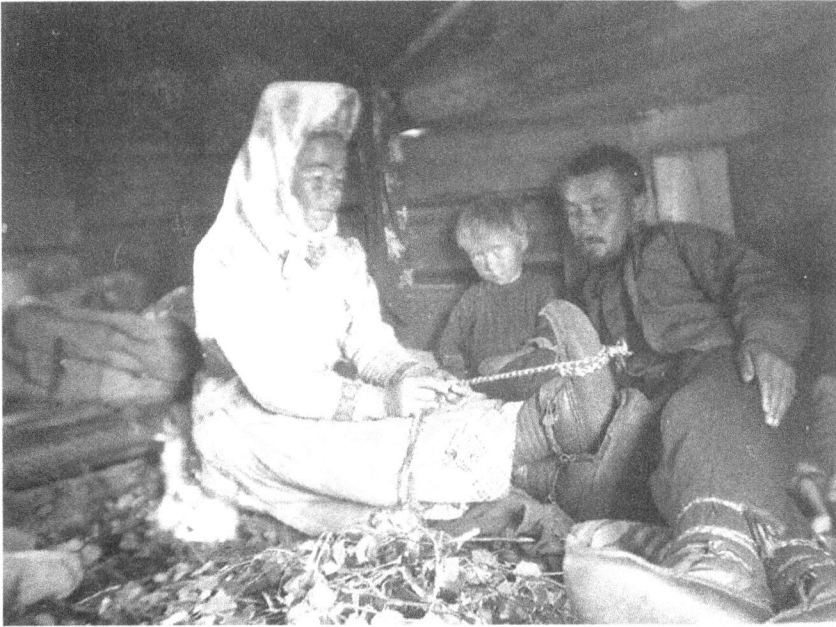

Figure 7.3 A Skolt Sámi family home in 1933. (Photograph: Karl Nickul. The Image
Collection of the National Board of Antiquities, Helsinki.)

for lying down, another bench or a table, a simple dish shelf and plenty of
hanging hooks on the walls. Their belongings were more or less in sight. To an
outsider, the dwelling could seem cramped (see Figure 7.3).[7]

Finnish observers could be highly critical of Sámi buildings. At the beginning of the twentieth century, the Evangelical Lutheran pastor of the Utsjoki
parish noted that Sámi dwellings were small and lacked base walls (Finnish
peasants had been instructed to build their log buildings on a base wall since
the eighteenth century). He was also appalled see open fireplaces without
smoke dampers to prevent heat loss. Rooms were small and unventilated,
and the heavy air was considered unhealthy.[8] Another report from the same
area stated that "Cleanliness is not common, it needs improvement. Cramped
dwellings, for example one room for a large family, make cleaning difficult.
Every house should at least have a sauna [steam bath]. I do not know of more
than seven in the whole municipality."[9]

Finns associated small and cramped living with bad health and impurity,
and considered a sauna a basic necessity. A Finnish family would commonly
start the construction of a farmhouse by first building a sauna, which was
regarded as essential for maintaining health and even for curing diseases.

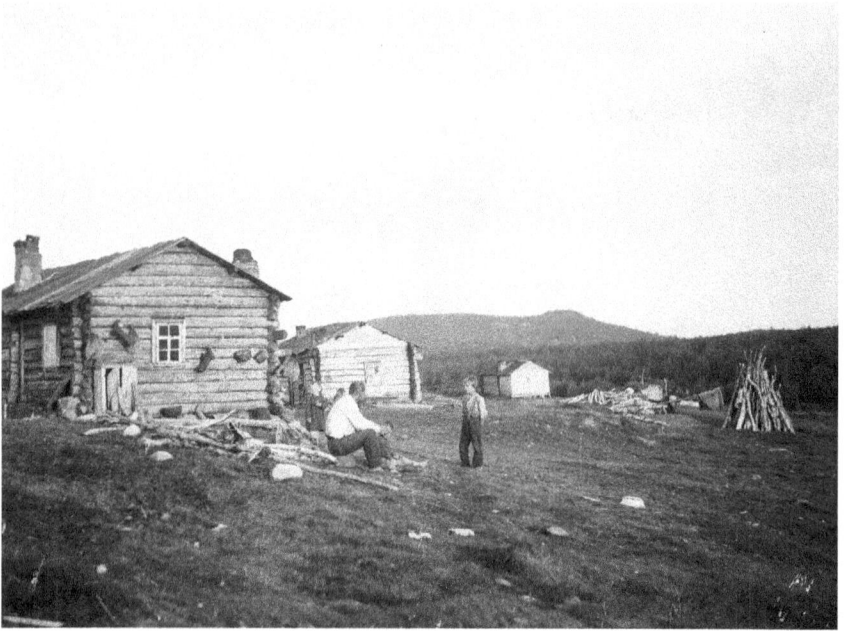

Figure 7.4 Sámi dwellings in Pechenga in 1930. (Photograph: Bernhard Åström. The Image Collection of the National Board of Antiquities, Helsinki.)

According to a stock phrase, "a person who cannot be cured by sauna, alcohol and tar is as good as dead." A report from Inari, written at the beginning of the twentieth century, noted approvingly that "Most houses already have a sauna, and the cleanliness in the wealthiest homes is very satisfactory."[10] Although by no means all educated Finnish observers regarded the Sámi as categorically unclean, many Finns did subscribe to this notion.

The buildings of a Finnish farmhouse were organized around a rectangular central yard. The placement of the buildings was influenced by the terrain and other considerations, for instance the need to minimize the amount of snow in the inner yard and the wish to have a broad view.[11] The Sámi way of building was also based on a long tradition, but it had different priorities. For the Sámi, practicality, durability, and wind and frost shields were more important than appearance in construction. The placement of the buildings lacked a regular plan (see Figure 7.4), which made them seem haphazardly scattered to Finnish observers. To the latter, Sámi dwellings, storage places and other structures appeared modest, the buildings seemed makeshift and ready to collapse, and constructed from little better than waste materials. The overall impression was often judged as untidy.

Finnish views on the Sámi (nineteenth and early twentieth centuries)

The Finns' image of the Sámi was formed over a long period of time. The oldest written documents are descriptions by civil servants and priests living in Lapland in the eighteenth and nineteenth centuries. They typically combine individual experiences with more general beliefs. As new settlements spread towards the north, it became more common to admire the agricultural way of life and regard farms as outposts of civilization in a hostile environment. The Sámi, in turn, were described as innocently child-like people, unburdened by civilization.[12]

The most influential early Finnish observer of the Sámi was Matias Aleksanteri Castrén (1813–1852), a folklore scholar and professor of Finnish and Uralian languages. He travelled in Lapland in 1838 and during 1841–1842. Castrén described the Sámi as a strange, dirty and uneducated, albeit fortunately humble, people. In describing their dwellings, he wrote, "The bunch of people passing through the low entrance hole of the *lávvu* is so full of dirt and vermin that you are scared to look at them."[13] The image that he draws of the Sámi village and its slow and sullen inhabitants is not flattering:

> A Lapp summer village is not a wonderful sight. Everywhere one sees fish bowels, fish scales, putrid fish, and other rotten trash on the ground, poisoning the air. A group of smudged people emerge from the *lávvus*, and they do not mind any of this.

Castrén's description found its way into an extremely influential work, *Boken om vårt land* ("A Book on our Land") (1875) by the author and historian Zacharias Topelius (1818–1898). In his chapter on the Sámi, Topelius relies heavily on Castrén's travel reports. Topelius, too, saw farming as a more highly developed form of life than nomadism. He praised the kindness and hospitality of the Sámi towards their guests but criticized their housing and their untidiness.[14] *Boken om vårt land* was crucially important to the development of the Finnish identity during the nineteenth century national revival, and it was used as a textbook in school geography and history classes as late as the 1950s, thus also influencing the Finnish view of the Sámi for generations.[15] Among other things, the book taught that the Sámi did not share Finnish standards of cleanliness and purity.

At the beginning of the twentieth century, educated Finns still approached the Sámi with these stereotypical images in mind. A 1905 report by the state committee for the economic development of Lapland praised the diligence of Sámi women but was concerned about the poor hygiene of the people, noting that:

> A Lapp is usually not clean or tidy in his lifestyle. The living conditions of the fell region Lapp (a reindeer herder) are such that cleanliness is

completely out of the question. A Lapp living by the river (a fisherman) is better positioned to keep clean, but he too is used to living in filth and does not, with some exceptions, yearn for anything better. Rooms are seldom washed or scrubbed.

The report found also Sámi eating habits wanting. The cooking utensils were not washed or cleaned, nor was the meat or fish served from a bowl; eating with fingers was seen as another sign of a primitive level of cleanliness. The report did not frame the low level of cleanliness as a racial feature but as a result of the nomadic way of life and cramped housing.[16] Crowded housing made it difficult to impossible to adhere to Finnish norms of cleanliness and purity.

Finns did not regard the Sámi as a homogeneous group, but rather saw differences in the tidiness of the different sub-sections of the Sámi society. For example, a book called *Suomenmaa* ("The Land of Finland") complimented the Sámi of the Utsjoki region for taking first place in cleanliness. It regarded the Sámi on the Muurman coast as tolerably clean. The Russian Orthodox Skolts, on the other hand, were looked down upon, partly because of the anti-Russian attitude prevalent in inter-war Finland. In the 1920s, the alleged Sámi untidiness, laziness and simplicity could also be cast as racial features.[17]

Finnish observers also made a note of differences between theirs and the Sámi interiors. According to a 1940s eyewitness, "reindeer herders in permanent dwellings […] have retained a whole set of nomadic habits and attitudes. It can be seen already from the interiors of their houses. They still retain a degree of the disorder characteristic of *lavvu* living."[18] The windows in Sámi dwellings usually lacked curtains, and a couple of boards on the wall were enough to serve as shelves. There were no large storage facilities, and commodities were often in plain sight. For example, a table in front of a window could be covered with varied utensils and materials, while a bench placed on the middle of the room could function as a seat and or even as a table.[19] In contrast, the ideal turn-of-the century Finnish farmhouse had well-lit rooms with curtained windows, painted furniture and separate storage space in chests, dressers or cupboards. Each item had its own place, and the common living area was divided into male and female sides, with men and women doing their chores in their own designated areas.[20]

Differences are also obvious with respect to the outlook of the yard. The Sámi yard missed the common planning features of Finnish farms or vernacular sites, such as a closed, symmetrical, rectangular form with clear boundaries that separated it from the environment. While the Finnish yard stood out in the landscape, the Sámi yard was integrated into the surrounding nature. The latter had many small storage places, structures and racks. The Sámi homestead was constructed appropriately and for practical reasons, but, to Finnish eyes, it appeared shapeless and dishevelled and signalled backwardness.[21]

Hygienic and health considerations and campaigns

The significance of cleanliness for maintaining health was stressed in Finland especially from the late nineteenth century onwards. A clean home was a social, moral and medical norm. Flies, bedbugs and other insects were seen as potential carriers of disease.[22] Since the beginning of the twentieth century, the aesthetic point of view gained in importance. Aesthetics is not merely a matter of individual taste, but an integral part of the social context. Aesthetic meanings are collectively shared, and non-compliance with aesthetic norms can lead to social disgrace, which is relevant from the point of view of the development of housing architecture and type-planned houses.

Tuberculosis, in particular, was regarded as a "dwelling disease." It was closely associated with industrialization and poorly nourished urban working-class people who were living in unsalubrious, overcrowded conditions. It was known that tuberculosis spread through droplets and sputum and it was believed that the bacteria could survive for a long time in dried household dust and domestic environmental conditions, thereby endangering the health of the occupants. Vigorous campaigns against poor ventilation, uncleanliness and inappropriate furnishings were an important part of European and Finnish anti-tuberculosis strategies.[23] These campaigns coincided with large-scale attempts to provide social housing as an aspect of public health and also with the emergence of architectural modernism. After the First World War, modernist architects in Europe were intent on looking for design solutions for low-cost social housing.

Another phenomenon that impacted notions of healthy housing was the household guidance movement. It emerged in Finland in the 1920s, with the overarching aim of rationalizing and modernizing households through counselling, education and guidance. It sought to alleviate problems such as poverty, ignorance and untidiness by giving practical advice aimed at facilitating everyday life and homemaking, especially in remote rural areas. Household guidance targeted "indolence, unconcern, untidiness, and envy."[24] The advice often revolved around cleanliness. Dirt and poverty were assumed to go hand in hand, and squandering and untidiness were considered a cause of poverty and suffering. Bad odour and an unkempt appearance indicated a lack of culture and a low level of civilization.[25]

The inter-war period saw both a significant rise in the membership of household associations and an expansion of the press. Magazines such as *Pellervo, Kotiliesi, Emäntälehti* and *Yhteishyvä* found their way into the hands of farmers' wives and offered ways to combine Finnish traditions with new homemaking ideals.[26] The message of purity that was so central to these magazines reached the people in Lapland, too, affecting the notions and norms of purity in Sámi homes. The ideals they propounded were often in conflict with Sámi traditions. The maintaince of the yard is one example of this. Homemaking magazines denounced messy yards, placing special emphasis on composting, which helped to keep the yard neat, and also contributed to household economy. They stressed that composting helped to keep the yard neat, and it also contributed to household economy. By recycling land-fill it was possible to produce good fertilizer and keep the environment tidy and animals away.[27] The Sámi yard, constructed with practical environment-specific considerations in mind, often failed to meet these standards.

Another route for the dissemination of Finnish homemaking ideals among the Sámi was the school. During the 1920s, primary schooling was extended to the whole of the population. However, in the northernmost municipalities travelling schools – a teacher moving from village to village, teaching the children of the community in a private house – remained popular with the municipal authorities, partly because the arrangement was cheap. Classes were given in Sámi houses, too, although their standard of hygiene was considered a problem. Teachers reported that children sat on the floor, "on which anyone could have spit." Lack of cleanliness was indeed used as an argument for founding proper schools in the region.[28] After the war, the travelling school system was abolished, even in the far north, where it was replaced by elementary boarding schools. The new school system offered Sámi children a better opportunity to acquire a full education. It also brought them into closer contact with Finnish culture and norms, including those concerned with purity and cleanliness (see Figure 7.5).[29] When researchers interviewed Sámi people

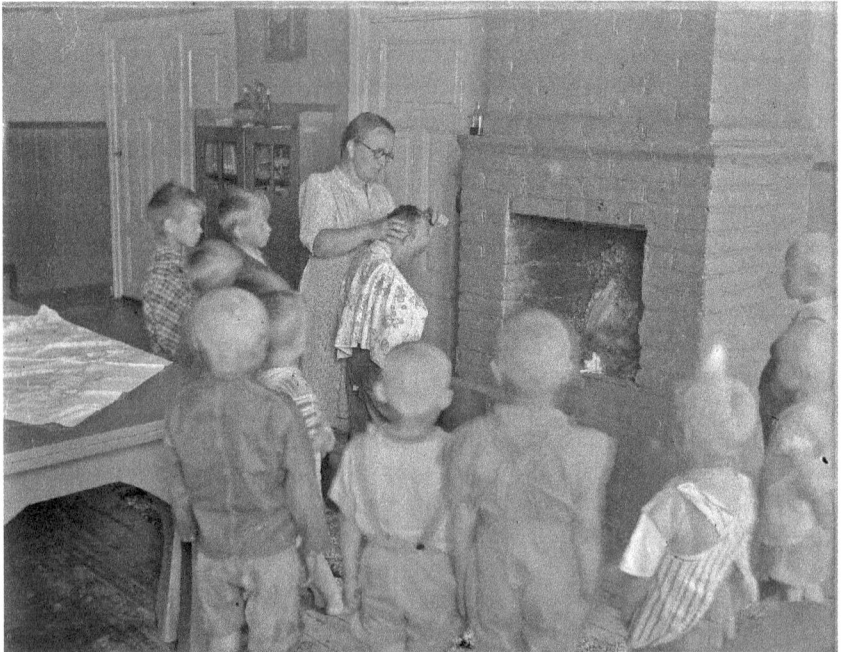

Figure 7.5 A haircut is taking place at Riutula Children's Home in 1949. Schools and children's homes did a lot to impart modern conceptions of hygiene on Sámi children. (Photographer unknown. Museum Centre Vapriikki, Tampere.)

about their childhood and upbringing in the1930s–1950s, they produced many memories of household chores, which largely consisted of cleaning and tidying both inside the house and in the yard.[30]

Architects' declaration of war against dirtiness and disorder

The idea of healthy living had already emerged in international architectural discussions in the late nineteenth century, and it was packaged in the form of a manifesto during the early modern movement (usually referred to in Finland as "functionalism"). The guiding principle of functionalism was to meet the changing needs of society. Social differences in housing were great, and both rural and the urban poor lived in cramped and modest conditions.[31] In Finland, discussions about hygiene and housing as a social issue entered the architecture in the 1910s.[32] At the time, a significant proportion of the population lived in tiny one-room flats, and an increasingly important objective of social policy and architecture was to solve the housing problem of the working population. One solution was type-planned housing projects, aimed at producing good-quality housing that the working class could afford.[33] After the Second World War, the class aspect became less pronounced. A modern dwelling was seen as a democratic right: everyone should have a kitchen, one or more bedrooms, a living room and a bathroom. The aim was to harmonize housing.

In the architectural discourse, too, lack of cleanliness was linked to the level of development and culture; the right kind of home was presented as a key to purity and tidiness. Inadequate housing conditions were pernicious to individuals but also a threat to social order, as disordered and dirty dwellings were thought to lead to crime, illness, indifference and decay. Clean homes, in turn, had an uplifting effect: they fostered purity, self-discipline and refinement. Modern housing was also linked to population policy. It was construed as a means of boosting population growth and as a tool for improving the quality of the population (and thus part of positive eugenics).[34]

The war and its aftermath presented planners and policy makers with new challenges. War veterans and invalids, as well as the over 400,000 resettlers from the areas ceded by the Soviet Union, had to be integrated back into society as productive members. Parts of the infrastructure had been damaged and great many buildings had been destroyed, especially in Helsinki and Lapland, leaving many people homeless. Along with the housing shortage and resettlement issues, the post-war planning projects addressed a lack of hygiene and purity, which were considered an integral part of the new planning ideals, alongside social equality and family life. The economy was another central issue. Post-war residential construction was, by necessity, practical and expedient, as both building materials and labour were in short supply. Type-planned houses were seen as a way to offer similar good quality housing to large parts of the population.

Standardized housing for the Sámi

In Finland, the period of the Second World War is usually divided into three separate wars: the Winter War (1939–1940), the Continuation War (1941–1944) and the Lapland War (1944–1945). The last was waged against the German troops that had been posted in the northern most provinces during the Continuation War. In the fall of 1944, when Finland signed an armistice with the Soviet Union, Germany turned from a co-belligerent into an enemy. The people of Lapland, including the Sámi, were then evacuated. Most Sámi spent the winter of 1944–1945 cramped in private homes in the Western province of Central Ostrobothnia. The time of evacuation brought the Sámi into contact with the Finnish way of life and culture in a new way. They received new impressions about clothing, cleanliness and agricultural practices.[35] After the war, most Sámi evacuees returned to their home communities. For the Skolt Sámi, however, the loss of the Pechenga area in the peace treaty meant they lost their traditional grounds and had to resettle in Finland.

More often than not, the evacuees had no homes to return to. Retreating towards the Arctic Ocean, the Germans had applied the scorched-earth tactic, destroying almost all the buildings in the province of Lapland. A major reconstruction was called for. Traditionally, the building of rural communities had been a slow process, with strong bonds to local nature and tradition. The post-war reconstruction, on the other hand, was conducted in a relatively short time as a top-down project, controlled at the national level. In this process, the locals were executors rather than partners.[36]

The reconstruction relied heavily on the use of type-planned model houses (see Figure 7.6). The type-planned houses of the reconstruction period were pitched-roofed, one-and-a-half-storey, one-family houses based on standardization and wood construction. People were provided with free blueprints and detailed instructions, and low-interest building loans were fairly easy to obtain. The architecture of these houses differed from the traditional Finnish building tradition and, even more clearly, from the Sámi building tradition. The outcome was influenced by the simple design and by the shortage of construction materials. The architecture of the post-war type-planned house loosely continued the principles of functionalism by providing more appropriate facilities for living. In differentiating the domestic space functionally, with each room – kitchen, living room, bedroom – having its own function, it brought a new kind of spatial experience to Finns and even more so to the Sámi.[37]

The reconstruction-era type-planned houses entailed changes in the Sámi way of life. For instance, whereas saunas had been rare in Sámi households prior to the war, they now became common. The new saunas were also equipped, in the Finnish way, with separate dressing rooms.[38] The type-planned house had a modern kitchen, a space closely associated with hygiene and cleanliness (although sometimes the water pipe and wastewater drain

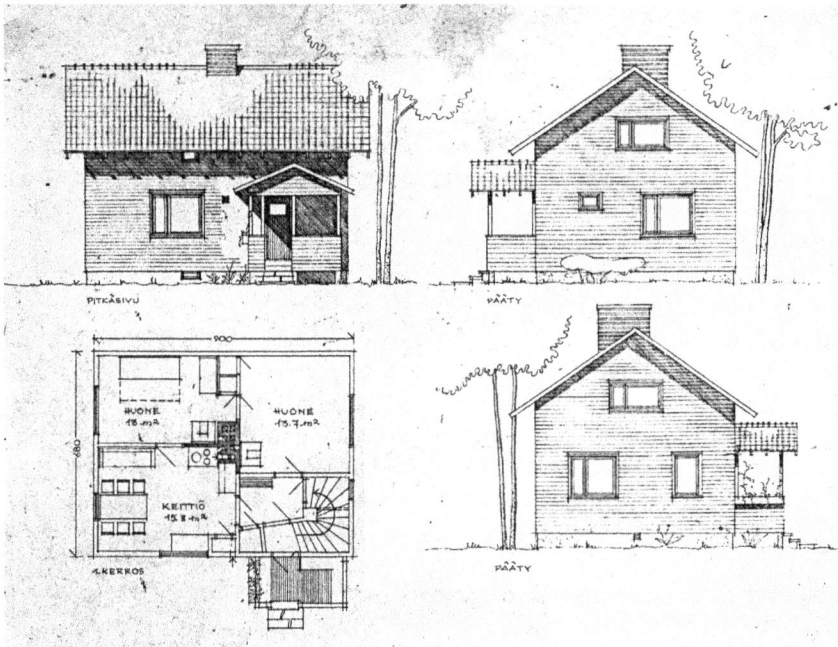

Figure 7.6 A typical type-planned house of the reconstruction period, from the end of the 1940s. (Image owned by the author.)

were missing). Appropriate kitchens or kitchen areas became distinct places designated for special kind of work and were equipped with a new type of countertop, cupboards and other storage spaces. Objects had their own places, often hidden in drawers or cupboards. Easy-to-clean surfaces were an important feature, and painted wooden fittings became common.[39]

The type-planned house of the reconstruction era provided a way to educate the common people into partially new forms of cleanliness. The houses came with manuals with several pages detailing ways of keeping the house clean and neat. For instance, a handbook instructed the readers to follow the interior design style associated with functionalism and Nordic modernism:

> Overly 'decorated' furniture should also be avoided, as well as bad paintings, gypsum objects, wooden sculpture imitations, paper flowers, and other things intended for home decorating but are cheap trinkets. Further, no postcards or other glossy papers should be hung on the walls, nor other multi-coloured papers, ten-year old entrance tickets, soap and perfume advertising posters etc. You should not put all your memorabilia on the walls, cabinets and desks; they only disturb the balance and gather dust.[40]

Window curtains became common also in Sámi houses, and table tops were now more likely to be covered with tablecloths than items in daily use. Instead of traditional open fireplaces, heat was now provided using convective fireplaces with small iron doors that could be shut.[41]

With the new house type came a new way of living which, together with impressions adopted during the evacuation period, at school and through the home guidance movement, transformed Sámi culture. The post-war period also saw an influx of new inhabitants from other parts of Finland to the Sámi regions, which consequently became more Finnish in outlook. As the building stock in Lapland became more homogenous and the everyday life and practices of the Sámi more Finnish, the boundary between the two cultures became less clear. Many old Sámi cultural practices were tested and some were discontinued.[42]

To take one example, the previously common habit of putting in shoe-hay indoors (see Figure 7.7) now became labelled as untidy.[43] As the new kitchen was equipped with a stove and drying cabinets, traditional outdoor cooking also became less common. The house came with storage facilities, and the dishes were now kept in a cupboard rather than on the table and clothes were hung in a closet rather than on the walls. Because the clean and warm interior was entered through the porch, it no longer felt natural to stalk inside with shoes on. The new houses were also warmer than the traditional ones, which made it possible to wear lighter clothing indoors; this had its own impact on everyday culture (see Figure 7.8).

The traditional, extensive Sámi yard with its many small buildings and structures, and with its non-distinct boundaries, was modified, to an extent, but it did not lose all its distinctive features. The placement of the new house and other buildings continued to resemble the way Sámi dwelling entities had traditionally been organized. According to the geographer Ilmari Hustich, who travelled in the Sámi regions in 1946, the loose assemblage of storage houses, cotes and racks reflected the "Lapps' unconscious pursuit to preserve something of the space and place around the *lavvus*." According to him, the Sámi had given up some of the practicality of their traditional living arrangements when they had adopted Finnish housing manners.[44] The traditional Sámi homestead had been an integral part of the environment and had reflected their livelihoods, with a strong connection to nature. Post-war yards continued this tradition, even when the building itself did not.

Conclusion

Finnish concepts of purity and cleanliness contributed to changes in Sámi housing and lifestyle. Culturally conditioned notions of purity influenced the way that outside observers appreciated the Sámi culture and assessed its level of development. This is apparent both in the texts of nineteenth-century scholars and in twentieth-century administrative and financial reports.

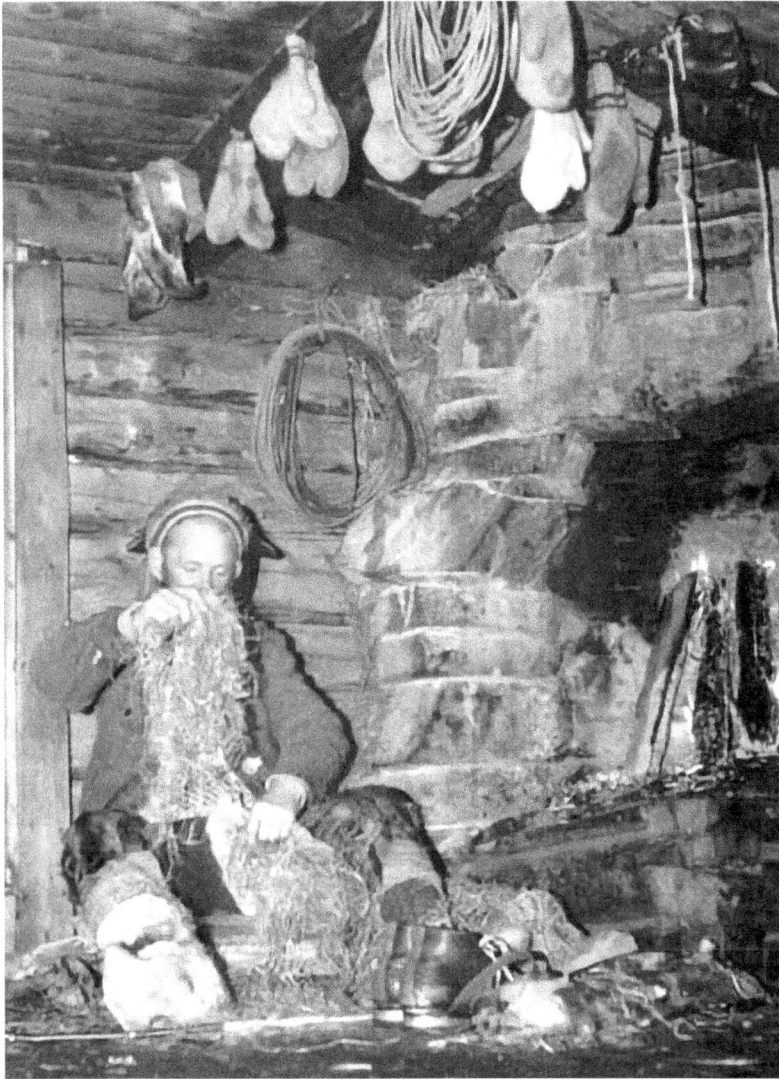

Figure 7.7 A Sámi man putting in shoe-hay. (Photograph: P. Eronen. The Image Collection of the National Board of Antiquities, Helsinki.)

During the first decades of the twentieth century, the way of life and values of the semi-nomadic Sámi still clearly differed from those of their Finnish farmer neighbours. The Second World War and especially the evacuation of 1944–1945 contributed significantly to the changes in their lifestyle. During the evacuation, the Sámi who were familiar with farming and spoke Finnish

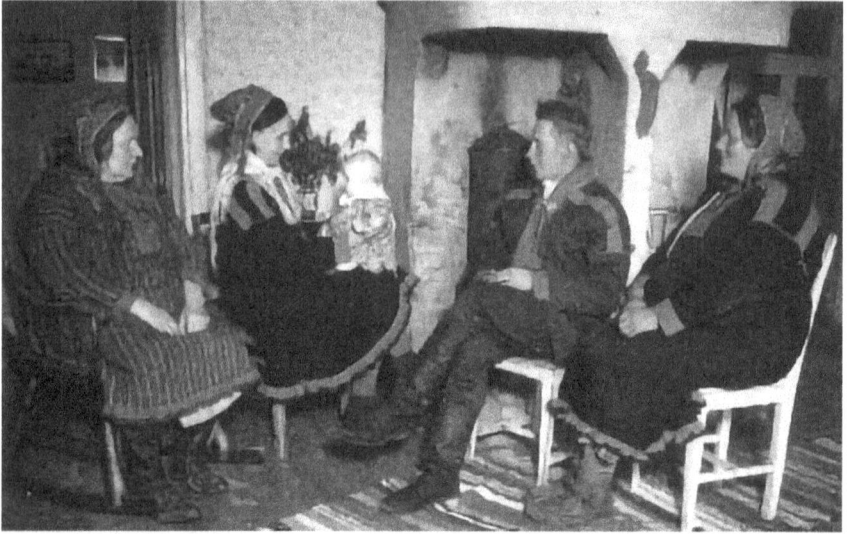

Figure 7.8 A visit taking place at the Harjula household, Nuorgam, in 1948. The owner of the house was a member of the regional reconstruction committee. (Photograph: Antti Hämäläinen. The Image Collection of the National Board of Antiquities, Helsinki.)

were treated better than the Skolt Sámi, whose nomadic lifestyle and Russian Orthodox faith made them seem alien to the Finns among whom they now resided. Their cleanliness was also judged to be poor. Many organizations worked to make the Sámi adhere to modern hygienic standards – although it should be noted that these organizations saw a lot of work to be done among the rural population in other parts of the country as well.

A popular encyclopaedia, first published in 1935, categorically stated that "The Lapps [i.e. Sámi] dwell in *lavvus*" and illustrated this notion with a photograph. The statement was published unchanged in the 1947 edition.[45] A few years later, in 1953, a non-fiction book on Lapland noted that "the last real *lavvu*-dwelling Lapp is dead and today they all have permanent places and houses."[46] The two different statements make use of a stereotypic image of the Sámi but they also reflect the rapid change that took place in Sámi housing arrangements during and because of the war, evacuation and reconstruction. In post-war Finland, the residential environment no longer merely responded to basic needs, but was accompanied by many political, aesthetic, and ethical objectives involved in building modern Finland. In the 1940s and 1950s, a bright, clean home was related to the ideal of the modern family and to the modernization of society. Design was guided by the idea of meeting the basic needs of all people on an equal basis and guided and justified by the needs of purity, hygiene and health.

The construction of type-planned houses accelerated the integration of the Sámi into Finnish society at large. The type house was a means of providing quality housing for the entire population, with no regard to differences in ethnic or cultural background. It was not the catalyst, but rather an indicator of a change that was already underway before the war. The residents made their new homes into lived places through everyday life and practices. They built it for themselves in cooperation with other people, using and decorating it, interacting with design and other ideas. At the same time, the changes undergone by Sámi housing during the reconstruction era also reflected the power of administrators, planners and architects. That power became particularly great during an era when the country was rebuilt materially and mentally. The regulation and determination of the nature of the Sámi home and its activities were part of the use of power related to the development of the housing culture.

Notes

1 Douglas 1966, 34–36.
2 See, e.g., Axelsson and Storm Mienna 2019, 13–22.
3 Lehtola 2012.
4 Magga 2015, 94; Huttunen 2015, 98.
5 A *lavvu* is a temporary dwelling built of three or more evenly spaced forked or notched poles that form a tripod. Traditionally, it was covered with reindeer hides or cloth.
6 A *goahti* is a dwelling with a structure in which the poles are enhanced with two semi-circular wooden extensions to provide increased space. It was traditionally covered with cloth, reindeer hides, sod or timber.
7 Nickul and Manker 1948, 21, photo plates I–LXIV; Paulaharju 1921, 54.
8 Soikkeli 2000, 83–84.
9 Lehtola 2012, 40.
10 Ibid., 43–43.
11 Kähkönen 2014, 37–38.
12 Lehtola 2015, 23–24.
13 Castrén 1878, 21.
14 Topelius 1910, 112. Topelius' description of the Sámi village is more detached than Castrén's, who expresses his own personal feelings of disgust. Topelius described the view in *Boken om vårt land* as if he, too, had been an eyewitness, which he was not.
15 Halonen and Aro 2005, 8; Raivo 2005, 187; Lehtola 2015, 25. See also Aikio-Puoskari 2010, 118.
16 Lehtola 2012, 107, 110.
17 Ibid., 233, 275, 265.
18 Hustich 1946, 36.
19 Lehtola 2012, 40.
20 Sirelius 1921, 297–302.
21 See, e.g., Sirelius 1921, 285, 293–94; Soikkeli 2000, 31–34.

22 Saarikangas 2002, 44–50, 59–62.
23 See, e.g., Härö 1992, 48–50: Hakosalo 2018; Mooney 2013.
24 Ollila 1993, 37.
25 Heinonen 1998, 138, 375–77; Ollila 1993, 37.
26 *Pellervo* and *Yhteishyvä* were the magazines of co-operatives and *Emäntälehti* was the magazine of a conservative women's association, while *Kotiliesi* was a commercial venture, a popular ladies' magazine. Korhonen 1999, 139–40.
27 Länsivuori 2017, 59–60.
28 Lehtola 2012, 287–88. It should be noted, however, that spitting on the floor was common in every part of Finland. At the beginning of the twentieth century, all schools in Finland were instructed to acquire a spit bowl, "without which a tidy school cannot cope" (*Kansakoulun opetusvälineet ja koulukuvasto* 1900, 48), and signs forbidding spitting on the floor could be seen in public places even after the Second World War.
29 Nikunlassi 2014, 180; Lehtola 2012, 274, 276.
30 Porsanger 2015, 49.
31 Vahtola 2003, 320.
32 Saarikangas 2002, 63, 65.
33 E.g. Malinen 2014; *Funkis: Suomi nykyaikaa etsimässä* 1980.
34 Saarikangas 1998, 206.
35 Lehtola 2012, 378–80.
36 Soikkeli 2018, 143–63.
37 Ibid., 157–59.
38 Lehtola 2012, 406.
39 See, e.g., Lakervi 1949, 457–58; Saarikangas 2002, 114–15.
40 Esti 1945, 105. Esti also delivered similar instructions in *Maaseudun rakentajat*, a magazine for settlers, in 1949. Esti 1949, 452–53.
41 Lehtola 2012, 406.
42 Ibid., 26.
43 Ibid., 27. Dried hay was used as insulation material in the traditional reindeer-skin footwear.
44 Hustich 1946, 55. See also Lehtola, 28; Lehtola 2012, 406.
45 *Jokamiehen tietosanakirja* 1947, 486.
46 Poutvaara 1953, 48.

References

Aikio-Puoskari, Ulla. 2010. "Saamelaisesta elämänmuodosta saamelaiseen kulttuuriin – isoäidin elämä muutoksen mittatikkuna." *Kylä kulttuurien risteyksessä. Artikkelikokoelma Vuotson saamelaisista,* edited by Ulla Aikio-Puoskari and Päivi Magga, 108–23. Sodankylä: Vuohcu Sámiid searvi.
Axelsson, Per and Storm Mienna, Christina. 2019. "Health and Physical Wellbeing of the Sámi People." In *Routledge Handbook of Indigenous Wellbeing*, edited by Christopher Fleming and Matthew Manning, 1–22. Abingdon: Routledge.
Castrén, Matthias Alexander. 1878. *Elämä ja matkustukset, nuorisolle kerrotut.* Helsinki: G.W.Edlund.
Douglas, Mary. 1966. *Purity and Danger: An Analysis of Concepts of Pollution and Taboo.* London: Routledge.

Esti, Armas. 1945. "Koti – ja sen kalustaminen". In *Siirtoväen käsikirja*, edited by Ilmari Vartiainen, 87–109. Helsinki: Kaski-Kirja.

Esti, Armas. 1949. "Viihtyisä koti." *Miten rakennan ja sisustan kotini. Maaseudun rakentajien ammattilehti* no. 10: 450–43.

Funkis: Suomi nykyaikaa etsimässä. 1980. Exhibition booklet. Helsinki: Museum of Finnish Architecture.

Hakosalo, Heini. 2018. "A Twin Grip on 'the National Disease': The Finnish Anti-Tuberculosis Associations and their Contribution to Nation-formation (1907–17)." *The Making of Finland: The Era of the Grand Duchy. Special issue of Journal of Finnish Studies* 21 (1–2): 208–36.

Halonen, Tero and Aro Laura Aro, ed. 2005. *Suomalaisten symbolit.* Jyväskylä: Atena-kustannus.

Härö, Sakari. 1992. *Vuosisata tuberkuloosityötä Suomessa: Suomen tuberkuloosin vastustamisyhdistyksen historia.* [Helsinki]: Suomen tuberkuloosin vastustamisyhdistys, 1992.

Heinonen, Visa. 1998. *Talonpoikainen etiikka ja kulutuksen henki: kotitalousneuvonnasta kuluttajapolitiikkaan 1900-luvun Suomessa.* Helsinki: Suomen Historiallinen Seura.

Hustich, Ilmari. 1946. *Tuhottu ja tulevaisuuden Lappi.* Helsinki: Kustannustalo.

Huttunen, Marko. 2015. "Salvoskota, hirsitupa ja hirsitalo – inarinsaamelaisten vanhat hirsiasumukset." In *Ealli biras – Elävä ympäristö. Saamelainen kulttuuriympäristöohjelma*, edited by Päivi Magga and Eija Ojanlatva, 98–109. Finland: Sámi Museum, Saamelaismuseosäätiö.

Jokamiehen tietosanakirja. 1947. Helsinki: Otava.

Kansakoulun opetusvälineet ja koulukuvasto. 1900. Helsinki: Otava.

Korhonen, Teppo. 1999. "Maaseudun elämäntavan muutos." In *Suomi. Maa, kansa, kulttuurit*, edited by Markku Löytönen and Laura Kolbe. Helsinki: SKS.

Kähkönen, Anu. 2014. "Apinoista ystäviin. Saamelaisten 'toiseus' 1800-luvun lopun valokuvissa." In *Jokapäiväinen valtamme. Kielen ja ajan politologiaa vai pelkkää retoriikkaa*, edited by Laura Mankki and Antti Vesikko, 12–55. Jyväskylä: Jyväskylän yliopisto.

Lakervi, Lauri. 1949. "Miten rakennan viihtyisän ja tarkoituksenmukaisen keittiön." *Maaseudun rakentajien ammattilehti* no. 10: 457–58.

Lehtola, Veli-Pekka. 2012. *Saamelaiset Suomalaiset, kohtaamisia 1898–1953.* Helsinki: Suomalaisen Kirjallisuuden Seura.

Lehtola, Veli-Pekka. 2015. *Saamelaiset. Historia, yhteiskunta, taide.* Päivitetty laitos. Inari: Puntsi.

Lehtola, Veli-Pekka. 2018. "Sielun olisi pitänyt ehtiä mukaan. Jälleenrakennettu Saamenmaa." In *Lappi palaa sodasta; Mielen hiljainen jälleenrakennus*, edited by Marja Tuominen and Mervi Löfgren, 259–82. Tampere: Vastapaino.

Länsivuori, Marjo. 2017. *Perheenemännästä kuluttajakansalaiseksi. Kuluttaminen ja ympäristö Marttajärjestön Emäntälehdessä 1953–1975.* Joensuu: Itä-Suomen yliopisto.

Magga, Päivi. 2015. "Saamelaisesta rakennusperinnöstä." In *Ealli biras - Elävä ympäristö. Saamelainen kulttuuriympäristöohjelma*, edited by Päivi Magga and Eija Ojanlatva. Inari: Sámi Museum, Saamelaismuseosäätiö.

Malinen, Antti. 2014. *Perheet ahtaalla. Asuntopula ja siihen sopeutuminen toisen maailmansodan jälkeisessä Helsingissä 1944–1948.* Helsinki: Väestöliitto.

Mooney, Graham. 2013. "The Material Consumptive: Domesticating the Tuberculosis Patient in Edwardian England." *Journal of Historical Geography* 42: 152–66.

Nickul, Karl and Ernst Mauritz Mankjer. 1948. *The Skolt Lapp Community Suenjelsijd during the Year 1938.* Stockholm: Hugo Gebers Förlag.

Nikunlassi, Laila. 2014. "Utsjoen kirkonkylän kansakoulu vuosina 1929–1939." In *Saamelaisen kansanopetuksen ja koulunkäynnin historia Suomessa,* edited by Pigga Keskitalo, Veli-Pekka Lehtola, and Merja Paksuniemi, 175–81. Turku: Siirtolaisinstituutti.

Ollila, Anne. 1993. *Suomen kotien päivä valkenee… Marttajärjestö suomalaisessa yhteiskunnassa vuoteen 1939.* Helsinki: Suomen Historiallinen Seura.

Paulaharju, Samuli. 1921. *Kolttain mailta. Kansantieteellisiä kuvauksia Kuollan-Lapista.* Helsinki: Kustannusosakeyhtiö Kirja.

Porsanger, Rosa-Maria. 2015. *"Rehellisyyttä arvostethin."* Hyveet kotikasvatuksessa 1930–1950 -luvulla Keski- ja Etelä-Lapin maalaiskylissä. Unpublished master's thesis. Rovaniemi: Lapin Yliopisto.

Poutvaara, Matti. 1953. *Lappi, keskiyön auringon maa.* Porvoo: WSOY.

Raivo, Petri. 2005. "Kamppailujen, muistojen ja unohduksen Karjala." In *Suomalaisten symbolit,* edited by Tero Halonen and Laura Aro, 184–89. Jyväskylä: Atena-kustannus.

Saarikangas, Kirsi. 1998. "Suomalaisen kodin likaiset paikat: hygienia ja modernin asunnon muotoutuminen." *Tiede & Edistys* 23 (3): 198–220.

Saarikangas, Kirsi. 2002. *Asunnon muodonmuutoksia. Puhtauden estetiikka ja sukupuoli modernissa arkkitehtuurissa.* Helsinki: Suomalaisen Kirjallisuuden Seura.

Sirelius, Uuno Taavi. 1921. *Suomen kansanomaista kulttuuria II.* Helsinki: Otava.

Soikkeli, Anu. 2000. *Suomen vanhat pappilat, menneisyyden tulevaisuus.* Oulu: Oulun yliopisto.

Soikkeli, Anu. 2018. "Tyyppitalojen aika; Lappilaisen asumisen muutos." In *Lappi palaa sodasta. Mielen hiljainen jälleenrakennus,* edited by Marja Tuominen and Mervi Löfgren, 143–63. Tampere: Vastapaino.

Topelius, Zacharias. 1910. *Maamme Kirja. Lukukirja Suomen alimmille oppilaitoksille.* Helsinki: S.W. Edlund.

Vahtola, Jouko. 2003. *Suomen historia jääkaudesta Euroopan unioniin.* Helsinki: WSOY.

Chapter 8

Health as living in tranquility

Dialogues with the Apurinã and Yaminawa in Indigenous Brazilian Amazonia

Pirjo Kristiina Virtanen and Laura Pérez Gil

Introduction

This chapter looks at the conceptualization of health and illnesses in Indigenous Amazonia that encompasses the sociality of humans and nonhumans such as agencies of animals and plants. We will discuss how Amazonian Indigenous peoples' ecology of relations,[1] in which different types of beings participate, is related to well being and "healthy lives." Meantime, we take into account that ethnographic studies on Amazonian Indigenous groups have drawn attention to corporality in the process of constituting social and moral human persons.[2] Consequently, here we are interested in a specific aspect of this process: what role does corporality play in achieving and maintaining health, and what then is the nature of the relationship with nonhuman entities as related to the health of persons?

The sources of this chapter were produced with two different southwestern Amazonian Indigenous peoples, representing two different language groups, whose histories in terms of contact with non-Indigenous people are quite different. The first is the Arawakan-speaking Apurinã, who live in several demarcated Indigenous territories in Brazilian Amazonia. Altogether they number approximately 8,000 persons, and they self-identify as *Pupỹkary.* The first author has worked mostly in the Tumiã River, where the communities' social organization is based on two patrilineal cross-marrying moieties: *Xiwapurynyry* and *Meetymanety*. The Tumiã is a tributary of the Purus River, and situated in the state of Amazonas, Brazil. Most of the Apurinã live in fishing, hunting, and gathering communities who practice swidden agriculture. People along the Tumiã River live days distant from the closest urban centres, and they have not had frequent contacts with non-Indians. Yet the Apurinã have been some of the first intermediators with the colonizers, and today a large number of them live in urban environments or close to urban areas.

The second group is the Panoan-speaking Yaminawa,[3] numbering around 3,000 persons, who are scattered across various Indigenous territories. *Yaminawa* is an ethnonym that emerged during the contact process with non-Indians, and includes several previous ethnonyms. Several different groups, very closely related culturally and linguistically, are known as Yaminawa. In general, they share memories of having lived along the Pixiya Piver (the Envira river, as identified by the state), and spreading out during the rubber (*caoutchouc*) boom, in the first decades of the twentieth century. Since the 1940s, these dispersed groups have gradually established contact with non-Indians. Living at the headwaters of the river, principally in the confluence of those of the Jurua, Purus and Envira Rivers, their mode of subsistence is also based on hunting and swidden agriculture, with fishing and gathering as complementary activities. The second author has worked primarily with the Yaminawa community of Raya, localized in Mapuya River, Ucayali Department, Peru. The Yaminawa live in Peruvian, Brazilian and Bolivian Amazonia, while the Apurinã live only in Brazilian Amazonia.

Our methods have been ethnography, including participant observation, conversational interviews and visual documenting. We have both also assisted in different governmental and non-governmental projects dealing with the well-being of Indigenous communities, and thus have experience of Indigenous peoples' encounters with the state through public policies, as well as with the current economic and extraction projects in the Amazon.

Our study points to an Amazonian conceptualization of health in which the body is a locus for living in tranquility with human and non-human subjects. The non-human subjects especially are social agents, and can be considered to constitute what is referred to as "the environment" in the Euro-American sense. In their turn, these social agents are crucial to forming personhood and health, or rather healthy persons. Meanwhile, these agents have to be considered in historical and political contexts, which have also to do with the politicization of certain non-humans of the Amazonian rainforest at certain historical times and periods, as well as being addressed strategically in some inter-cultural contexts.

Historical and political context of southwestern Amazonia

The turning points in the histories of the Indigenous communities living in the Amazonian rainforest environment have been, among others, climatic changes even in the pre-colonial period, settler-colonization, involving several massacres, assimilation, and movement towards civil society, and consequent demarcation of territories, and the recent extraction of natural resources in the Amazon region. There is rich evidence that shows how Amazonia was largely inhabited before the colonisation, at least 10,000 bp.[4] Our study region has been occupied by so-called earthwork building societies since 3000 bp, and they contributed greatly to the rainforests.[5] The reasons for the collapse of Amazonian pre-colonial civilizations are still not well known, but new diseases and climate changes could have been some of the factors causing their decline.[6] Since the sixteenth century onwards, once the colonizers arrived in the Amazon basin, the Indigenous lifestyles and political and economic institutions altered radically. Within the Positivist paradigm and state assimilation attempts, Indigenous populations were not regarded as fully human, nor were their onto-epistemological differences recognized.[7] Later human rights discourses aimed to deconstruct the racial ideas that had established social hierarchies, and opened a space for diversity.

Since the 1970s, the Amazonian Indigenous movement has been pointing to the dominated positions of the Indigenous peoples and the pressing need to protect their rights. Indigenous people have gained a voice in public debate and a specific place in public policies, through the work of the Indigenous movement as well as non-governmental organizations, local social movements and activists. The international environmental movement played a big role in bringing attention to Amazonian Indigenous groups in the 1980s, and at that time many people talked about the greenhouse effect and the Amazon as the lungs of the world that would save it from destruction. The environmental debates presented the Indigenous population as saviours of the planet, which was othering for them, and amidst the global media attention Amazonian Indigenous people were seen as exotic peoples.[8] Then it was Sting and many other famous figures who spoke for the Kayapós, among other Amazonian Indigenous peoples. Since the 1990s, an increasing number of Indigenous leaders and spokespeople have occupied political positions at different levels, even in the highest positions of the state, and spoken for their communities.

Indigenous peoples' collective rights become recognized in the Brazilian constitution of 1988 and in the Peruvian Constitution of 1993. Among other things, their territorial rights become recognized, which was fundamental for those whose ancestral lands were demarcated or for those who obtained new territories demarcated for them. When acting in state politics, they often incorporate the discourses of the state politics. Yet, several Indigenous leaders talk about their differing views on economic development, education, and health. Apurinã have not yet taken up these highest state political roles, but they have been candidates, as well as gaining positions in Indigenous organization at state level. They have also been active, even as leaders, in the local Indigenous movement since the 1980s.

The experiences of the Apurinã and Yaminawa have been quite different. The Yaminawa, not only the Raya community, had little contact with ONGs and even with Indigenous organizations, in comparison with other Indigenous groups. In Peru, since they established permanent contact with non-Indians in the 1960s, their principal interlocutors have been loggers, extracting precious wood near their territory, and missionaries, both Catholics and Evangelists. Because of the stinginess of logger bosses and the exploitative character of large-scale wood extraction, both of people and the environment, the Yaminawa have been reluctant to engage with loggers. Nevertheless, due to the remoteness and the low density of population in the region where they live in the Peruvian-Brazilian border area, it was just recently that they have begun to be conscious of the impacts that these deforestation and timber business activities have, principally for the disappearance of certain woods and the consequent rarity of animals in the environment, such as white-collar peccaries.

In the 2000s, there have been many changes for Indigenous people. Both the Peruvian and Brazilian governments designed special Indigenous territorial, health, and educational policies, but their actual implementation still lacks resources. Furthermore, state development projects, increasing large-scale resource extraction and pollution have resulted in deforestation, a decrease of biodiversity, and forced removals from ancestral lands. Even though both countries have ratified ILO Convention 169, Indigenous peoples are rarely truly consulted about the economic activities taking place in their ancestral lands. The exploitation of natural resources has also increased the scale of human disturbances and caused environmental and climate changes that pose huge challenges for the future of the region's Indigenous people, especially for those who live in rural areas.

Approaches to "the environment" in Amazonian thinking

In the forest, we human beings are the "ecology." But it is equally the *xapiri*, the game, the trees, the rivers, the fish, the sky, the rain, the wind, and the sun! It is everything that came into being in the forest, far from the white people: everything that isn't surrounded by fences yet.[...] The white people call these things 'ecology'! As for us, we say *urihi* a, the forest, and we also speak of the *xapiri*, for without them, without 'ecology,' the land gets warmer and the epidemics and the evil beings get closer. Davi Kopenawa.[9]

One of the most prominent theoretical proposals in contemporary anthropology in the course of the last two decades has been the ontological turn. Among its main concerns was a critical reconsideration of "nature" and "culture" as analytical concepts: instead of ontological provinces, they "rather refer to exchangeable perspectives and relational-positional contexts; in brief, points of view."[10] Based mainly on ethnographical works among Amazonian Indigenous groups, perspectivist and animist theories have showed that the forest "constitute[s] theaters of a subtle sociability within which, day after day, humans engage in cajoling beings distinguishable from humans only by their different physical aspects and their lack of language."[11] Non-humans have human attributes, such as agency, intentionality, soul or consciousness. These aspects turn them into social beings with whom humans must interact regularly. As Philippe Descola (2013) has pointed out, in the Amazonian ontology there is continuity *in* the interiority of the beings, and discontinuity in the exteriority that is in their physicality. In other words, there is symmetry between humans and non-humans because of their common intentionality and asymmetry because of their different bodies. The interactions between humans and non-humans are extremely varied and concern all life spheres, which we will show to be the case among the Apurinã and Yaminawa.

It is not our intention here to present an overall discussion of perspectivism and animism, but merely to point out the repercussions that the perspectivist character of Amazonian cosmologies have when we describe and think about health and the environment. Those concepts, in *multiculturalistic* ontology, imply contrasts such as those of object/subject, nature/culture, body/soul, which are not appropriate to Amazonian *multinaturalistic* ontologies.[12] Thus, as in most Amazonian cosmologies, among both the Apurinã and Yaminawa, certain animals, birds, fish, trees, plants, and meteorological phenomena are regarded as subjects with whom people establish relations that can take different forms: alliance, predation, transmission of knowledge, help, infatuation, or revenge, among others. We will focus here on those aspects more directly associated with health in order to show that individual well being is about coexistence within the collective well being and that the maintenance and restoration of people's condition of health depends on the management and care of relations with a wide grouping of human and nonhuman agencies.

Relationality with non-humans

As mentioned, for the Apurinã, various beings living in the forest, such as certain animals, trees, plants, as well as meteorological phenomena, are conceived as persons, and they have their own master or chief spirits. Some are known by their proper names with their individual histories, while others are known just as the chiefs or masters of certain entities known as *awĩte*. The master-spirits share a humanity similar to people and sometimes these beings are seen in their human forms, especially during dreams and rituals. Certain non-humans have contributed to the Apurinã's human form and health over many generations by providing resources, protection and knowledge, and in exchange the Apurinã respect the master spirits by among other things, not hunting, fishing, or extracting more than what is necessary, and not making too much noise in the places of master spirits. Without these exchanges and mutual relations, humans can neither maintain their lives nor their health. Therefore, several non-humans are so embedded with the formation of the Apurinã that one does not precede another. The non-humans and chief spirits of different kinds play an important role in knowledge production. Relationality with master-spirits is crucial in hunting and in the dream-world, where the master-spirit can show where game can be found or if it useful to leave for a hunting trip at all. Ignoring them could have direct consequences: they are known for shooting invisible darts at people, which cause fatal illnesses. They must be consulted and respected whenever people seek to exploit forest resources. Some of the master spirits are Apurinã ancestors who have taken an animal form and now guide now contemporary Apurinã. Ancestor messenger animals (the shamans transformed into animals, often birds) communicate any number of things, such as the presence of edible animals, arrival of people to the village, impending storm, rain, or illness.[13]

In the case of Yaminawa cosmology, the polysemic concept of *yuxin* connects all living beings. In some contexts, *yuxin* is somewhat vague and diffuse. Any corporeal element is impregnated by *yuxin*, but it is particularly powerful and dangerous in some of them, like blood. In other contexts, *yuxin* takes a more precise shape, showing up – in myths, dreams or ayahuasca visions, for example – in human form, and would resemble more closely our concept of soul or spirit. Human beings have, for instance, the "soul of the eyes" (*wero yuxin*) and the "soul of the shadow" (*dia waa*), which have different destinies after death. But animals, plants, places or trees also have *yuxin*, and it is this that gives things and beings their particularities and attributes.[14] In some contexts, it seems just a vague energy – it could be said that most hunted animals have *yuxin* because of their blood – but some species or places have powerful *yuxin*. The better defined and shaped a *yuxin* appears, the more agentivity and intentionality is attributed to it, and the more powerful it will be considered. Ceibas, anacondas, river dolphins, jaguars or tobacco and ayahuasca plants are beings with particularly powerful *yuxin*.

Although the Yaminawa sometimes refer these beings as *ihu* (owner, master), unlike the Apurinã they do not have the concept of a master-spirit of an animal with whom they would negotiate their hunting activities, nor the notion that an excess of hunting and fishing may lead to revenge from animals. This does not mean that they overhunt or overfish, as the Yaminawa are very critical of the non-Indians in the area for abusing and unnecessarily exploiting natural resources.

Spirit beings are complex and ambiguous for both the Apurinã and Yaminawa. In certain contexts and circumstances, they are remarkable and crucial allies. During Yaminawa shamanic initiation, for example, the spirits of anaconda and jaguar as well as tobacco, ayahuasca plant and other vegetable species transmit their knowledge and power to apprentices, as long as they are strong and can withstand the hard and painful process of learning from non-human spirits. Traditionally among the Yaminawa, almost all men engaged in a period of shamanic initiation during their youth. Accompanied by one or two recognized *ñuwë* who acted as teachers, a group of young men isolated themselves in the forest. During this period of seclusion, sexual intercourse or indeed any interaction with people outside the group, was forbidden. The principal aspects of shamanic initiation were several ordeals consisting mainly of making different species of ants and wasps sting specific parts of the body; a rigorous diet; continual consumption of various shamanic substances; and learning the *kuxuiti* healing songs. The insertion in the body of substances pertaining to or associated with powerful beings (boa's saliva, tobacco, ayahuasca beverage, etc.) permits communication between these beings and the apprentices, setting off the transmission of knowledge and the transformation of their bodies. These transformations must be controlled and directed to be productive in terms of development of shamanic power and knowledge. In fact, outside this context, any contact with those beings may lead to illness and eventually even death, because the nature of these non-human beings is inherently ambiguous and too strong.[15]

Among the Apurinã, shamanic knowledge and powers also comes from the environment and via personal experience. In order to obtain this knowledge, certain qualities must be evident in the person, but diet, seclusion, and the consumption of curing and purifying plants, which in themselves are considered to transmit knowledge, are also crucial parts of shamanic training. There are various traditionally recognized techniques that can be followed, such as focusing on the sucurucu snake's spirit and its knowledge during the rainy season, or the jaguar spirit in the dry period. Once the person is ready for personal growth in shamanic knowledge and interactions with the spirit world, the sucurucu or jaguar appears in a human form, usually has a physical fight with the shaman novice, and then eventually gives the shamanic stones to the new shaman. Even if there are a few people recognized as shamans, like the Yaminawa, shamanic knowledge exists in various forms, as it relates to hunting and healing skills, and generally maintaining life, thus this type of knowledge is also communally shared. Overall, individual experiences in tropical forests and rivers, hunting, or other secular moments are also an important source of knowledge.

What does it mean to be a healthy person in Amazonia?

Earlier works on ethnomedicine in Amazonia have shown how relationships with diverse non-humans constitute health and illnesses, as well as personhood, in the region.[16] Personhood and corporality are major issues in Amazonian ethnography. Over the last three decades, ethnologists have shown the centrality of body production in the constitution of sociality and personhood. Bodies are produced in daily activities, such as caring, feeding or working as much as in ritual contexts, and thus this continued corporeal making is coextensive to the constitution of social relations. Here, the body is not just a physical and organic component of the person, but also an existential ground for social life: its productive and gendered capacities, ways of moving, shape, character, memories, knowledges, morality or affections are closely associated with corporeal qualities, substances, parts and processes.[17] Even if each Amazonian Indigenous society has its own particularities on this point, two common aspects should be highlighted. The first is the fact that health is something people must continually work at, it is never a given, especially in relation to non-humans. This view differs from the Euro-American view, in which frequent exercise would maintain the health of a person. The second is the fact that health is not defined by the mere absence of illness, but also depends on emotional states, and on the individual's capacity to contribute to sociality and social reproduction. In other words, health is crucially about balanced social relations with both non-human and human beings.

As the social universe includes both humans and non-humans, when we describe and analyse the processes by which corporality is constructed, it is necessary to consider the actions of all these agents and their effects on the Amazonian Indigenous conceptualization of health. The body is related to several entities and a healthy body is largely a result of these relations. For many of the activities related to natural resources and activities, a certain type of healthy body is needed. It means that an individual, constituted as a relational being, should have good relationships with others. Morality is thus crucially included in the production of health, as immoral acts towards others, both humans and non-human, would harm a person. In the case of the Yaminawa, the outcome of hunting activities depends on the proper and moral care of the hunter's own body. Some of the social and moral qualities that the Yaminawa most appreciate in a person are generosity, hard work and a good mood. To be active, diligent and tough in hunting, fishing or garden activities means to be able to support one's own family, and to contribute generously to village social life by organizing *masato* (manioc beer) parties or distributing meat or fish after a profitable day. The condition for such activities is to have a hard (*kërëx*) body. Women have hard bodies that enable them to carry wood or heavy baskets packed with manioc or corn from the garden, to give birth to their babies or to accomplish the exhausting activities of housekeeping. Men, besides a hard body that enables them to lay down trees to make an extensive garden, for example, must preserve the qualities required to be successful hunters.

When unlucky in hunting, both the Apurinã and Yaminawa would say that it has happened because of immoral acts. When a man is unable to kill animals, both would say that he is with *panema*, and several measures must be taken. They might have disrespected the non-human beings. For the Yaminawa, it has also to do with the type of body the hunter has. For example, it is commonly thought that residues of food accumulate in the stomach, and this has harmful consequences for health in general, and for hunting efficacy in particular. In order to be in good health and to improve their capacity to find animals, men regularly use certain plants with emetic effects. Similarly, the *kapu* frog's exudation is applied to the index finger to ameliorate aim.

There are also emotional levels that are considered morbid and potentially lethal. For both of our interlocutors, one such emotional state is sadness. For the Yaminawa, there are certain culturally defined moments and methods for the expression of sorrow, such as the *yama yama* songs. The act of singing in these cases is motivated by a feeling of longing (*xina bitsai*) for a relative who is far away or by someone's death. Nevertheless, when sorrow turns into a condition, it is considered an illness and generates concern. Generally, a profound sentiment of sadness is attributed to the agency of someone else, as the *yuxin* of a close relative recently deceased, or a rejected lover. If this is the case, ritual treatment by a specialist becomes necessary to restore health. On the contrary, cheerfulness, embellishment of bodies, and sociability promotes the well being of people, and these characteristics distinguish humans from some kinds of non-human *yuxin*, described as ugly, solitary, stinking and eaters of raw meat. In the same way that bodies are produced, emotional states are also managed in this respect, and the Yaminawa and Apurinã know and use various plants to avoid being angry, violence from spouses, or any sentiment that could threaten individual and social harmony. Furthermore, both the Apurinã and Yaminawa are careful that their children do not become scared of anything, as being scared can have permanent consequences for the health of a child. That would cause the spirit of the baby not to be in harmony with her or his body, thus making them weak.

When Apurinã people aim to exploit forest resources, the entities associated with dangerous transformations in mindful bodies must be respected, as ignoring them could have dire consequences for the mindful bodies of persons, thus engendering illnesses. Human presence in places associated with master or chief spirits is strictly controlled; babies, children and pregnant women are forbidden to pass in their vicinity. However, the master spirits are also understood to provide people with game, fish and knowledge and, in addition to making forest resources available, they (re)produce health and personal growth as they supply vitality and strength. It is vital to produce strong, resistant bodies, and the older kin participate in that production. In the production of healthy persons, several immaterial and material aspects of Apurinã traditions are used. They include the practice of artwork, such as in body paintings and the use of *awiri* snuff, their most common shamanic substance, protector and medicine, which is even used by children. The songs can also be protectors of people from entering into relations with harmful entities or in their interactions with them, by making their bodies strong. In other words, they create and strengthen relations with certain non-humans, making certain kinds of bodies. They alter the relation between a person and others, thus the body paintings, chants and medicines, which are taken before the illness takes over, have transformative powers. The songs themselves are entities that are considered subjects that affect people and their development. The different forms of art are about special skills of perception, of sounds and geometric images, which point to the parallel invisible worlds and materialize their non-human interactions; they are thus crucial parts of the dynamic and personal reflective construction of healthy persons. The non-human beings manifested and interacted with in different art forms are part of the communities' oral histories, myths and personal stories, transmitted through the generations.

Illnesses in Amazonian lived worlds

An overall description of nosological theories of the Apurinã and Yaminawa is beyond the scope of this text, so we will restrict our account to those related to interaction with different human and non-human subjectivities. Among the Apurinã and Yaminawa, several illnesses are provoked by other humans, but they can involve animated entities. Previous literature concerning the taxonomy of Amazonian native conceptions of illnesses has shown how several illnesses are considered the result of an aggressive spirit taking over a person. This is usually said to occur at the point when one becomes frightened or cannot control one's emotions, or because of jealousy, feelings of disgust, or irresponsibility related to gender-related roles.[18] In this view, certain substances are released into a person, changing the person's body, and thus his/her behaviour towards others. Social relations thus involve other non-human animated entities. Donald Pollock (1999) has pointed out that illnesses make people less caring or less intimate in relation to other people, distancing them from their community. In general, illnesses affect people in various ways, including being unlucky in hunting and fishing trips.

The illnesses are also caused by non-humans and living in forest and rivers, as relationality with animal, plant and spirit subjectivities may harm people. Illnesses are of various types, linked to the social relations which make people and their bodies. The illnesses are transmitted by non-humans, especially master spirits, and by their aggression towards people who do not respect them. They are called *mapitxiri* and are about reformulating social relations and thus people. In its metaphysical form, illness for them is a substance, such as a small stone (shamanic stone) or spirit arrow, which has to be removed to heal a person. *Mapitxiri* can be gained from these particles released by certain powerful tree agencies, such as moriche palm trees (*Mauritia flexuosa*), buritirianas (*Mauritiella martiana*), murmurus (*Astrocaryum murumuru*), and tabocas (*Guadua*) if they are not respected. Therefore the Apurinã approach these with the utmost caution. Animist thinking is manifested in the idea that, according to the Apurinã along the Tumiã River, the master spirits of these entities shoot their shamanic small stones, with their invisible poisonous arrows. These cause permanent transformations, mapitxiri illnesses, in people. Mapitxiri is like an infection, an everlasting pain in the back, arms, or ears that can usually take years before it manifests itself. Eventually it can even lead to death. It is a transformation that does not heal by itself, unless manipulated by shamans, as will be explained in the next section.

Children are particularly vulnerable to the entities present in the forest and the transformational powers of its non-human entities. Taking care of their development begins even before birth. This is similar among the Apurinã and Yaminawa. Apurinã mothers avoid eating certain types of fish, such as those with spiky skin, in order to have an easy birth. A father should not kill snakes or cut down big trees, so that their spirits do not affect the foetus. Among the

Yaminawa, both, mothers and fathers – all men who had sexual relations with the mother during pregnancy – must avoid eating certain animals. The *yuxin* of the animal might transmit its characteristics to the child, causing illness or even death. For example, if the parents eat sloth, the *yuxin* of the animal might attack the child with its powerful claws, or if they eat red howler, the child might develop mange, which is typical of this animal. Illness and death among young children is frequently attributed to inappropriate food ingestion by the parents. Similarly, during the post-natal period, certain foods affect not only the baby but also the mother: for example, she should not eat guans or trumpeters because she may become skinny like those birds or red tail catfish or tapir to avoid becoming paunchy.

For Apurinã children, who are still forming their subjectivity, several protective rites are performed. These include enjoying different foods and substances, being given herbal baths, as well as receiving ornaments and a variety of body painting, depending on the type of relationality desired. The paintings can manifest fish, jaguar, anaconda, different snakes, tortoises and so forth. Herbal baths and plants are taken, digested or consumed to avoid harmful relationships and create new ones that will defend people. When starting out on a journey, contact with a protective herb is required by stepping onto it or rubbing it into the baby's body. Furthermore, when movement assumes the form of water travel, a small boat from a piece of bark or leaf is prepared and placed in the river in order for the baby's spirit (*isanyka*) to travel well. Pouring breast milk into the river is another of these protective rites. The baby might otherwise acquire a fatal relation to overly foreign subjectivities. Attentiveness to these matters is fundamental in taking care of children who have not yet reached puberty. For instance, when entering a forest for the first time with a baby, one has to inform the forest's non-human beings that, "Here is my child who is my kin." Then the forest spirits will not regard the newly arrived person as a stranger. In turn, small children should not pass close to specific earth formations or certain other powerful entities. If they do, the spirits of these non-humans will draw the child in.[19]

Analogous precautions are taken by Yaminawa in order to protect their children. It is crucial to keep *yuxin* and *diawaa* (spirits of dead people who remain near the place where they were buried) away from children; to do this, different preventive measures are performed, such as painting their bodies with jenipa to strengthen them; putting necklaces and bracelets made of specific plants that ward off spirits on their necks and wrists; or avoiding places where dead people were buried or that are inhabited by powerful beings, like the ceiba trees, or river pools, where anacondas and river dolphins are said to live. Certain times, spaces and meteorological phenomena are considered particularly dangerous for children because they might be affected by *yuxin* or *diawaa*. When night falls, all mothers hurry their children to stay inside the house. Similarly, rainbows, associated with the anaconda spirit, or wind, may carry *diawaa* and put people's health at risk; everyone hurries to take cover from them.

In Amazonia, food is traditionally an essential substance and a means to produce health and healthy balanced relations. Among the Apurinã, certain food taboos have to be followed in order to avoid *mapitxiri* illnesses. The members of the Xiwapurynyry (of all ages) avoid eating tinamous (*iũku*), uru birds (*puturu*), and certain types of fish in particular. The Meetymanety abstain from collared peccary and coati. The people of the Tumiã River assert that if the Xiwapurynyry eat an uru bird, they will feel a tapping or prickling sensation in their lower back, while certain fish cause a biting pain on one side of the lower back or a strong pain in the ears. In a similar way, if a Meetymanety consumes peccary or a coati, s/he starts to feel pain in their lower back. This is an illness called *mapitxiri* and it is, in fact, most often caused by violating the moiety food taboos, which follow along patrilineal lines. Owing to exogamous marriages between the moieties, couples follow different dietary rules.

Not being attentive to one's food can also make predators follow a person, or they will start to hear sounds and voices when there is nothing there. One may also start behaving like an animal and begin to lose one's mind. Such people become *mapitxiri-ta* or – in other words – crazy. Apurinã's two moieties and their foods protect them from becoming *mapitxiri-ta* (crazy, lost), and position themselves clearly, according to their moiety, in the web of human and non-human actors.

Apurinã diets have a crucial role in constructing Apurinã personhood and avoiding illnesses that would break their intimate relations with their kin and the ideal of forming new relations. As we have seen, human social relations are also concerned with non-human elements. Misfortune in human relations is always linked to the non-human world, because people incorporate power from non-human entities (such as from the plants used for *awiri* snuff). In human-animal relations, the powers of non-human forces can be tamed and incorporated within certain limits.

Among Yaminawa, food avoidance is not related to social moieties, but to specific vital conditions. Throughout their life, a person goes through situations of body instability, precarity or transformation[20] during which precautions regarding food are crucial to preserve health and body capacities that are socially valued. There are several other contexts and situations where people must be scrupulous about what they eat: during illnesses, shamanic initiation, menstruation and pregnancy. Old people often explain that, in ancient times, the number of foods avoided was greater than today. Inappropriate foods often cause illness, conceptualized as the revenge (*kupĩ*) of the animal's *yuxin*, but also undesirable body transformations that are considered aesthetically unpleasant; many of these are associated with anti-social behaviour, such as laziness or feebleness. Loss of shamanic power, inefficacy in hunting and the weakening condition of a patient are usually explained as a failure of dietary control. In all the contexts mentioned, bodies are in an unstable and critical condition, and thus more easily influenced by the *yuxin* of other beings. Sometimes, this openness to other beings may be sought, as in shamanic initiation, because it is a way of incorporating their knowledge and power, but it is always crucial to control the transformations that these situations generate. In Amazonian Indigenous thinking, alterity is a necessary element in the social production of persons and for the reproduction of society.[21] Nevertheless, this in-corporation of alterity must always be controlled and directed to transform it into a productive element and avoid its lethal potentiality. The control of food is a crucial element at this point, and points to the central role of the body[22] as a locus for interactions and making a healthy person.

Balancing relationships with non-humans – practices of curing

Both humans and non-humans are the authors of several illnesses among the Apurinã and Yaminawa, but taking into account the role of the non-humans often requires attention to the invisible aspects of reality. *Yuxin* and Apurinã owner spirits are recognized as being present in various everyday activities, such as fishing, trekking, extracting and so forth. But they are especially related to using chants and movements, and eventually they can become a source of shamanic power and knowledge. This is an example of predatory incorporation of powers from the outside by a person who can master and control the power of others.[23] The non-humans are also important allies in the healing practice, and shamans in particular work with those entities from whom they have received their shamanic powers.

Special shamanic knowledge is required to cure several illnesses. For the Apurinã, *mapitxiri* is an illness that can be healed only by shamans, as for them there is no pharmaceutical cure. It can be removed, replaced and sent away by shamans (*mỹyty*). They usually inhale *awiri* snuff or chew dried coca leaves, *katsupary, with (kixinintaari*– a certain type of vine), and the burned bark of the cacao tree in their healing rituals to enable them to diagnose the cause of illness. The illness may be a result of a person being present in the wrong place, or disrespectful acts, but may also be due to witchcraft. The use of just *awiri* snuff is also common in healing, and it helps the shaman to suck or pull out the illness, which, in the form of a stone, can be blown away. A shaman can place the shamanic stones in a snuff inhaler, a *mexikana*, and blow them out to cause witchcraft. The Apurinã shaman's powers (*ithapara*) have a very similar metaphysical form to illnesses: they are small stones (*hỹtykelisuruke*) of different colours, received most commonly from jaguars or boas during shamanic initiation. These are the principal animal masters for those learning shamanic skills. The shamanic stones of master spirits (*awĩte*) of big trees or other powerful creators can also be used. The shaman retains these in his body, and his *awiri* snuff container (*mekaru*).

Yaminawa, as well, affirm that in the past there were shamanic specialists (*tsibuya*) among them who also had a sort of "stone" (*tsibo*) inside their bodies, which allowed them to suck illness out, or harm someone by introducing a stone into his body. They received these stones from the jaguar, who introduced them into the apprentice body during initiation. Nowadays, the main shamanic technique is the *kuxuiti* song. In order to treat a sick person, the shamanic practitioner (*kuxuitia*) consumes a tobacco and ayahuasca brew and chants *kuxuiti* over the patient. Frequently, various men participate in curing sessions, even if not all of them have a great power. Each session is also an opportunity to learn and develop their shamanic faculties. The *kuxuiti* lyrics are connected to the visions produced by ayahuasca. The songs enumerate elements of the disease, such as its symptoms or the agents who provoked it, in order to neutralize them. The allusion to each element is metaphorical and frequently makes reference to mythology because it is in myths where the qualities and attributes – that is to say the *yuxin* – of things and entities are revealed.[24] By naming them, *koxuitia* act upon their *yuxin*.

Another frequent practice of curing is the use of *disa* plants, whose leaves are boiled in water and placed on the diseased part of the body. Here, too, it is through their *yuxin* that the plants are effective. Both *koxuiti* songs and *disa* plants are knowledges that anaconda transmitted to men.

Even if these curing practices are still present in daily life in Raya, it is frequently affirmed, especially by the elders, that their health became worse and their bodies weaker after contact with outsiders. Several factors contribute to this. One of them is food. Although they like foods from the city, like sugar, rice or paste, these make their bodies softer, affecting their abilities and capacities in productive activities. Working for loggers was also considered something that negatively affected men's health. During the first years after contact, in order to obtain manufactured goods, many Yaminawa men worked for logging enterprises near their territories. However, exploitative working conditions, excessive exposure to the sun, and managing machines such as motors or electric saws were felt to damage their bodies, which was one of the reasons why they abandoned these activities.

Another major cause of body deterioration and disease is alcohol. After contact with other Indigenous people in the region they adopted the habit of consuming manioc beer. Yaminawa affirm that, before contact, when their vegetable drinks fermented, they threw them out because of their prejudicial effect on shamanic power. In fact, the consumption of alcohol, bought either in the city or brewed in the village, is today considered the cause of great social distress and the decline of shamanic power. People say that it is because they eat sugar and drink manioc beer and firewater that the efficacy of their shamanic practices is poor, and they must resort to shamanic specialists in the city.

Conclusion

In this chapter we have presented the views of two different Amazonian Indigenous peoples on their environment. We hope it has made evident the Amazonian Indigenous view that the environment and health are inseparable elements, and the construction of the person is closely situated and drawn from sociality and interactions with different non-human subjects. Yet, it is not just about the external healthy environment making healthy individuals. A central point here is that the Amazonian Indigenous peoples' concept of health emerges from healthy relationships with both non-humans and humans, and their health is tied to constant learning and aimed at living in tranquility with certain non-humans.

Over recent decades, the environmentalist struggle for the protection of Amazonia has found Indigenous political leaders to be exceptional allies. As we have pointed out, various anthropologists[25] have discussed this alliance in the light that environmentalists and Indigenous leaders mobilized conceptions quite differently. Tensions eventually arose in these relationships, resulting from the divergence in their ways of conceptualizing the environment and including different Indigenous points of view, but they remain largely ignored and unrecognized. The recent forest fires in the Amazon in 2019 is a good example. Many non-Amazonian people have signed petitions against fires in and deforestation of the Amazon. Scientific organizations, such as the World Anthropological Union (2019), have denounced the Brazilian government for ecocide, accusing it of crimes against humanity and the planet: extensive destruction of ecosystems, oxygen production and global cycles of sweet water. There are some similarities in the discourses in the 1990s when the greenhouse effect was raised, but the state of emergency is now higher because the Anthropocene is coming to an end. Unlike the 1990s, however, Indigenous peoples now have space to talk for themselves. Amazonian Indigenous organizations have also raised their voices to stress the fact that these fires put their lives and survival at stake, and refer to several international legal frameworks protecting Indigenous rights and even to their SDGs.[26] We hope this chapter has contributed to propagating the Indigenous views on the environment as a subjective and animated milieu, inhabited by non-human entities with whom humans constantly aim to relate through addressing or avoiding, and that crucially contribute to the very existence of the humans and consequent health becoming even more visible. Degradation of the socio-natural spaces where the intertwined and embedded lives of the humans and non-humans play out have a direct and immediate impact on their health, bodies and way of life.

Notes

1 Descola 2013.
2 Seeger et al 1979; Erikson 1996; Vilaça 2005; Londoño Sulkin 2012.
3 Jaminawa and Yaminahua are also spellings used for this ethnonym.

4 Heckenberger and Neves 2009.
5 Watling et al. 2017; Saunaluoma et al. 2018.
6 See, e.g., Räsänen et al. 1987; Pärssinen et al. 2003.
7 See, e.g., Ramos 1998.
8 Conklin 2002; Conklin and Graham 1995.
9 Kopenawa and Albert 2013, 393.
10 Viveiros de Castro 2012, 47.
11 Descola 2013, 5.
12 Viveiros de Castro 2012.
13 Virtanen 2015.
14 Townsley 1993.
15 Pérez Gil 2006.
16 See, e.g., Pollock 1999.
17 Jones 1993; Lagrou 2007; Londoño Sulkin 2012; Taylor and Viveiros de Castro 2006.
18 Garnelo and Buchillet 2006; Overing 1989; Pollock 1999.
19 See Virtanen 2016.
20 Vilaça 2005.
21 Fausto 1999
22 See also Vilaça 2004 and 2005.
23 Fausto 2012; Viveiros de Castro 1992.
24 Déléage 2009; Townsley 1993.
25 Conklin 2002; Conklin and Graham 1995; Albert 2002.
26 See, e.g., COICA 2019.

Bibliography

Albert, Bruce. 2002. "O ouro canibal e a queda do céu. Uma crítica xamânica da economia política da natureza (Yanomami)." In *Pacificando o branco: cosmologias do contato no norte-amazônico*, edited by Bruce Albert and Alcida Rita Ramos, 239–74. São Paulo: UNESP.
COICA. 2019. "Carta abierta de los pueblos indígenas. Declaratoria de emergencia ambiental e humanitaria." COICA 22 April 2019. At https://coica.org.ec/pueblos-indigenas-de-la-cuenca-amazonica-nos-declaramos-en-emergencia-ambiental-y-humanitaria/
Conklin, Beth A. 2002. "Shamans versus Pirates in the Amazonian Treasure Chest." *American Anthropologist* 104 (4): 1050–61.
Conklin, Beth A. and Laura R. Graham. 1995. "The Shifting Middle Ground: Amazonian Indians and Eco-Politics." *American Anthropologist* 97 (4): 695–710.
Déléage, Pierre. 2009. *Le chant de l'anaconda. L'apprentissage du chamanisme chez les Sharanahua (Amazonie occidentale)*. Nanterre: Société d'Ethnologie.
Descola, Philippe. 2013 [2005]. *Beyond Nature and Culture*. Chicago: The University of Chicago.
Erikson, Philippe. 1996. *La Griffe des Aïeux. Marquage du corps et démarquage ethnique chez les Matis d'Amazonie*. Paris: Editions Peeters.
Fausto, Carlos. 1999. "Of Enemies and Pets: Warfare and Shamanism in Amazonia." *American Ethnologist* 26 (4): 933–56.

Fausto, Carlos. 2012. *Warfare and Shamanism in Amazonia*. New York: Cambridge University Press.

Garnelo, Luiza and Dominique Buchillet. 2006. "Taxonomias Das Doenças Entre Os Índios Baniwa (Arawak) e Desana (Tukano Oriental) Do Alto Rio Negro (Brasil)." *Horizontes Antropológicos* 12 (26): 231–60.

Heckenberger, Michael and Eduardo Góes Neves. 2009. "Amazonian Archaeology." *Annual Review of Anthropology* 38: 251–66.

Hugh-Jones, Stephen. 1993. "'Food' and 'Drugs' in Northwest Amazonia." In *Tropical Forests, People and Food: Biocultural Interactions and Applications to Development*, edited by A. Hladick, O. F. Linares, C. M. H. Pagezy, and H. Pagezy, 533–48. Paris: Unesco.

Kopenawa, Davi and Bruce Albert. 2013. *The Falling Sky: Words of a Yanomami Shaman*. London: Harvard University Press.

Lagrou, Elsje. 2007. *A fluidez da forma: arte, alteridade e agência em uma sociedade amazônica (Kaxinawa, Acre)*. Rio de Janeiro: Topbooks.

Londoño Sulkin, Carlos David. 2012. *People of Substance: An Ethnography of Morality in the Colombian Amazon*. Toronto: University of Toronto Press.

Overing, Joanna. 1989. "Styles of Manhood: An Amazonian Contrast in Tranquility and Violence." In *Societies at Peace: Anthropological Perspectives*, edited by Signe Howell and Roy Willis, 79–99. London: Routledge.

Pérez Gil, Laura. 2006. "Metamorfoses yaminawa: Xamanismo e socialidade na Amazonia peruana." PhD thesis. Federal University of Santa Catarina.

Pollock, Donald. 1999. "Personhood and Illness among the Kulina." *Medical Anthropology Quarterly* 10 (3): 319–41.

Pärssinen, Martti, Alceu Ranzi, Sanna Saunaluoma, and Ari Siiriäinen. 2003. "Geometrically Patterned Ancient Earthworks in the Rio Branco Region of Acre, Brazil: New Evidence of Ancient Chiefdom Formations in Amazonian Interfluvial Terra Firme Environment." In *Western Amazonia. Multidisciplinary Studies on Ancient Expansionistic Movements, Fortifications and Sedentary Life*, edited by M. Pärssinen and A. Korpisaari, 97–133. Helsinki: University of Helsinki, Renvall Institute.

Ramos Alcida, Rita. 1998. *Indigenism – Ethnic Politics in Brazil*. London: The University of Wisconsin Press.

Räsänen, Matti, Jukka Salo, and Risto Kalliola. 1987. "Fluvial Perturbance in the Western Amazon Basin: Regulation by Long-Term Sub-Andean Tectonics." *Science* 238 (4832): 1398–1401.

Saunaluoma, Sanna, Martti Pärssinen, and Denise Schaan. 2018. "Diversity of Pre-colonial Earthworks in the Brazilian State of Acre, Southwestern Amazonia." *Journal of Field Archaeology* 43 (5): 362–79.

Seeger, Anthony, Roberto DaMatta, and Eduardo Viveiros de Castro. 1979. "A construção da pessoa nas sociedades indígenas brasileiras." *Boletim do Museu Nacional*, no. 32: 11–29.

Taylor, Anne-Christine and Eduardo Viveiros de Castro. 2006. "Un corps fait de regards." In *Qu'est-ce qu'un corps?*, edited by Stéphane Breton, 148–99. Paris: Musée du Quai Branly / Flammarion.

Townsley, Graham. 1993. "Song Paths: The Ways and Means of Yaminahua Shamanic Knowledge." *L'Homme* 33 (2–4): 449–68.

154 Pirjo Kristiina Virtanen et al.

Vilaça, Aparecida. 2002. "Making Kin Out of Others in Amazonia." Journal of the Royal Anthropological Institute 8 (2): 347–65.
Vilaça, Aparecida. 2005. "Chronically Unstable Bodies: Reflections on Amazonian Corporalities." Journal of the Royal Anthropological Institute 11 (3): 445–64.
Virtanen, Pirjo Kristiina. 2015. "Fatal Substances: Apurinã's Dangers, Movement, and Kinship." Indiana 32: 85–103.
Virtanen, Pirjo Kristiina. 2016. "The Death of the Chief of Peccaries – The Apurinã and Scarcity of Forest Resources in Brazilian Amazonia." In Hunter-gatherers in a Changing World, edited by V. Reyes-García and A. Pyhälä, 91–105. New York: Springer.
Viveiros de Castro, Eduardo. 1992. From the Enemy's Point of View: Humanity and Divinity in an Amazonian Society. Chicago: University of Chicago Press.
Viveiros de Castro, Eduardo. 2012. Cosmological Perspectivism in Amazonia and Elsewhere. HAU Journal of Ethnographic Theory.
Watling, J., J. Iriarte, F.E. Mayle, D. Schaan, L.C.R Pessenda, N.J Loader, F.A. Street-Perrott, R.E. Dickau, A. Damasceno, and A. Ranzi. 2017. "Impact of pre-Columbian 'Geoglyph' Builders on Amazonian Forests." Proceedings of the National Academy of Sciences of the United States of America 114 (8): 1868–73.
World Anthropological Union. 2019. "Denouncement of the Brazilian government for *ecocide*: crime against humanity and the planet by deliberate destruction of the rainforest ecosystem, causing loss of biodiversity and genocide of indigenous peoples and other traditional communities." At www.iuaes.org/statement/WAU%20Letter%20Amazonia%20Forest%20190830%2005.pdf

Part III

Environmental and medical knowledge

Chapter 9

Local environmental knowledge, cultural go-betweens and Linnaean scientists in the Dutch colonial world

Kalle Kananoja

Introduction

The aim of early modern natural historians was a universal system of classifi-cation encompassing the natural resources of the whole world. The only feas-ible way to write global natural histories was through networks of collectors. The creation of the Linnaean Taxonomic system was achieved through a knowledge network that included correspondents and field workers sent out to explore the natural resources of different parts of the world. Recent schol-arship has shown how indigenous and enslaved people's botanical, geograph-ical, and pharmacological expertise was central to knowledge-making in various European empires.[1] Although historians of science have remarked on Linnaeus' and his students' proclivity to rely on local knowledge and adopt its elements, for the most part this historiography is a celebration of European conquest over nature.

This chapter argues that, at the heart of this conquest lays an uneasy rela-tionship between local indigenous and universal scientific epistemologies, which ultimately turned into a moral question of authority. It examines how Linnaeus and his disciples set out to solve these disparities by silencing dis-sonant voices in the writing of global natural history. Yet, they could not camouflage the crucial role of cultural go-betweens in providing local envir-onmental and medical knowledge to scientists, who were essentially outsiders in the multiple spaces of natural historical investigation.

Historians of science have in recent years turned increasingly towards studying local knowledge in the making of early modern European empires. This shift in emphasis from scientists to informants has brought to the fore-ground the tensions of empire; race, gender, and the cultural politics of exclusion were all important components in the making of early modern nat-ural history.[2] Indigenous medical and botanical experts, women, and slaves were effectively marginalized when global natural histories were being set on paper. This chapter focuses on the strategies of inclusion and exclusion in the Atlantic networks of Linnaeus and his apostles. It analyses the works of Daniel Rolander, Anders Sparrman and Peter Thunberg, whose field work took place in Dutch colonial enclaves in Suriname and the Cape colony in South Africa.

Despite growing evidence of the contributions of indigenous and enslaved individuals to the formation of scientific knowledge outside Europe, most narratives of Enlightenment science still argue that the scientific revolution took place in Europe. The voices of slaves and indigenous peoples were often marginalized or silenced completely in accounts of natural history. Thus, finding these local authorities in published texts remains a methodological challenge while they are easier to detect in private journals and correspondence. Publicly, very few natural historians of the Enlightenment were prepared to admit that a substantial amount of the collected information came from enslaved or indigenous individuals. In the Atlantic world, scientific racism was on the rise at the time, and enslaved blacks were often portrayed as less able and intelligent both physically and morally – in a word, unreliable. Therefore, what follows is partially a methodological exercise in how to detect the contributions of slaves in early modern knowledge making.[3] By focusing on Linnaean networks, this chapter discusses how local and slave knowledge became incorporated into Swedish natural history. It shows how, in their quest for global scientific knowledge, Linnaeus' disciples constantly employed local people for longer periods or purchased specimens from lay collectors they encountered.

Linnaeus, slavery and colonialism

Rolander, Sparrman and Thunberg's ending up in Dutch colonies is not surprising as their teacher, Carl Linnaeus, had made a name for himself in the Netherlands in the 1730s. At that time, Holland was still one of most celebrated centres of natural history in Europe, although it was already losing its place to Great Britain and France. Nevertheless, Holland was still a popular destination for Swedish students who sought to complete their doctoral studies.[4] Linnaeus had defended his doctoral thesis on malarial fevers, which he had already written before arriving in Holland, at the University of Harderwijk. Before Holland, however, was Lapland. Linnaeus' expedition to the northern parts of Sweden in 1732 had an important role in building his empirical credibility.[5] In Lapland, Linnaeus first encountered and described plants such as *Angelica archangelica*, which held an important role in Sámi phytotherapies and diet. Describing the indigenous Sámi, Linnaeus maintained that they were relatively healthy. When they fell ill, the Sámi relied on herbal medicines, leading Linnaeus to write admiringly about traditional Arctic medicine.[6] In recent years, historians and archaeologists have taken a critical stance towards colonial projects in Lapland, placing Linnaeus, among others, in the context of colonial encounters and the colonization of indigenous knowledge.[7]

As Thomas Gieryn has argued, Linnaeus was able to establish his own scientific truth through field work in Lapland. The location was central in his rise to fame, allowing him to compile a unique collection in a place where no other contemporary scientist had access to. Timing mattered, as this was also a moment when collecting and identifying natural historical samples was about to reach its high point. By travelling to Lapland, Linnaeus took a risk that forced him out of his easy chair – the perils of travel could be detailed in the travel account, where a natural historian created his own prowess. Linnaeus and his apostles travelled at a time when the laboratory had not yet become the primary site for creating scientific knowledge. Laboratory research brought out the limits of field work. Wild and pristine nature was unpredictable and uncontrollable. A scientist in the field was prone to make misperceptions and misinterpretations that could not be tested again, unlike in the laboratory. Moreover, human influence – nay, colonial influence – spread wider; Sparrman and Thunberg were faced with this in South Africa. In Linnaeus' time, however, the trust in natural historical field work, and on the observations made in the field, was still strong. When posing for the portrait painted in Holland, Linnaeus chose to dress in indigenous clothes he had acquired in Lapland, holding a shaman's drum and attaching trinkets to his belt. For a modern observer, these details would perhaps speak of cultural appropriation, but in the eighteenth-century Netherlands they were meant to show that Linnaeus was worth all the attention the world was ready to give him.[8]

Besides the plant specimen and the doctoral thesis, Linnaeus brought several manuscripts to Holland, one of which dealt with a new system to classify plants. *Systema Naturae* (1735) soon began to assert its place as the most important taxonomical work and was adopted everywhere in Europe, and later around the world. Linnaeus, however, returned to Sweden, leaving further field work to his students, the so-called "Apostles of Linnaeus." It is obvious that some of them benefited directly from their teacher's connections in the Netherlands. Although Linnaeus did not leave Sweden after his return there, he relied not only on his Apostles, but also on correspondence with numerous contacts throughout Europe. *Systema Naturae*, which Linnaeus constantly revised, and which appeared in new editions, was eagerly adopted by Dutch and English naturalists, whereas the French still continued to rely on the authority of Buffon and Adanson. Rejecting the earlier "Great Man" narratives, the new network-orientated research on Linnaeus has shown his reliance – even dependency – on collaborators, partners, students, amanuenses, and his own son. They all helped the master to cope with the information overload, with which Linnaeus suffered from the 1750s onwards, when the study of natural history practically expanded to a level that was out of control. The flood of natural historical specimens was ceaseless and merciless, leading Linnaeus to constantly revise and supplement his publications. This has been described as a repeating publication strategy, which not only helped to spread his fame, but also led to immediate feedback and comments from correspondents. The strategy bore fruit scientifically and economically.

Although Linnaeus was overwhelmed with information, the flood of knowledge was a positive problem.[9]

Despite its scientific merits, Linnaean science has occasionally been portrayed in a more critical light. According to Mary-Louise Pratt, Linnaean-inspired natural history asserted an urban, lettered, male authority over the whole of the planet – a learned world to which very few women had access in the early modern period. Men like Anders Sparrman elaborated a "rationalising, extractive, dissociative understanding which overlaid functional, experiential relations among people, plants and animals," creating an innocent vision of European global authority, to which Pratt refers to as anti-conquest. Pratt asserts that Indigenous peoples were rarely allowed to make their voices heard in European scientific travel writing.[10] In other words, whereas Linnaean science focused on the taxonomies of the world's fauna and flora, local indigenous peoples had a practical relationship with natural products. Plants were used as food, medicines, for making clothing, ropes, soap and skin-care products. If they were not used, they were not disturbed.

The multi-dimensional personality of Carl Linnaeus discoursed in botany, ethnography, economy, medicine and theology. His meditations on the relationship between nature and culture marked him for life. In *Systema Naturae* (1735), Linnaeus placed the human being at the top of the animal kingdom, heading the classification of quadrupeds. Without description, justification or explanation, humans were crudely classified into four categories: European, defined as white; American, defined as red; Asiatic, defined as dark; and African, defined as black. In later editions, his descriptions became more sophisticated, and Linnaeus added two other categories of human beings: the wild man, defined as four-footed, mute and hairy; and the monstrous man, "varying by climate and air." In this way, humans were integrated into nature and related to other animals in an implicit hierarchy. The hierarchy of human beings was established by skin colour, from white to black. He described the Africans as phlegmatic, relaxed, indolent, negligent, crafty and governed by caprice, while the supposedly superior Europeans were muscular, inventive and acute.[11]

Despite this hierarchical classification, it is well-known that Linnaeus valued the knowledge of common people without formal botanical training. When he assumed the title of professor of medicine at the University of Uppsala in 1741, he recommended the study and travel within Sweden before turning, if at all, to foreign countries. For practical reasons, then, Linnaeus relied on a wide network of people to provide him with specimens from all over the world. One of his relied correspondents was Eric Brander (Skjöldebrand), the Swedish consul in Algiers, who eagerly studied natural history during his first years in the Maghreb. On his way to Algiers, Brander had been trained in Linnaean natural history in 1753 by Mårten Kähler in Marseille. In 1756, Brander wrote Linnaeus describing how he devoted all his spare time to natural history. In the letter, Brander revealed that he had employed several moors and slaves to seek out curiosities in places where he could not go personally. Thanks to them, he had cabinets full of seashells, insects, fossils and plants, which he sent to Sweden by sea. Revealing this in a letter was easy for Brander, but what happened when the specimens were put to use by Linnaeus, is telling. The correspondence between the two lasted from 1754 to 1761 and Linnaeus, in the twelfth edition of *Systema naturae*, described about 60 specimens collected by Brander, or rather by the slaves employed by him. The subalterns' role in the making of the Brander collection was nowhere to be seen. It was effectively erased from the pages of history. Even for Brander, the moors and slaves were an anonymous mass rather than individuals with names, personalities, families and interests.[12] This was symptomatic of Linnaeus' apostles.

Rolander in Suriname

Linnaeus and his apostles connected with the Dutch colonial world during a period when it was already in decline. The Dutch East India Company (VOC) had lost its hegemony in the Indian Ocean world, and in the Atlantic, the West Indian Company (WIC) was a small operator compared to the English, French and Luso-Brazilian slave empires. Nevertheless, the Dutch companies could still offer a ride to exotic locations around the world, and this was the main goal of the Swedes. Daniel Rolander took advantage of opportunities for field work in Suriname, and Daniel Sparrman and Carl-Peter Thunberg ended up in South Africa, with the former joining Captain Cook's globetrotting expedition, and the latter sailing from Cape Town to Java and Japan with the Dutch. Despite the different locations and cultures they encountered, the work of all three naturalists speak to the problems of moral authority and "tensions of empire" inherent in the Dutch colonial system.

Daniel Rolander spend a little over six months in Suriname between 1755 and 1756. His return to Sweden was marked by a conflict with Linnaeus because Rolander refused to share his collection. Infuriated, Linnaeus even broke into Rolander's house, and the two never spoke to each other again. Due to this, Rolander's sojourn in Suriname remained poorly studied for a long time. His diary *Diarium Surinamicum, quod sub itinere exotico conscripsit Daniel Rolander, tomus I & II, 1754–1756* was published posthumously only in 1811. An English translation was published in 2008 and will be used here.[13] Rolander, however, was not the only Swede who could give Linnaeus access to Surinamese collections. In fact, his short visit has to be placed in a larger context, where Carl Gustav Dahlberg (1721–1781), a Swedish lieutenant-colonel, held a central role. Historiography has largely focused on the Apostles of Linnaeus and forgotten other, academically untrained amateur naturalists such as the aforementioned Brander and Dahlberg, who were in correspondence with Linnaeus. In fact, these lay informants were often better positioned to serve as collectors because they lived for long periods in the local communities, whereas traveling naturalists worked in the field for a shorter time.

Rolander's journal provides a detailed exposé of the naturalist's reliance on slaves and indigenous peoples as sources of knowledge. This reliance already began in Sweden before Rolander's trip began. Dahlberg, in Dutch service in Suriname, was instrumental in guiding Rolander's trip. Rolander joined Dahlberg as the former was preparing to return from Sweden to Suriname in 1755. As Rolander's journal makes clear, the two Swedes were constantly accompanied by Dahlberg's slave Primo, whose presence was a source of wonder to many Swedes unaccustomed to the presence of blacks in their towns. Primo acted as Rolander's first informant. Before leaving Sweden, the naturalist learned that tobacco was regarded as a sacred pleasure of the blacks in Suriname.[14]

Suriname's natural history was not a blank slate before Rolander's field trip and Dahlberg's collecting activities. African slaves' and indigenous Americans' environmental knowledge was central in guiding the Dutch to take advantage of Suriname's natural products. Pursuing healthy environments meant first and foremost the pursuit of local healing knowledge, namely phytotherapies, used by the non-European population. In the Dutch Atlantic, this can clearly be detected in the work of Maria Sibylla Merian (1647–1717), a famed artist-naturalist who, in 1699, travelled to South America with her daughter Dorothea. Merian is best-known for her observations on insects, which she published in *Metamorphosis Insectorum Surinamensium* after her return to Holland. Her trip was in many ways exceptional, not least because she was interested in something other than sugar-planting. Surinamese plantation owners probably regarded Merian as an eccentric fool. However, she adapted to her surroundings by becoming a slave owner almost as soon as she landed.[15]

In early modern natural history, it was not unusual that, in addition to plant, animal and mineral specimens, naturalists collected people. Focused on her observations and data recording, Merian had more use for Africans and Amerindians than for European plantation owners. She often quoted her slaves and joined them in search of new larva in her own garden and outside of Paramaribo. She conversed about insects and plants with the indigenous and Africans, and they brought her novel specimens to study. Illustrating her observations was central to Merian's work and, together with her daughter, she painted the insects and their metamorphosis on parchment. Contemporaries regarded Merian's paintings as the most beautiful illustrations ever made in America. Anyone reading the *Metamorphosis* today can attest that beauty was also translated to the published work.[16]

Rolander's contact with Atlantic slavery intensified gradually as he travelled in Dahlberg's company. They embarked on a Dutch ship in the port of Texel in April 1755. For the first month of the Atlantic journey, the ship headed to Suriname was accompanied by another ship heading to West Africa to purchase slaves. The slave ship was captained by a Swede named

Westerdal, whom Rolander identified as very knowledgeable and genuinely interested in natural history. Westerdal promised to share whatever specimens he came across on the Gold Coast, which Rolander held in esteem since ship captains did not usually appreciate scientists on board.[17] It was upon arrival in Suriname, however, that Rolander started to constantly refer to slaves and slavery. On 21 June 1755, he described the creole society of Suriname in some detail, writing also of blacks and slavery:

> The black people have black bodies, black curly hair, dark eyes, flat noses with upturned and enlarged tips. They constitute the second variety of man common in this land. A large part of them are bought in Africa and brought here, and their descendants begotten here constitute the other part. They are held in such a great number that they fill up all the streets and houses of the city. The whites have imposed the yoke of slavery upon all of them, so that they do all the work in the houses, at the plantations, and all the whites' doings; these wretched people, whose Lady Fortuna is but a stepmother, labour all the way into their graves. Happy are those born here and used to slavery from early childhood whom the cruel desire of recuperating liberty does not oppress.[18]

Rolander clearly felt pity for the African slaves who had lost their freedom and had been brought forcibly to the Americas. He acknowledged that slaves were treated harshly by the whites. Yet, his first impression was that slaves sought solace in singing and dancing when not working. Rolander's first nights in Suriname were disturbed by the high-pitched singing of animals, fragile health, and not being used to sleeping in a hammock. He was also disturbed by little sparks flying around the streets and courtyards and even inside the houses. On his fourth night onshore, Rolander could no longer contain his curiosity. Since nobody knew for sure what the sparks were, Rolander went "running about till late in the night together with some slaves to catch them." The attempt failed since nothing could be seen in the dark of the night once the sparks were extinguished. This demonstrates, however, that a natural historian's interaction with slaves could be quite intense and certainly differed from the norm in Suriname's hierarchical society. Sometimes Rolander payed random black slaves to catch things for him. A lizard, *Lacerta mutabilis*, or *angulata*, was caught by an anonymous slave passing by, who climbed a tree to chase the chameleon. He then went on to argue with the white and black onlookers about the reasons why a chameleon changed its colour.[19]

In the following days and months, Rolander continued to report on the uses of local flora by Suriname's black inhabitants. He observed constantly and relied on the word of people passing by, trying to ascertain what he heard from various sources. In Rolander's scientific work, local knowledge reigned supreme. Any person with empirical knowledge of the local environment could become a trusted informant, regardless of skin colour. One day, when venturing to have a closer look at the small yards surrounding residences in the city, Rolander remarked of *Scoparia dulcis* that "the daily repeated experiments of the blacks indicate that this plant enjoys medicinal potency." Knowledge of medicinal plants, therefore, was not only based on ancient indigenous traditions or African pharmacological heritage but also on constant experimentation with new substances. In a word, new healing knowledge was constantly created through experimentation.[20]

While the specific source of information is often unclear in Rolander's journal, it is clear that in many cases it must have been an Indian or a black slave. In some passages this was expressed directly: "The Surinamese Indians and black servants say…" Information was also provided by whites who knew the ways of blacks and Indians intimately. For example, Rolander referred to the daily use of *Ricinus vulgaris*, or *communis*, among the Indians and slaves, and went on to describe a specific way in which its leaves were used by blacks. Because its leaves wrapped around the head were said to remove headaches, slaves were thought to wrap the leaves around their heads and pretend to have a headache in order to avoid unpleasant work. The wording here suggests that this piece of information came from slave masters. The majority of local informants remained anonymous in Rolander's journal whether they were black or white.[21]

Given the large number of informants at Rolander's disposal, anonymity in his travel journal is understandable. After all, the journal went through an editorial process before it was published. Another facet of anonymity is that pharmacological knowledge-formation in Suriname cut through divides of class, race and gender. While most medical knowledge might have originated from the experiments of blacks and Indians and the exchanges between the two (especially in maroon communities), white slave owners eagerly sought to profit from this knowledge and put it to use. Lodging with a white lady, Rolander brought a poisonous plant into the house. His landlady ordered them to be thrown out and warned Rolander that he should not bring them inside. A few days later, however, the lady allowed Rolander to examine plants in his own room, and also, accompanied by two blacks, brought some plants to him. She advised the natural historian to store them safely and not to kill anyone with them. Rolander then added that the lady made a habit of learning from the blacks who had medical knowledge about the properties of the plants Rolander brought home, in order to appropriate their conclusions and judgments about their qualities.[22]

The anonymity of informants in Rolander's account can also be explained by his habit of validating information from various people. Although he wrote extensively about the healing practices of Suriname's Indians and blacks, it is as if Rolander did not want to take only their word when explaining the uses of individual plant medicines. When describing a small bush common to meadow and grove that the Dutch called *slaapers*, Rolander wrote that both whites and blacks informed him how, each evening, the bush pops together, collapses, and sleeps the night away, only to revive in the morning. In another instance, after being provided with a lengthy first-hand explanation on the nutrient value of a berry of a common tree by a black slave, Rolander hastened to add that whites had testified that they had the same experience.[23]

The best-known and oft-cited example of Rolander's reliance on slave knowledge is the story of the *Quassia amara* (Linn) or Quassy root. Although the use of the Quassy had been known in Suriname for a long time and it had been used by the natives as a stomach remedy, Rolander learned about it and purchased the knowledge from a black named Graman Quassi, who used it to treat fever.[24] Later, in 1761, Dahlberg brought specimens of the wood and of the fructification to Linnaeus, who drew up a botanical description of the plant, with an account of its virtues. Later experiments by Mr Farley, a practitioner in Antigua, and medical thesis by Dr Ebeling, confirmed its medical powers. The Quassy was added to many pharmacopeias, but Dahlberg was infuriated with Linnaeus for giving the credit to Quassi and for naming the plant after a black slave. In Linnaeus' words, Dahlberg "wanted to be great but he was not."[25]

Besides Quassi, Rolander's native and enslaved informants had a very limited effect on the naming of plants. This influence was often indirect, as in the case of *Coccolobis emetica*. Rolander named it thus because a decoction of its flowers and inner bark was used by both the Indians and blacks as an effective emetic. Rolander went on to divide the medicinal plants used by Suriname's natives into two primary classes: the emetics, with purging properties; and the others, with astringent and tonic properties. At the onset of common fevers, Indians drank plant-based emetics. Their experiments had revealed the properties of a great number of emetic plants in Suriname.[26]

Graman Quassi was part of Suriname's plural medical culture, in which European physicians and surgeons had a small role. Although the methods of indigenous Americans and African slaves were often regarded as mere superstition and quackery, they were Suriname's primary healers. Amerindians and Africans understood that illnesses were caused by natural reasons, but this did not reveal why illness struck a certain person. This question was usually explained through a spiritual framework, in which ancestral and nature spirits played a central role. Healing disease was based on herbal remedies. Many people commonly shared this kind of everyday knowledge, but certain healers had more extensive knowledge of phytotherapies that could be used to treat a wide variety of ailments. Besides the natural historians discussed above, some physicians described local healing knowledge in detail.[27]

Surinamese folk remedies did not consist solely of plants native to the Americas, but Old World plants also spread to the New through the Columbian exchange. Watermelon, sesame and oil palm were some of the indigenous African plants that arrived in the Americas. Slave healers could also make use of Asian plants that had earlier spread to Africa and eventually came to be used in the Americas. Slaves had their own plots on the plantations, where they could grow African food plants for their own use. For medical use, slaves adopted a number of plants related to medicinals that grew in Africa. Some Surinamese plant medicines were given African names after those that were in use in the slaves' homelands. In other words, Africans recognized many plant families without any kind of scientific taxonomy. What the slaves could not figure out among themselves, they found out from the indigenous Americans.[28] According to Rolander, Africans were always the first to ask the Amerindians about the uses of local plants, as they were trying to tap into Caribbean healing knowledge. Generally, Europeans were the last to start to use local remedies, after first seeing their slaves use them.[29] In this way, Suriname's nature was gradually turned into a healing, if not a healthy, environment.

Sparrman and Thunberg in South Africa

In the second half of the eighteenth century, the Cape Colony in Southern Africa was one of the most important settings for natural historical research. Two Apostles of Linnaeus, Anders Sparrman (1748–1820) and Carl Peter Thunberg (1743–1828), spent time in the Cape during the 1770s. Sparrman arrived in South Africa in 1771, then joined James Cook's second expedition between 1772 and 1775, after which he briefly returned to Cape Town. Thunberg stayed in the Cape colony for three years from 1772 to 1775, after which he headed to Japan via the Dutch East Indies.

Although Europeans had first made their way to southern Africa by the end of the fifteenth century, permanent colonization did not begin until 1651, when the VOC decided to establish a base in Table Bay in order to provision the ships sailing to the East Indies. Cape Town provided water, medicinal plants and food for the fleets, giving the ships' crews a chance to recover from illness before the second leg of their journey. Ships sailing under other nations' flags also began to use Table Bay as an anchorage point, but VOC ships remained in the majority until the 1770s. In the VOC infrastructure, Cape Town was clearly linked to the Indian rather than the Atlantic Ocean world. Batavia, VOC's headquarters in Asia, developed its own colonial culture, which was also reflected in South Africa. As VOC's operations grew, the Cape Colony also changed from a rather insignificant outpost to an extended settlement, which had a significant influence on the Khoi and the San, or South Africa's indigenous population, referred to by the Dutch as *Boschjesmens* (Bushmen). The latter established trading relations with the Dutch and provided them with cattle. Meat protein did not suffice for the ocean-going ships, which also needed grain, vegetables and fruit. Soon after its establishment, the settlement transformed into an agricultural colony, when the VOC gave land grants to some of its employers.[30]

Carl Peter Thunberg's voyage to South Africa was made possible by Johannes Burman, an old Dutch contact of Linnaeus. Following his doctoral disputation, Thunberg travelled to Paris, after which he headed to Amsterdam, where Burman arranged for him a surgeon's contract with a VOC expedition to Japan. Anders Sparrman, in turn, was an experienced traveller before ending up in South Africa. He had made a two-year trip to China in the mid-1760s with a Swedish East India Company's ship.[31]

Cape Town drew naturalists partly because of its mild Mediterranean climate, which made its interior more attractive and much more accessible than other parts of tropical Atlantic Africa. In Angola and Mozambique, the Portuguese had managed to extend their settlements to the interior of the continent, but Portuguese colonies remained closed to foreigners. The VOC had an interest in exploring the southern African interior, and sent out scouts to map the region's economic potential. The results of these expeditions remained thin and they rarely, if ever, made news in Europe.[32] Scientific research, however, had different goals. Sparrman and Thunberg were not only interested in biodiversity but also made observations about local populations and their cultural practices.

However, scientific research at this time was not free of Eurocentrism. Sparrman and Thunberg were well aware that Linnaeus had classified indigenous South Africans as the lowest level of humanity, barely human monsters (*Monstrosus*).[33] In other words, they were not regarded as part of the civilized world. This is of note especially because naturalists traversing southern Africa in the late eighteenth century hardly encountered untouched African communities. Cultural interaction with the Dutch had continued for over a century and resulted in sociocultural change. Isolated communities who wanted to remain so had to keep retreating deeper into the interior to avoid European influence. In these frontier settlements, travelling naturalists encountered whites who had adopted African practices and had sometimes taken indigenous women as their partners. For travellers, these cross-cultural go-betweens served as useful informants and guides, introducing them to local environmental practices and medical botany.

As we have seen in Suriname's case, Linnaeus and his apostles were not the first to take an interest in extra-European natural products. European settlers were extremely interested in indigenous knowledge that could have practical applications. In Europe, as Alix Cooper has shown, this led to the invention of the indigenous, whereby naturalists began to seek out the local knowledge of peasants, the primary botanical experts, who employed this environmental knowledge in their everyday lives. Of course, the practical knowledge of peasants did not make them scientists; this role was reserved for scholars. Peasants sharing their knowledge did not become celebrities, but natural historians did. With a significant discovery, the fame of a naturalist potentially spread across Europe.[34]

The practice of European natural history in Africa in the 1770s can be examined in the light of these European precedents. Although masculine and rationalizing authority was central to the literary representations of the extra-European world, this literary genre should not be over-simplified. Scientific knowledge of southern Africa – and the globe generally – was in a formative state, and it did not develop in isolation from multiple sources of knowledge. The Cape Colony's geography, vegetation and fauna was very diverse. Knowledge about this diversity drew from multiple sources, including indigenous and colonial informants, who spoke different languages, practiced different trades and lifestyles, and had their own environmental conceptions. Sparrman and Thunberg's writing reflects this multiplicity and, at the same time, offers a view of Cape society in the 1770s.

Knowledge about Cape's environment and natural products was formed by multiple linkages between observers and oral informants. Since the seventeenth century, Khoisan had worked as shepherds and servants on Dutch farms. By the time Sparrman and Thunberg made their way to the region, many of these indigenous inhabitants were at least partially dependent on income from agricultural work. Khoi women, in turn, took up employment as domestic servants in Dutch households. Environmental knowledge was made and exchanged in these everyday settings, in which whites were in a commanding position, and could also acquire information by force.[35]

European botanists, travellers, and hunters spent time with farmers and settlers in the backlands of the Cape colony. Settlers offered food and shelter, of course, but also provided local knowledge. Travelers also met Khoisan along the way, although in communicating with them they had to rely on interpreters. Khoisan also served as guides and servants for the naturalists, offering further opportunities for the acquisition of local experience and knowledge. Indigenous Africans, in turn, learned new skills from Europeans. In addition to language skills, they learned to fire guns and ride horses. The use of wagons spread from the Dutch to Africans, helping people to move between different places. Mobility led to increased knowledge about local environments.[36]

Cross-cultural interaction in southern Africa was not an experience in racial equality. European naturalists exploited the Cape's hierarchic society similarly to other whites, and they never questioned the subordinate role of African assistants and informants. This did not obstruct camaraderie, especially on longer expeditions to the interior, when Europeans as outsiders were more dependent on local help. Power was further checked by the realization that African assistants would simply abandon the expedition or lead it astray if they were treated too harshly. In other words, leading a trip to the interior meant that Europeans had to constantly negotiate with rather than whip their African assistants.

In South Africa, both the Dutch and Africans were of great value to natural historians. They were familiar with the safest passages, the best watering holes, and the whereabouts of flora and fauna. In contrast to the coastal farmers, the settlers in the interior possessed lots of local environmental knowledge, even if the Khoisan were unwilling to share their knowledge with foreign intruders. Local knowledge became not only marketable, but also a form of political power and resistance. Europeans noted that indigenous southern Africans were often secretive about medicinal plants and healing methods.[37] Healing knowledge was easier to hide than knowledge related to hunting, watering and pasturing.

Cape fauna was extremely rich and had already fascinated European hunters in the seventeenth and eighteenth centuries. Hunting was not only a source of animal protein and monetary wealth, but also cleared space for farming. Khoisan use of arrows and spears lost some of their significance as firearms spread to the region, but indigenous hunting techniques, including the digging of hunting pits, were still being used when Sparrman and Thunberg travelled there. Khoisan taught the Dutch that it was worthwhile to wait for animals at the watering holes. Horses were a Dutch import which facilitated hunting and especially the tracking of injured animals. However, in the 1770s, Sparrman still encountered remnants of the past when he saw "the hottentots" riding their bulls. Khoikhoi had a habit of taming wild bulls by piercing their nostrils. Bulls were used not only for riding but also as beasts of burden. They also facilitated the Khoikhois' mobile and pastoral lifestyle. These human-animal relations were given new significance when the Dutch introduced wagons in southern Africa. Sparrman was in awe of the Cape servants' unmatched skill in keeping the ox-wagons on the move.[38]

The tracking of animals was another indigenous skill that some Dutchmen admired. Khoisan hunters were occasionally forced to rely on tracking because of the ineffectiveness of their traditional weapons compared to firearms. Families living on the frontiers often had domestic animals to track. Cattle could take off on its own or be stolen. Catching lost animals could take a lot of time. According to Sparrman, Africans' observational skills were of great use in demanding tracking expeditions. Although the Khoikhoi impressed Europeans with their hunting skills, the Dutch were not willing to imitate everything. One of these habits was the Khoi practice of smearing their bodies with grease from the killed animals. The Dutch, however, learned that some parts of animals could be used for the preparation of healing ointments. Sparrman learned that the heart of an eland could be used to prepare fat for eating on bread.[39]

Such environmental knowledge easily translated to medical practices in pastoralist Khoikhoi societies, where medicine, health and nursing were deeply rooted and valued long before the arrival of the Dutch. As Viljoen has shown, concerted efforts were made to prioritize health and control common disorders. The Khoikhoi sought to prevent illnesses by lubricating themselves with sheep's fat mixed with soot and ash, as Thunberg reported. Sparrman, in turn, described that a mix of grease, soot and powder ground from the leaves of the *buchu* plant shielded indigenous bodies "from the influences of the air."[40] *Buchu*, indeed, was their principal healing herb, regarded by the Khoikhoi as a magic plant.[41]

One of the most remarkable ways the Dutch sought to recreate a healthy environment in the western Cape was the establishment of a warm bath facility called Hottentots Holland's Bath, which Sparrman visited in July 1775. Given the widespread use and popularity of mineral baths in European medicine in the early modern period, this should come as no surprise. Perhaps more surprising is the variety of patients using the bath, as Sparrman reported it. According to a list Sparrman saw at the establishment, the annual number of patients was between 150 and 200 persons. Only eight people were bathing at the time of his visit during the cold season. Sparrman encountered at least two slaves who had been sent by their masters to seek a cure at the bath. One of them was dead within a few hours of his first bathing. The other was a young slave from Madagascar, who accompanied Sparrman to the bath, and who had been given over as incurable by a surgeon at the Cape. This anonymous slave had an inveterate ulcer in his leg, and he claimed to have been healed of a similar ulcer before his enslavement in Madagascar by means of a certain bark. Like the African slaves taken to the Americas, the Malagasy slave had sought the tree in South Africa after arriving there, but had not been able to find it.[42] Directing his words at "[t]he Christians who arm the natives of Madagascar against each other," this set Sparrman on a tirade upon the usefulness of indigenous knowledge:

> The Peruvian *bark, senega, ophiorbiza, sarsaparilla, quassia,* with many other useful remedies, calculated for preserving millions of our species, have not we learned them all from those we call Savages? and perhaps might learn still more, if our tyranny had not already, I had almost said, entirely extirpated them, and together with them lost the result of their useful experience.[43]

The establishment at Hottentots Holland's Bath consisted of a brick house, which Sparrman found very unhealthy due to dampness, for accommodation of guests and to serve as housing for the overseer of the bath. The bathing house was located about 100 paces from the welling house, and it had a cistern or pit. Warm water ran from its underwater source to one of the gables of the house, and from there into an open channel to the cistern, where it came pouring down. Patients lay down or sat in the cistern until the water reached their chin. Due to the warmth, it was recommended that bathing should take between eight and ten minutes; patients who stayed longer sometimes passed out and drowned. After taking a bath, the patients lay down, in their clothes, at the other end of the room to sweat. The cistern could be emptied by turning a cock in the interval between each person's bathing, if required. Each patient usually bathed once or twice a day, or very seldom three times. At the site, there were two other baths used by slaves and free blacks. Sparrman did not specify whether the slaves who had been sent to the facility by their masters were allowed to use the bathing house.[44]

Although Sparrman was familiar with the use of warm and mineral baths in Sweden and elsewhere in Europe, the southern African variant did not convince him. Patients generally did not follow the methodical advice of physicians in using the bath, because they hardly ever had an opportunity to consult a physician there. Therefore, they used the bath at their own whim and convenience, without any regular order, without the least attention to diet, or any distinction of disorders. Patients often went into the bath directly after meals, which Sparrman found troubling. According to common lore, rheumatism and contractions of the limbs were usually cured in three or four days, but, in the case of gout, bathing was not regarded as a powerful remedy. Sparrman encountered a girl patient who was using the bath for the second year for a swelling and ulcers in her leg. She had also used a herbal remedy of mallows and other plants which had brought no relief. Sparrman, however, suggested to her another folk remedy, namely a salve made of wax and honey. This remedy healed the ulcer. In Sparrman's opinion, the cures of the bath depended very little on the minerals in the water, and instead proceeded from the repeated mutations of the humours by sweating.[45] Therefore, he suggested that the bath might be used more efficiently with a more suitable diet and course of medicine. More benefit, Sparrman claimed,

> would perhaps be found by making use of the natural baths at the Cape with a more moderate degree of warmth, which would allow of the water being absorbed in the body; and likewise by using them with addition of herbs: as for example, of *bucku* (*diosma*) and wild *dacka* (*phlomis leonurus*) which are known both by the colonists and the Hottentots to be as efficacious as they are common, and of the powerful effect of which, in pains and contractions of the limbs, when used in the form of baths, I myself have seen instances.[46]

A balanced diet of milk, plant foods and water kept the Khoikhoi in relatively good health. Thunberg believed that unseasoned and unsalted food was a key to low susceptibility to disease.[47] Khoikhoi practitioners made use of botanic medicine, some surgery and cupping. The environment played an essential role in how medicines were devised, and the ingredients and the methods used by indigenous healers were rarely debated. What mattered was the experience of their desired effects.[48] Like in Suriname, southern African healers guarded their secrets and did not reveal the contents of their medicines easily. How, then, did Sparrman and Thunberg go about making their medical observations? Their travel narratives were published well after their return to Europe, and gave hardly any clues about their methods of gathering information. However, it is clear that, like Rolander in Suriname, Sparrman and Thunberg constantly talked with resident Boers, Dutch settlers and indigenous inhabitants, or, as Sparrman noted, had their observations "confirmed… by so many Hottentots as well as Christians."[49] Yet, in their travel accounts, these individuals often remained an anonymous mass, whether they were white or black. African slaves were invariably anonymous but whites were sometimes recorded using their last names. In the Cape, as Marie-Christine Skuncke has argued, Thunberg practised a system of exchange with Dutch colonists and VOC officials, reciprocating help in his collecting activities with medical services.[50]

Conclusion

Like many other earlier European collectors and botanists in Africa and the Black Atlantic world, the disciples of Linnaeus recognized the central role of subaltern informants in guarding medico-botanical knowledge and practicing healing in their everyday lives. Yet, with the exception of Graman Quassi, few Amerindian or black informants had a place in publications regarding scientific discoveries. Their role was downplayed and silenced. Eighteenth-century European men were reluctant to show their intellectual debt to blacks and Indians, some of whom were women. In his private journal, Rolander could reveal his admiration for local informants, but in published accounts, these anticipated and fruitful encounters were often left without a mention. Similarly, in the Cape, Sparrman and Thunberg constantly talked with settlers and indigenous southern Africans, but the majority of these individuals remained anonymous and faceless in the accounts. The wealth of environmental knowledge Linnaeus' Apostles were able to record is nevertheless remarkably rich. Medicinal plants formed the bulk of observations, but indigenous and folk practices related to diet and hygienic practices were also noted. In the Cape, Sparrman and Thunberg also recorded the use of warm baths as a major form of health seeking in the interior, clearly an attempt by the Dutch settlers to recreate European bathing culture in southern Africa as a form of health-seeking practice.

Notes

1 Parrish 2006; Cook 2007; Safier 2008.
2 Schiebinger 2004; Cagle 2012.
3 Schiebinger 2005; Schiebinger 2017; Cagle 2012.
4 Boerman 1978.
5 Koerner 1999, 56–81.
6 Kylli 2019.
7 Nordin and Ojala 2018. However, see Staffan Müller-Wille 2005, 34–36.
8 Gieryn 2018, 35–52.
9 Charmantier 2018, 32–33.
10 Pratt 1992, 38.
11 Bethencourt 2013, 252–53.
12 E. Brander to Linnaeus, 23 August 1756. Letter 611 in Fries 1909, 304; Skuncke.
13 Rolander 2008.

14 Rolander 2008, 1224.
15 Davis 1995, 167–75; Schiebinger 2004, 30–35.
16 Davis 1995, 175–77.
17 Rolander 2008, 1245.
18 Ibid., 1260.
19 Ibid., 1262, 1278–82.
20 Ibid., 1263–64, 1267, 1270.
21 Ibid., 1270, 1295.
22 Ibid., 1293–94.
23 Ibid., 1344, 1363–64.
24 Lantjouw and Uittien 1935–36.
25 Linnaeus to Abraham Bäck, 4 September 1764, Letter 1048 in Fries 1911, 127.
26 Rolander 2008, 1357–58.
27 Andel 2016, 690–91.
28 Ibid.
29 Rolander 2008.
30 Penn 2005; Ross 1999.
31 Skuncke 2014, 15–37.
32 Huigen 2009, 3–8.
33 Bethencourt 2013, 252–53.
34 Cooper 2007.
35 Beinart 2003, 28–42.
36 Ibid.
37 Hokkanen 2019, 131–33.
38 Beinart 2003, 32.
39 Ibid., 34.
40 Viljoen 1999, 516–18.
41 Low 2007.
42 Sparrman 1783, 146–47.
43 Ibid., 144.
44 Ibid., 139–42.
45 Ibid., 144–45, 148–49.
46 Ibid., 145.
47 Thunberg 1788, 217.
48 Viljoen 1999, 519–20.
49 Sparrman 1786, 155.
50 Skuncke 2014, 76, 92

References

Andel, Tinde van. 2016. "The Reinvention of Household Medicine by Enslaved Africans in Suriname." *Social History of Medicine* 29: 676–94.

Beinart, William. 2003. *The Rise of Conservation in South Africa: Settlers, Livestock, and the Environment 1770–1950*. Oxford: Oxford University Press.

Bethencourt, Francisco. 2013. *Racisms: From the Crusades to the Twentieth Century*. Oxford: Oxford University Press.

Boerman, A.J. 1978. "Linnaeus and the Scientific Relations Between Holland and Sweden." *Svenska Linnésällskapets årsskrift* 1978: 43–56.

Cagle, Hugh. 2012. "The Botany of Colonial Medicine: Gender, Authority, and Natural History in the Empires of Spain and Portugal." In *Women of the Iberian Atlantic*, edited by Sarah E. Owens and Jane E. Mangan, 174–195. Baton Rouge: Louisiana State University Press.

Charmantier, Isabelle. 2018. "Notebooks, Files and Slips: Carl Linnaeus and His Disciples at Work." In *Linnaeus, Natural History and the Circulation of Knowledge*, edited by Hanna Hodacs, Kenneth Nyberg, and Stéphane van Damme, 25–56. Oxford: Voltaire Foundation.

Cook, Harold J. 2007. *Matters of Exchange: Commerce, Medicine, and Science in the Dutch Golden Age*. New Haven: Yale University Press.

Cooper, Alix. 2007. *Inventing the Indigenous: Local Knowledge and Natural History in Early Modern Europe*. Cambridge: Cambridge University Press.

Davis, Natalie Zemon. 1995. *Women on the Margins: Three Seventeenth-Century Lives*. Cambridge, Massachusetts: Harvard University Press.

Davis, Natalie Zemon. 2016. "Physicians, Healers, and their Remedies in Colonial Suriname." *Canadian Bulletin of Medical History* 33: 1–34.

Fries, Theodor Magnus, ed. 1909. *Bref och skrifvelser af och till Carl von Linné*. Första avdelningen, Del III. Upsala: Upsala Universitet.

Fries, Theodor Magnus, ed. 1911. *Bref och skrifvelser af och till Carl von Linné*. Första avdelningen, Del V. Upsala: Upsala Universitet, 1911.

Gieryn, Thomas F. 2018. *Truth Spots: How Places Make People Believe*. Chicago: University of Chicago Press.

Hokkanen, Markku. 2019. "Contestation, Redefinition and Healers' Tactics in Colonial Southern Africa." In *Healers and Empires in Global History: Healing as Hybrid and Contested Knowledge*, edited by Markku Hokkanen and Kalle Kananoja, 115–48. Cham: Springer.

Huigen, Siegfried. 2009. *Knowledge and Colonialism: Eighteenth-Century Travellers in South Africa*. Leiden: Brill.

Koerner, Lisbet. 1999. *Linnaeus: Nature and Nation*. Cambridge, Massachusetts: Harvard University Press.

Kylli, Ritva. 2019. "Traditional Arctic Healing and Medicines of Modernisation in Finnish and Swedish Lapland." In *Healers and Empires in Global History: Healing as Hybrid and Contested Knowledge*, edited by Markku Hokkanen and Kalle Kananoja, 27–53. Cham: Springer.

Lantjouw, J. and H. Uittien. 1935–36. "Surinaamsche geneeskruiden in de tijd van Linnaeus." *De West-Indische Gids* 17: 173–90.

Low, Christopher H. 2007. "Different Histories of Buchu: Euro-American Appropriation of San and Khoekhoe Knowledge of Buchu Plants." *Environment and History* 13: 333–61.

Müller-Wille, Staffan. 2005. "Walnuts at Hudson Bay, Coral Reefs in Gotland: The Colonialism of Linnaean Botany." In *Colonial Botany: Science, Commerce, and Politics in the Early Modern World*, edited by Londa Schiebinger and Claudia Swan, 34–48. Philadelphia: University of Pennsylvania Press.

Nordin, Jonas M. and Carl-Gösta Ojala. 2018. "Collecting, Connecting, Constructing: Early Modern Commodification and Globalization of Sámi Material Culture." *Journal of Material Culture* 23: 58–82.

Parrish, Susan Scott. 2006. *American Curiosity: Cultures of Natural History in the Colonial British Atlantic World*. Chapel Hill: University of North Carolina Press.

Penn, Nigel. 2005. *The Forgotten Frontier: Colonist and Khoisan on the Cape's Northern Frontier in the 18th Century*. Athens: Ohio University Press.

Pratt, Mary Louise. 1992. *Imperial Eyes: Travel Writing and Transculturation*. London: Routledge.

Rolander, Daniel. 2008a. "The Suriname Journal: Composed during an Exotic Journey, 1754–1756." In *The Linnaeus Apostles: Global Science and Adventure*, Vol. 3, Book 3, edited by Lars Hansen, 1215–1569. London: IK Foundation & Company.

Rolander, Daniel. 2008b. "Daniel Rolander's Journal." In *The Linnaeus Apostles: Global Science and Adventure*, Vol. 3, Book 3. Translated from Latin by James Dobreff, Claes Dahlman, David Morgan, and Joseph Tipton. London and Whitby: The IK Foundation and Company, 2008.

Ross, Robert. 1999. *Status and Respectability in the Cape Colony, 1750–1870: A Tragedy of Manners*. Cambridge: Cambridge University Press.

Safier, Neil. 2008. *Measuring the New World: Enlightenment Science and South America*. Chicago: University of Chicago Press.

Schiebinger, Londa. 2004. *Plants and Empire: Colonial Bioprospecting in the Atlantic World*. Cambridge, Massachusetts: Harvard University Press.

Schiebinger, Londa. 2005. "Prospecting for Drugs: European Naturalists in the West Indies." In *Colonial Botany: Science, Commerce, and Politics in the Early Modern World*, edited by Londa Schiebinger and Claudia Swan, 119–33. Philadelphia: University of Pennsylvania Press.

Schiebinger, Londa. 2017. *Secret Cures of Slaves: People, Plants, and Medicine in the Eighteenth-Century Atlantic World*. Stanford: Stanford University Press.

Skuncke, Marie-Christine. "Eric Skjöldebrand." In *Svenskt biografiskt lexicon*. At https://sok.riksarkivet.se/Sbl/Mobil/Artikel/6017/

Skuncke, Marie-Christine. 2014. *Carl-Peter Thunberg, Botanist and Physician: Career-Building across the Oceans in the Eighteenth Century*. Uppsala: Swedish Collegium for Advanced Study.

Sparrman, Anders. 1783. *Resa till Goda-Hopps-Udden, södra Pol-kretsen och omkring jordklotet, samt till Hottentot- och Caffer-Landen, åren 1772–76*, Vol. I. Stockholm: Anders J. Nordström.

Sparrman, Anders. 1786. *A Voyage to the Cape of Good Hope, towards the Antarctic Polar Circle, and around the World: But Chiefly into the Country of the Hottentots and Caffres, from the Year 1772, to 1776*, Vol. I. 2nd edition. London: G.G.J. and J. Robinson.

Thunberg, Carl Peter. 1788. *Resa uti Europa, Africa, Asia, förrättad åren 1770–1779*, Vol. I. Uppsala: Joh. Edman.

Viljoen, Russell. 1999. "Medicine, Health and Medical Practice in Precolonial Khoikhoi Society: An Anthropological-historical Perspective." *History and Anthropology* 11: 515–36.

Chapter 10

Promotion of a modern holistic vision of hygiene

E.W. Lane's hygienic medicine in the British medical market, 1850s–1880s

Min Bae

Introduction

Hygiene in the nineteenth century was as complex a concept as the concept of medicine itself. It was used in a wide variety of contexts and, throughout the course of the nineteenth century, the concept was given different meanings and emphases. Historians of nineteenth-century medicine have scarcely paid sufficient attention to the relationship between hygiene and medicine. The historical importance of Edward Wickstead Lane's (1823–1889) medical philosophy comes from his attempt to combine the amorphous concept of hygiene with that of medicine. Until the 1880s, when he published his last book on hygienic medicine, Lane consistently promoted the holistic vision of hygiene as the essence of medical philosophy. However, his medical theories on hygiene did not receive much attention as a new medical system, not even with his massive advertising efforts, nor did he manage to theoretically reform hydropathy's stagnant state, which began in the 1860s.

In this chapter, I focus on the topic of "medical reconciliation" that Lane raised in his book and relate it to the concept of the medical market and to his efforts to find recognition for his medical theory and philosophy both from the professional and the lay public. In this respect, I attempt to present a combined approach to Lane's hygienic medicine through his medical philosophy and the medical market. The chapter consists of three parts. After a historiographical discussion, I first explain the relationship between hygiene and medicine in the nineteenth century, particularly regarding the medical market. Second, I introduce the characteristic features of Lane's medical thinking, and third, I investigate how Lane viewed the medicine and the medical market of his day.

Hygiene and hydropathy in the historiography of medicine

When Lane entitled his book "hygienic medicine," he was thinking of "hygiene" in the classical holistic sense rather than as public hygiene or personal cleanliness. Medical historians have largely recognized hygiene as an embodiment of the holistic tradition of Western medicine,[1] and they have also recognized the stronger holistic inclination of British medicine compared with that of Europe during the nineteenth century.[2] However, among studies that have investigated the Victorian concepts of hygiene,[3] few have taken the perspective of medical philosophy. An exception is Virginia Smith's *Clean* (2007). She approaches nineteenth-century personal hygiene based on both the markets and the medico-philosophical trends of the time.

Most studies on hydropathy, the heterodox healing system closest to the classical form of hygiene, have investigated services and goods rather than its intellectual aspects. For instance, Marland and Adams' "Hydropathy at Home" (2009) draws on patient records and popular manuals, arguing that enthusiasm for domestic hydropathy did not abate when institutional hydropathy began to lose its "curative thrust" in the late nineteenth century.[4] However, given their lack of interest in distinguishing the use of water for healing and for health, it is not easy to see whether their study is about the history of domestic hydropathy or about the history of bathing in water at home. In her most recent book *Healing with Water* (2015), Adams seems to attempt to confine the historical meanings of hydropathy.[5] She views hydropathy merely as one of the types of special expertise provided in the health resorts of the nineteenth century, which chronologically represented a certain period of trends in water cures, along with balneology, hydrotherapy and medical hydrology.

A similar situation is also visible in the studies of the medical market. The marketplace in the history of medicine has been studied by many scholars, but few of them have attempted to associate the medical market with the intellectual history of medicine. Since the 1980s, when economic aspects became one of the main concerns in the history of medicine,[6] historians have investigated the relationship between the medical market and the medical profession in the nineteenth century.[7] They mostly agree that pluralistic or unidentifiable medical practitioners with widespread dissension among them developed into a unified profession[8] as "free markets" changed to "restricted" and "diminished" markets in the course of the century.[9] Regarding the concept of the medical market itself, however, there has been little consensus among historians who have used the term. Mark Jenner and Patrick Wallis (2007) observe that the term "medical marketplace" has been used in a confusing manner by medical historians depending on their own perceptions. Jenner and Wallis emphasized "the socially embedded nature of economic relationships" in medicine,[10] such as co-operation and social networks, in opposition to profit-orientated competition and argued that the concept of markets in the history of medicine should be confined to "the markets for medical goods and services," criticizing the "long-established narratives of the development of modernity and of capitalism" associated with the concept.[11] However, a view of markets as confined to medical services and goods may lead to separating medical theories and philosophies from patients' choices and expectations. Patients in the nineteenth century not only chose their treatments within the limits of their financial means and their social conditions but also chose them according to their beliefs and lifestyles. Sarah Cant and Ursula Sharma (1998) saw this period as one of the very rare times in the history of medicine when plurality could develop and compete in relatively even relations and conditions.[12]

Lane's heterodox medical views as a physician are closely related to the theme of the medical profession, particularly the boundaries of the profession. As a medically qualified hydropath, Lane is an example of the type of a medical practitioner familiar to historians of the nineteenth century: doctors on the fringes. Since Ian Inkster's (1977) and Thomas Gieryn's (1983) innovative studies,[13] "marginal men" and boundary-work in medicine have been studied mostly in relation to the heterodox healing systems of the period.[14] For instance, Bradley and Dupree (2003) focused on the economic and social views of medically qualified hydropaths. They identified a heterogeneous group of about 40 individual doctors (including Lane) who ran their own hydropathic establishments and they also statistically analysed the educational and career patterns of these doctors.[15] Bradley and Dupree analysed not only the subtle marginality of doctors excluded from the circle of the metropolitan elite but also their intellectual efforts, "their translation of Priessnitz (the founder of hydropathy)." However, the authors paid little attention to contemporary British medical thought and to the difficulties that physician hydropaths experienced in combining their hydropathic practice with orthodox medical knowledge. Bradley's "Medicine on the Margins?" (2002) was more concerned with the intellectual aspects, particularly when it comes to hydropathy's relationship with orthodox medicine and the differences between lay and medically qualified hydropaths. He noted the importance of the concepts of hygiene and medical holism in the nineteenth century but did not discuss the changes undergone by the theoretical features of hydropathy during the latter part of the century.

Hygiene in the medical market

Hygiene was a symbolic part of traditional Western medicine which represented its holistic aspect.[16] As Marc Regenmortel and David Hull have noted, "Reductionism Rules" in present-day biomedical sciences in the developed world.[17] Especially during the nineteenth and twentieth centuries, as Christopher Lawrence and George Weisz have indicated, "medicine became increasingly reductionist in orientation and increasingly dominated by laboratory research and technology."[18] In comparison, the Greek concept of hygiene, often called "dietetics" (a way of life) in Hippocratic medicine, later developed into the concept of the "six non-naturals" by Galen. The latter were (1) air, (2) food and drink, (3) sleep and watch, (4) motions and rest, (5) evacuations and repletion and (6) passions of the soul.[19] "Non-natural" meant that the factors were not innate or part of a person's constitution.

The doctrine of "non-naturals" remained as the crystallized form of Western hygienic tradition, especially in relation to the rationalism and individualism since the Enlightenment era.[20]

This traditional view of hygiene was significantly challenged by the French physician Jean Noël Hallé (1754–1822), who attempted to redefine hygiene, promoting the concept of "public hygiene," which he distinguished from "private hygiene."[21] The division into the two separate spheres was accompanied by important changes in the medical conception of disease. The Parisian clinical and statistical methodology challenged previous medical individualism by reducing the patient to a clinical object,[22] which led many doctors to regard poverty as a fundamental cause of poor hygiene.[23] However, during the second half of the nineteenth century, the earlier trend of environmental hygiene was gradually replaced by a new trend, resulting in "a narrowing and focusing of public health."[24] This new reductionist trend in public hygiene, one that Erwin Ackerknecht regarded as "modern hygiene," began to develop in Europe around 1848.[25]

Doctors in the second half of the nineteenth century who were interested in hygiene had, in principle, three ways to relate their medical philosophies or knowledge. The first was to focus on the public dimension of hygiene, seeking to make Victorian towns and cities cleaner primarily through improvements in sanitation.[26] The second was to focus on the personal dimension of hygiene. Washing with hygienic products increasingly became the core of a new "hygienic individualization" reflecting the modernization of Victorian society.[27] This approach, closely connected to the significant role of the "consumer" in the medical market, was a characteristic feature of British hygiene.[28] The third way was to emphasize the medical dimension of hygiene. Doctors played a significant role here. As "fear of infection" became an increasingly decisive factor in social attitudes towards hygiene,[29] medical hygiene was gradually orientated towards infection control.[30] By the 1870s, through the discovery of certain pathogens and the surgical revolution, medical hygiene became almost exclusively concerned with micro-organic germs and asepsis. In general, as Tom Crook has noted regarding personal hygiene, late nineteenth-century hygiene was "intensified," "reanimated" and more "formalized" than in the previous era.[31]

Unlike mainstream reductionist approaches, holistic views of hygiene were held by a small number of doctors, one of whom was Lane. These doctors attempted to apply certain traditional values of hygiene to their therapeutics, which were often, if not always, inclined towards medical heterodoxy, for instance hydropathy. It was Andrew Combe (1797–1847) who affected young Lane the most. Combe is the best example of a physician who exploited the increased public interest in physiology, which was regarded as almost another name for hygiene, particularly in Edinburgh.[32] Lane, unlike Combe, chose hydropathy as his main therapeutic measure. This new therapeutic and hygienic system advocated the external application of cold water in various ways and was often combined with other regimens aimed at strengthening the vital force. In the mid-nineteenth century, hydropathy was constituted by "a range of reforming health and lifestyle approaches"[33] and was deeply related to the Romantic spirit of the return to nature.[34]

The place of hydropathy in the nineteenth-century medical market was complex. Amidst the rapid growth of the resort business, specialist water cure resorts were prosperous well beyond the level of the medical market,[35] and hydropathy occupied a small section of both the leisure and medical markets. When Lane set up his own hydropathic establishment in 1854, he could not escape the bitter atmosphere between hydropaths and medical practitioners,[36] but this period was also when hydropathy was "new and at its most distinctive."[37] Towards the end of the century, hydropathic institutions relied increasingly on their resort facilities, most often combined with spas.[38] Most historians have considered that hydropathy, at least among medically qualified practitioners, was significantly in eclipse by the 1870s.[39] The decline of hydropathy was not a coincidence. Although the 1858 Medical Act did not enforce certain orthodox approaches as legitimate by law, it helped the "intellectual balance" to incline towards medical orthodoxy.[40]

Lane's medical philosophies

Lane's *Hydropathy: or Hygienic Medicine* (1859) was the second edition of his *Hydropathy: Or, the Natural System of Medical Treatment* (1857).[41] The second edition represented the extended and final version of his medical philosophy in an era when medical theory and practice were largely regarded as chaotic, characterized by loss of trust in the traditional humoural and vitalist concepts and by criticism of the prevalent heroic procedures.[42] In the preface, Lane clarified his two aims, setting forth "the rational grounds of hygienic medicine" and "the present position of the medical art." He specified the main audience of his book as medical practitioners.

In Lane's hygienic medicine, traditional hygiene, which had been a significant part of medicine for a long time, became newly "re-medicalized" through intellectualization based on theoretical and philosophical reasoning. While his view of hygiene was certainly distinctive, it also reflected certain features in both medicine and hygiene from the 1850s to the 1880s. Lane shared with Combe the classical holistic concept of hygiene. Both adopted the notion of the "laws of health." Andrew Combe's concept of the laws of health was clearly influenced by his brother George, whose *Constitution of Man Considered in Relation to External Objects* (1828) acquainted the expanding reading public with the philosophy of natural laws (physical, organic and moral).[43]

It is regarding the pathological aspect of blood physiology where Lane's medical theory most explicitly demonstrated his efforts at the medicalization of hygiene. In Lane's hygienic medicine, all diseases were divided into two groups based on the state of vitality: Class 1 was characterized by a superabundance of vital power and Class 2 by a deficiency of vital power. Such binary theoretical frameworks had been used since the preceding century by medical teachers, most notably William Cullen (1710–90), for whom treatments were fundamentally aimed at restoring normal bodily functions through stimulating or depleting measures.[44] However, Lane developed his own aetiological model on the basis of "modern pathology," or new experimental accounts of the functions of blood. He incorporated both vitality and humours into the concept of "quality of the blood,"[45] while attempting to accommodate John Hughes Bennett's (1812–1875) and Charles Williams' (1805–1889) pathological findings. Lane held that "quality of blood" was the decisive factor in the contraction of disease and that that quality was significantly influenced by diet and digestive powers.

However, in Lane's blood physiology, the elements associated with Combe, such as its prescriptive and humoural features, conflicted with Bennett's and Williams' more descriptive and solidist blood physiology. Although Lane sought to harmonize them, the conflict between the two reflects the unstable, transitional state of mid-nineteenth century physiology. Lane lived in an age when, as Lois Magner has described, the "fundamental philosophical questions" were becoming increasingly marginalized in physiology. Towards the end of the century, physiology became inclined towards "experimental methods and concepts" based on chemistry and physics.[46]

The important difference between Lane and other contemporary British physicians was Lane's strong belief in nature cures and his radical view of the relationship between vitality and hygiene, as he saw a causal link between disease and wrong habits. From the perspective of mid-nineteenth century medical philosophy, the nature cure was often related not only to an outdated obsession with hardy regimens or fashionable spa services for the upper-class but also to empiricism, stigmatized by medical professionals as the practice of unqualified heterodox healers.[47] In contrast, the medical mainstream was predominantly interventionist. According to the renowned Scottish physician John Forbes (1787–1861, MD Edinburgh 1817), who was one of a small number of orthodox physicians openly subscribing to and promoting the nature cure philosophy, the interventionist tendency was more visible among young practitioners.[48] Even though most physicians of the time were well aware of the necessity of controlling vital forces with regimens and of the importance of hygiene,[49] they gave hygienic factors a minor etiological role compared with more specific causative factors and the natural constitution.

It is highly likely that Lane developed his nature cure philosophy by incorporating the philosophical tradition of Romantic medicine. Lane's approach to vitality was strongly influenced by Andrew Combe, whose view on vitalism, as reflected in his *The Art of Preserving Health* (1833), was substantially influenced by Hufeland's *The Art of Prolonging Life* (*Die Kunst das menschliche Leben zu verlängern*, 1804). Hufeland was a major representative of the *Naturphilosophie* of the Romantic era,[50] and his medical philosophy significantly influenced European vitalists, who attempted to tackle the debility of the urban poor by hygienic measures, such as moderate exercise, diet and domestic baths.[51]

Lane's view of the medical profession

Lane viewed the medical art as slowly going through a "large reform" based on the medical profession's awakening to the importance of hygiene. He considered that, in contemporary medicine, "hygiene [...] is regarded merely in the light of an adjunct in the treatment of disease, waiting upon drug medication as its handmaid."[52] He criticized the problems of drug medication using binary frameworks, such as progressivism versus conservatism and rationalism versus empiricism. Lane considered the establishment of Brompton Hospital as "an omen of a still further professional advance, in the future establishment of kindred institutions in the vicinity of all our large towns, for the treatment of every form of chronic disease on the broad and infallible basis of hygienic principles."[53] For Lane, physicians related to Brompton Hospital, such as John Forbes, Charles Williams and Richard Quain (MD, University College, London, 1842), symbolized changes in the medical trends towards hygienic medicine. Apart from the establishment of Brompton Hospital, he saw the plan to establish a Chair of Hygiene at King's College and the launching of *Journal of Public Health and Sanitary Review* (1855) as signs of a "large reform."

However, the reality was more complex than Lane's hopes. The reform that Lane expected was thwarted by the conservatism of the medical profession. He was also aware that even the Brompton Hospital physicians did not share exactly the same view of hygiene as he did. According to Lane, Williams and Forbes approved of the hygienic approach but regarded it "rather in the light of an auxiliary to drug medication at best, and as being adapted to but a limited number and kind of cases."[54] As for Quain, his involvement with hygiene did not seem to continue. He became the chairman of the pharmacopoeia committee of the General Medical Council (GMC) in 1874 and he left Brompton Hospital the next year. He was elected president of the GMC in 1891.[55] The medical licence of Thomas Richard Allinson (1858–1918), another doctor who publicly promoted "hygienic medicine," was revoked by the GMC in 1892, a year after Quain's inauguration.

Lane considered the problems of drug medication to be interrelated with the lack of rational approach to treatment. He cited John Stuart Mill's *Logic,* in which he discussed "the action of mercury in disease."[56] Furthermore, he argued that the prevalent empiricism in contemporary medicine resulted in the rampant adulteration of drugs, noting that "some important medicines are so often falsified in the market, and others so often mis-made in the laboratory," that "it is next to impossible to procure medicines of genuine quality and strength."[57]

Lane sought the fundamental cause of the prevalence of conservatism and empiricism in the profession in the realities of medical practitioners, asking rhetorically: "How is he to get his bread?"[58] The medical practitioners' struggle to make a living hampered all rational and progressive awakenings in medicine, particularly troubling young practitioners: "Young graduates in medicine have no choice but to enlist themselves for the pure sake of a livelihood."[59] Lane saw humans as "creature[s] of circumstance" and believed that the fundamental problem of the medical profession and medicine was rooted in the situation of the medical market, where the consumers did not realize the value of more progressive and rational medicine.

Lane's view of the medical market

Lane shared general practitioners' common views about the competition with irregular practitioners. He argued for high standards in medical education and for strict qualifications in medical practice. The 1858 Medical Registration Act was a watershed in the progress towards what sociologists have regarded as the monopolization of the medical market by the medical profession in the latter part of the century,[60] but irregular practitioners remained able to practice unless they broke common law.

However, the medical profession's animosity was not limited to irregulars but also included heterodox medical ideas. John Harley Warner has suggested that nature-trusting doctors drew criticism from other doctors because the former were seen to undermine the social position of the latter by denying the utility of their procedures, which mostly relied on drug medication.[61] Lane was clearly aware that the factionalism surrounding the Medical Act involved not only medical politics but also medical theory and philosophy, as seen in his praise of Williams's recognition of the value of hydropathy:

> It is gratifying to recognise the love of truth which, in an age of transition, with all its perplexities and jealousies, prompted the writer fairly to admit, even so far, the existence of a scientific and highly curative principle in a system of therapeutics hitherto considered as rank quackery by the professors of what has been termed par excellence legitimate medicine.[62]

Lane's attitude towards the medical market is most obviously expressed in his view of the Medical Act 1858. Regarding heterodox medical ideas and systems, he wrote: "It is hardly necessary to state that the provisions of the New Medical Act are a boon, and will be a protection, to the practitioners of Hydropathy, as well as every other branch of Medicine."[63] This is where his opinion of the Act differed from that of contemporary general practitioners, who were concerned about the threat posed by heterodox healing systems. Lane looked forward to the day "when all such designations will no longer be needed [...] and when under the wholesome influences of a more mature reflection [...] and, above all, a more enlightened professional candour, the whole medical world will be united together."[64] "When that day does arrive," he stated, "reconciliation [...] shall have been realized," and "the simple term *physician* may be held sufficient to designate a qualified member of the medical profession."[65]

Although he mentioned unification, Lane's medical view was not monistic. The ideal medical market for him was not a place where the winner monopolized all medical philosophies and theories under the name of unification. Rather, Lane's ultimate goal was to protect medical professionals' autonomy regarding their theories, philosophies and practices: "It may be left to the judgment and discretion of each such member to treat his patients to the best of his conscientious conviction, without incurring thereby the jealousy [...] of his fellow-practitioners, and without being dubbed by some narrow and quasi characteristic title supposed to represent his particular *pathy*."[66] For him, the ideal medical market and medical profession were characterized more by reconciliation and mutual tolerance than by uniformity.

Lane's strategies in the market of medical philosophies

Lane's broad definition of medical art also reflected his view of the medical market. He argued that "the term [medical art] must be held to include every species of attempt to modify or control disease, whether such attempt consist in the administration of powerful drugs, or [...] the systematic use of all those natural agents which we group together under the one title of hygiene."[67] As already mentioned, medical historians have hardly studied the marketplace from the perspective of the intellectual history of medicine. However, medical theories and philosophies are at the core of the medical market. As Roy Porter put it, "sufferers are fertile in their resources,"[68] but patient choice was restricted by the hegemony of certain medical philosophies in the medical market.

In mid-century Britain, the medical market was a battle field between competing medical philosophies.[69] Before the 1858 Act, the market had been almost completely free.[70] Medical knowledge and philosophy published in books enabled their authors to establish their reputations within medical circles and the public. As Porter has noted, "popularization" had a significant role in the medical enterprise.[71] Heterodox healing ideas were more organized and systematic than ever before.[72] Healers were armed with rational doctrines, moral earnestness and were associated with a wide range of political causes from conservatism to atheism.[73] It was also not always easy to distinguish heterodox practitioners from regular practitioners, given the ambiguity of medical orthodoxy at the time.[74]

Lane considered public education about hygiene as necessary for the acceptance of his hygienic ideas by medical professionals, since he believed that patients who received physiological education would choose professionals whose approach was hygienic. He was convinced that "when the clear and broad doctrine of hygienic medicine have once fairly been taken hold of by the public at large, woe to the practitioner who fails to give them their due weight in the rationale of his medical treatment."[75] This strategy regarding medical knowledge differed overtly from that of the physicians of the previous century, for whom medical knowledge was something to be "kept as trade secrets" rather than shared with "professional rivals" in the competition for patronage from the higher classes.[76]

Lane seemed optimistic about the future of the medical market, as can be seen in his expectation that physiological instruction would soon take "a systematic form as a necessary branch in the curriculum of an ordinary education."[77] The situation of the book market may also have encouraged him. The constant decline in book prices resulted in low-price books (3s 6d or under) dominating the market from the mid-1850s, allowing a wider public than ever before to enter the book market.[78] In addition, as Terrence Nevett noted, the nineteenth-century market evolved from a seller and product orientation towards a buyer and sales orientation, which might also have encouraged Lane to invest more in advertisements (see Figures 10.1 and 10.2).[79]

Lane actively advertised his book, which was published not long after the abolition of the duties on advertisements (1853) and newspapers (1855).[80] Regarding the low number of advertisements of hydropathic books during the late 1850s and early 1860s, the frequency with which Lane advertised his book was outstanding. Particularly in intellectual magazines, such as *The Athenaeum* and *The Saturday Review*, Lane might have been the hydropath whose name appeared most frequently. The second edition was advertised in a wide range of media, from *The Times* and *The Athenaeum* to *Bell's Life in London and Sporting Chronicle*[81] and *The Malvern Advertiser*. In contrast, he hardly ever advertised in major medical periodicals.

Lane's professional arguments in his book and his efforts to promote his medical ideas among the public might also be related to his desire to establish his position in medical circles. As Mark Weatherall has indicated, the meaning of the medical discourse at the time was significant for physicians, who were cautious not to express differences of medical opinion "in less than erudite terms."[82] Although Lane held heterodoxical views, he was a promising young physician with good networks in intellectual circles when he graduated from the Edinburgh medical school.[83] He may have been looking for ways to put forward his hygienic medical system in authoritative and logical terms, and therefore painstakingly combined his prescriptive and vitalist concepts with the latest patho-physiological knowledge. In this respect, Lane's philosophical and theoretical arguments presented a combination of professional and plebeian elements. His plea for reconciliation may have been an attempt to appeal to a wider range of doctors.

Lane's involvement in a well-known divorce case heard in the London Court for Divorce in June 1858 severely tainted his social reputation and

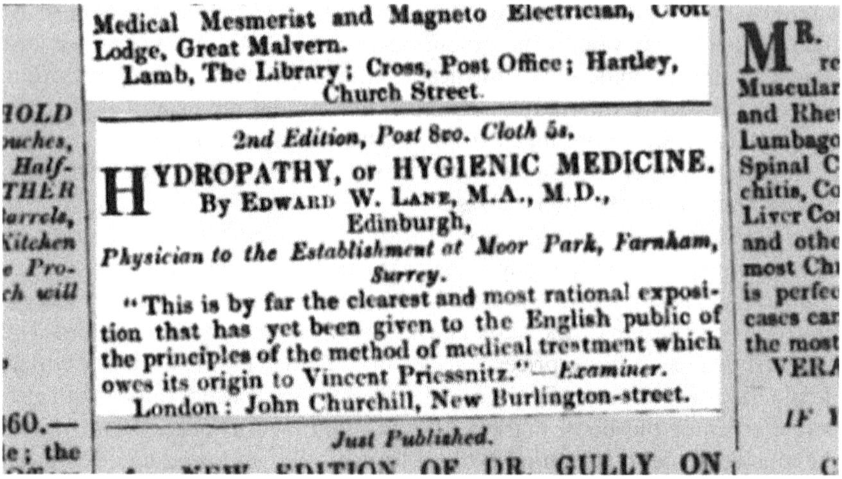

Medical Mesmerist and Magneto Electrician, Croft
Lodge, Great Malvern.
Lamb, The Library; Cross, Post Office; Hartley,
Church Street.

2nd Edition, Post 8vo. Cloth 5s.

HYDROPATHY, or HYGIENIC MEDICINE.
By EDWARD W. LANE, M.A., M.D.,
Edinburgh,

*Physician to the Establishment at Moor Park, Farnham,
Surrey.*

" This is by far the clearest and most rational exposition that has yet been given to the English public of
the principles of the method of medical treatment which
owes its origin to Vincent Priessnitz."—*Examiner.*
London : John Churchill, New Burlington-street.

Just Published.

Figure 10.1 An advertisement for E.W. Lane's 1859 book in the *Malvern Advertiser* on 5
May 1860. This is one of the last advertisements showing the name of his Moor
Park establishment. He began to advertise his new Sudbrook Park establishment only two weeks later. The *Malvern Advertiser* (1855–1907) was founded
by a hydropath in Great Malvern, Dr Ralph Barnes Grindrod (1811–1883)
and was rivalled in Great Malvern by the *Malvern News*, launched by Dr James
Gully in 1860.

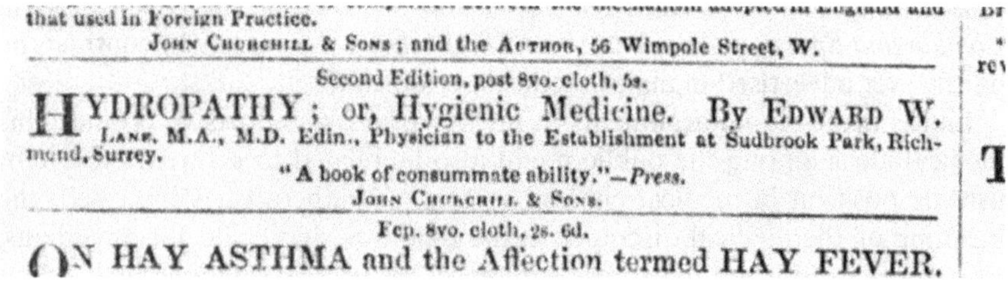

JOHN CHURCHILL & SONS ; and the AUTHOR, 56 Wimpole Street, W.

Second Edition, post 8vo. cloth, 5s.

HYDROPATHY ; or, Hygienic Medicine. By EDWARD W.
LANE, M.A., M.D. Edin., Physician to the Establishment at Sudbrook Park, Rich-
mond, Surrey.
" A book of consummate ability."—*Press.*
JOHN CHURCHILL & SONS.

Fcp. 8vo. cloth, 2s. 6d.

ON HAY ASTHMA and the Affection termed HAY FEVER.

Figure 10.2 One of the last advertisements for E.W. Lane's 1859 book, published in *The
Saturday Review* on 22 May 1869.

influenced the view of the media on his hygienic medicine.[84] The patterns of
the advertisement for the first and second editions of his book were similar
but the reduction in the number of media reviews of his second edition might
have been one of the signs of his tainted reputation. The reviews in medical
journals were mostly less favourable than those in the general media, while
some of the latter were misleading because the reviewers had misunderstood
Lane's ideas. The reaction of the former group was marked less by criticism

than by lack of interest in understanding his book, attributable to a variety of reasons, including differences in theoretical and philosophical perspectives.

Conclusion

Within the interventionism of medicine and the reductionism of hygiene in the second half of the nineteenth century, Lane promoted hygienic medicine. He attempted to medicalize hygiene, which was increasingly treated as an element external to orthodox medicine. He painstakingly accommodated modern pathological findings in the theorization of hygiene, although his view was contrasted with the trend of medical hygiene in the latter period of the century, in which the concept of hygiene was reduced to pathological infection control. Lane's naturalistic and Romantic medical beliefs, which led him to hygiene and hydropathy, also led him to face the reality of the medical profession and the medical market.

Lane defined medicine in a broad and comprehensive way regarding what he called a "large reform in medicine." He hoped that more medical professionals would change their minds and adopt the principles of hygienic medicine. Following Lane, I also took a broad perspective of the medical market to analyse Lane's view of the Medical Act 1858. The ideal picture of the medical market for Lane was a place where the autonomy of medical professionals regarding their medical theories, philosophies and practices were protected in the spirit of medical reconciliation and mutual respect. From Lane's perspective of the market of medical philosophies, both pursuing reform in medicine and establishing his reputation as a physician were based on the professional and lay recognition of his medical theory and philosophy. In promoting his idea of hygienic medicine, Lane relied almost entirely on advertising his book, but he did not sufficient attention from the media, particularly medical journals, whose views on hygiene and medicine differed from Lane's.

Few people today remember the name of E.W. Lane, or his Hygienic Medicine. Today, reductionism prevails in medicine and other scientific fields and we no longer seem to appreciate the value of natural wind and fresh air for our health, instead relying heavily on the comfort from closed windows and chemical products. Although doctors emphasize the importance of washing hands, brushing teeth and regular check-ups, a "hygienic" way of life still seems to be missing from most people's daily lives and today's monopolized medical market.

Notes

1 Wear 1993; Rosenberg 2003; Smith 2007; Bergdolt 2008.
2 Weisz 2003.
3 Whorton 1978 and 2000; Reiser 1985; Wear 1993; Thomson 2001; Rosenberg 2003.

4 Marland and Adams 2009.
5 Adams 2015.
6 Loudon 1985; Porter 1986; Cook 1986.
7 Loudon 1986; Digby 1994; Davies 1996; Davies 1999; Loeb 2001; Jenner and Wallis 2007; Ueyama 2010.
8 Loudon 1986, 3–6. Loudon argued that the compulsory registrations and educational standards were critical in professional unification.
9 Pickstone 2006, 306; Wear 1992, 8.
10 Jenner and Wallis 2007, 3.
11 Ibid., 16.
12 Cant and Sharma 1998.
13 Inkster 1977; Gieryn 1983.
14 Brown 1987; Winter 1997.
15 Bradley and Dupree 2003.
16 Lawrence and Weisz 1998. In terms of etiology, medical holism can be associated with identifying disease as a general disorder with underlying fundamental causes, whereas reductionism focuses on histopathological findings and anatomical localizations.
17 Regenmortel and Hull 2002; Reiss and Ankeny 2016; Marcum 2008.
18 Lawrence and Weisz 1998, 1.
19 Albala 2002, 115; García-Ballester 1993.
20 Coleman 1974.
21 Niebyl 1971, 492.
22 Hardy 1983.
23 Bynum 1979, 108–10.
24 Hamlin 1994, 140.
25 Ackerknecht 1948.
26 Cassedy 1962; Broich 2013.
27 Crook 2016, 247.
28 Smith 2007, 264, 55; Cant and Sharma 1998.
29 Wear 1993, 1303.
30 Morris 1976; Durey 1979.
31 Crook 2016, 245–86. He considered that such changes accompanied changes in the other sphere of hygiene which became centralized and bureaucratic than ever before.
32 Thomson 2001.
33 Marland and Adams 2009, 503.
34 Price 1981.
35 Walton 1983.
36 Browne 1990. The number of hydropathic establishments in Britain was between 20 and 30 by that time.
37 Bradley and Dupree 2003, 174.
38 Price 1981, 279. Such a tendency began to grow explicitly from the 1870s.
39 Metcalfe 1906; McMenemey 1952; Price 1981; Brown 1991.
40 Barrow 1991, 174.
41 The term "hygienic medicine" appeared many times in the first edition although it was not the title.
42 Rosenberg 1977; Lawrence 1985; Warner 1986; Bynum 1994; Weatherall 1996; Worboys 2011: Carter 2012.

43 Wyhe 2004.
44 Wear 1993,164.
45 Lane 1859, 69.
46 Magner 2002, 197.
47 Whorton 2002, 12.
48 Quoted in Lane 1859, 134.
49 Smith 1987.
50 Poggi and Bossi 1994.
51 Smith 1987, 187.
52 Lane 1859, 157.
53 Ibid., 94.
54 Ibid., 133.
55 Davenport-Hines 2004.
56 Lane 1859, 139.
57 Ibid., 141, 142.
58 Ibid., 144.
59 Ibid.
60 Saks 2002; Harrison et al. 2002; Larkin 1995. Sociologists have awarded special
    meanings to this event as the first state intervention in the division of labour in any
    occupation.
61 Warner 1977.
62 Lane 1859, 113.
63 Ibid., 15.
64 Ibid., 18, 19.
65 Ibid., 19.
66 Ibid.
67 Ibid., 129.
68 Porter 1985.
69 Bradley and Dupree argued that "therapeutics were one of the most important
    battlegrounds of mid-nineteenth century medicine." See Bradley and Dupree
    2003, 180.
70 Pickstone 2006.
71 Porter 1992, 2.
72 Bivins 2007, 35.
73 Lawrence 1994, 37, 38.
74 Winter 1997, 26.
75 Lane 1859, 146.
76 Jewson 1974.
77 Lane 1859, 145.
78 Eliot 2007.
79 Nevett 1982, 42–49. Nevett associated this market evolution with the removal of
    the stamp duty on newspaper advertising in the mid-nineteenth century.
80 Hewitt 2013.
81 *Bell's Life in London and Sporting Chronicle* (1822–86) was a weekly magazine
    that introduced general news and sports, particularly famous for its reports on
    horse-racing. In the mid-1850s, its circulation was at its peak (about 30,000 copies
    a week).
82 Weatherall 1996, 177.

83 Sato 1978.
84 Regarding the divorce case, see Colp 1981 and Allan 2010.

References

Ackerknecht, Erwin H. 1948. "Hygiene in France, 1815–1848." *Bulletin of the History of Medicine* 22: 117.
Adams, Jane M. 2015. *Healing with Water: English Spas and the Water Cure, 1840–1960*. Manchester: Manchester University Press.
Albala, Ken. 2002. *Eating Right in the Renaissance*. Berkeley, CA: University of California Press.
Allan, Janice M. 2010. "Mrs Robinson's 'Day-Book of Iniquity': Reading Bodies of/and Evidence in the Context of the 1858 Medical Reform Act." In *The Female Body in Medicine and Literature*, edited by G. Depledge A. Mangham, 169–81. Liverpool: Liverpool University Press.
Barrow, Logie. 1991. "Why Were Most Medical Heretics at Their Most Confident around the 1840s?" In *British Medicine in an Age of Reform*, edited by A. Wear R. French, 165–85. London: Routledge.
Bergdolt, Klaus. 2008 [1999]. *Wellbeing: A Cultural History of Healthy Living*. Translated by Jane Dewhurst. Cambridge: Polity Press.
Bivins, Roberta E. 2007. *Alternative Medicine? A History*. Oxford: Oxford University Press.
Bradley, James and Marguerite Dupree. 2003. "A Shadow of Orthodoxy? An Epistemology of British Hydropathy, 1840–1858." *Medical History* 47 (2): 173–94.
Broich, John. 2013. *London: Water and the Making of the Modern City*. Pittsburgh: University of Pittsburgh Press.
Brown, P.S. 1991. "Medically Qualified Naturopaths and the General Medical Council." *Medical History* 35 (1): 50–77.
Brown, P.S. 1987. "Social Context and Medical Theory in the Demarcation of Nineteenth-Century Boundaries." In *Medical Fringe and Medical Orthodoxy 1750–1850*, edited by W.F. Bynum and Roy Porter, 216–33. London: Croom Helm.
Browne, Janet. 1990. "Spas and Sensibilities: Darwin at Malvern." *Medical History* 34 (10): 102–13.
Bynum, William F. 1979. "Hospital, Disease and Community: The London Fever Hospital, 1801–1850." In *Healing and History: Essays for George Rosen*, edited by Charles E. Rosenberg, 97–115. New York and London: Dawson.
Bynum, William F. 1994. *Science and the Practice of Medicine in the Nineteenth Century*. Cambridge: Cambridge University Press.
Cant, Sarah and Ursula Sharma. 1998. *A New Medical Pluralism? Complementary Medicine, Doctors, Patients and the State*. London: Taylor & Francis.
Carter, K. Codell. 2012. *The Decline of Therapeutic Bloodletting and the Collapse of Traditional Medicine*. New Brunswick, NJ: Transaction Publishers.
Cassedy, James H. 1962. "Hygeia: A Mid-Victorian Dream of a City of Health." *Journal of the History of Medicine and Allied Sciences* 17 (2): 217–28.
Coleman, William. 1974. "Health and Hygiene in the 'Encyclopédie': A Medical Doctrine for the Bourgeoisie." *Journal of the History of Medicine and Allied Sciences* 29 (4): 399–421.

Colp, Jr. Ralph. 1981. "Charles Darwin, Dr. Edward Lane, and the 'Singular Trial' of Robinson V. Robinson and Lane." *Journal of the History of Medicine and Allied Sciences* 36 (2): 205–13.

Cook, Harold J. 1986. *The Decline of the Old Medical Regime in Stuart London*. Ithaca, NY: Cornell University Press.

Crook, Tom. 2016. *Governing Systems: Modernity and the Making of Public Health in England, 1830–1910*. Berkeley, CA: University of California Press.

Davenport-Hines, Richard. 2004. "Quain, Sir Richard, Baronet (1816–1898)." In *Oxford Dictionary of National Biography*. Oxford: Oxford University Press, 2004.

Davies, Owen. 1999. "Cunning-Folk in the Medical Market-Place During the Nineteenth Century." *Medical History* 43 (1): 55–73.

Davies, Owen. 1996. "Healing Charms in Use in England and Wales 1700–1950." *Folklore* 107: 19–32.

Digby, Anne. 1994. *Making a Medical Living: Doctors and Patients in the English Market for Medicine, 1720–1911*. Cambridge: Cambridge University Press.

Durey, Michael. 1979. *The Return of the Plague: British Society and the Cholera, 1831–32*. Dublin: Gil and Macmillan.

Eliot, Simon. 2007. "From Few and Expensive to Many and Cheap: The British Book Market 1800–1890." In *The Blackwell Companion to the History of the Book*, edited by Simon Eliot and Jonathan Rose, 291–302. Malden, MA: Wiley-Blackwell.

García-Ballester, Luis. 1993. "On the Origin of the 'Six Non-Natural Things' in Galen." *Sudhoffs Archiv; Zeitschrift fur Wissenschaftsgeschichte, Beiheft*, 32: 105–15.

Gieryn, Thomas F. 1983. "Boundary-Work and the Demarcation of Science from Non-Science: Strains and Interests in Professional Ideologies of Scientists." *American Sociological Review* 48 (6): 781–95.

Hamlin, Christopher. 1994. "State Medicine in Great Britain." In *The History of Public Health and the Modern State*, edited by Dorothy Porter, 132–64. Amsterdam: Rodopi.

Hardy, Anne. 1983. "The Medical Response to Epidemic Disease During the Long Eighteenth Century." *Medical History* 27: 111–38.

Harrison, Stephen, Michael Moran, and Bruce Wood. 2002. "Policy Emergence and Policy Convergence: The Case of 'Scientific-Bureaucratic Medicine' in the United States and United Kingdom." *The British Journal of Politics & International Relations* 4 (1): 1–24.

Hewitt, Martin. 2013. *The Dawn of the Cheap Press in Victorian Britain: The End of the 'Taxes on Knowledge', 1849–1869*. London: Bloomsbury Publishing.

Inkster, Ian. 1977. "Marginal Men: Aspects of the Social Role of the Medical Community in Sheffield, 1790–1850." In *Health Care and Popular Medicine in Nineteenth-Century England*, edited by John Woodward and David Richards, 128–64. London: Croom Helm.

Jenner, Mark and Patrick Wallis. 2007. "The Medical Marketplace." In *Medicine and the Market in Early Modern England and Its Colonies, c. 1450 – c. 1850*, edited by Mark Jenner and Patrick Wallis, 1–23. Basingstoke, UK: Palgrave Macmillan.

Jewson, Nicholas D. 1974. "Medical Knowledge and the Patronage System in 18th Century England." *Sociology* 8 (3): 369–85.

Lane, Edward. W. 1857. *Hydropathy: or the Natural System of Medical Treatment*. London: John Churchill.

Lane, Edward. W. 1859. Hydropathy: or, Hygienic Medicine. London: John Churchill.

Larkin, Gerry. 1995. "State Control and the Health Professions in the United Kingdom." In *Health Professions and the State in Europe*, edited by G. Larkin, T. Johnson and M. Saks, 25–30. London: Routledge.

Lawrence, Christopher. 1985. "Incommunicable Knowledge: Science, Technology and the Clinical Art in Britain 1850–1914." *Journal of Contemporary History* 20 (4): 503–20.

Lawrence, Christopher. 1994. *Medicine in the Making of Modern Britain, 1700–1920*. London: Routledge.

Lawrence, Christopher and George Weisz. 1998. "Medical Holism: The Context." In *Greater Than the Parts: Holism in Biomedicine, 1920–1950*, edited by George Weisz and Christopher Lawrence, 1–22. Oxford: Oxford University Press.

Loeb, Lori. 2001. "Doctors and Patent Medicines in Modern Britain: Professionalism and Consumerism." *Albion: A Quarterly Journal Concerned with British Studies* 33 (3): 404–25.

Loudon, Irvine. 1986. *Medical Care and the General Practitioner, 1750–1850*. Oxford: Clarendon Press.

Loudon, Irvine. 1985. "The Nature of Provincial Medical Practice in Eighteenth-Century England." *Medical History* 29 (1): 1–32.

Magner, Lois N. 2002. *A History of the Life Sciences*. Revised and expanded. London: CRC Press.

Marcum, James A. 2008. *An Introductory Philosophy of Medicine: Humanizing Modern Medicine*. Dordrecht: Springer.

Marland, Hilary and Jane Adams. 2009. "Hydropathy at Home: The Water Cure and Domestic Healing in Mid-Nineteenth-Century Britain." *Bulletin of the History of Medicine* 83 (3): 499–529.

McMenemey, William H. 1952. "The Water Doctors of Malvern, with Special Reference to the Years 1842 to 1872." *Proceedings of the Royal Society of Medicine* 46 (1): 5–12.

Metcalfe, Richard. 1906. *The Rise and Progress of Hydropathy in England and Scotland*. London: Simpkin, Marshall, Hamilton, Kent & Co..

Morris, Robert John. 1976. *Cholera 1832: The Social Response to an Epidemic*. London: Croom Helm.

Nevett, Terrence R. 1982. *Advertising in Britain: A History*. London: Heinemann, 1982.

Niebyl, Peter H. 1971. "The Non-Naturals." *Bulletin of the History of Medicine* 45 (5): 486–92.

Pickstone, John V. 2006. "Medicine, Society and the State." In *The Cambridge History of Medicine*, edited by Roy Porter, 260–97. Cambridge: Cambridge University Press.

Poggi, Stefano, and Maurizio Bossi. 1994. *Romanticism in Science: Science in Europe, 1790–1840*. London: Kluwer Academic Publishers.

Porter, Roy. 1985. "The Patient's View: Doing Medical History from Below." *Theory and Society* 14 (2): 175–98.

Porter, Roy. 1986. *Patients and Practitioners: Lay Perceptions of Medicine in Pre-Industrial Society*. Cambridge: Cambridge University Press.

Porter, Roy. 1992. *The Popularization of Medicine, 1650–1850*. London: Routledge.

Price, Robin. 1981. "Hydropathy in England 1840–70." *Medical History* 25 (3): 269–80.

Regenmortel, Marc V. and David L. Hull. 2002. *Promises and Limits of Reductionism in the Biomedical Sciences*. Chichester, UK: John Wiley & Sons, Ltd., 2002.

Reiser, Stanley J. 1985. "Responsibility for Personal Health: A Historical Perspective." *The Journal of Medicine and Philosophy* 10 (1): 7–17.
Reiss, Julian and Rachel A. Ankeny. 2016. "Philosophy of Medicine." In *The Stanford Encyclopedia of Philosophy*, edited by Edward N. Zalta. At https://plato.stanford.edu/archives/sum2016/entries/medicine/.
Rosenberg, Charles E. 2003. *Right Living: An Anglo-American Tradition of Self-Help Medicine and Hygiene*. Baltimore, MD: Johns Hopkins University Press.
Rosenberg, Charles E. 1977. "The Therapeutic Revolution: Medicine, Meaning, and Social Change in Nineteenth-Century America." *Perspectives in Biology and Medicine* 20 (4): 485–506.
Saks, Mike. 2002. *Orthodox and Alternative Medicine: Politics, Professionalization, and Health Care*. London: Sage.
Sato, Tomo. 1978. "E.W. Lane's Hydropathic Establishment at Moor Park." *Hitotsubashi Journal of Social Studies* 10 (1): 45–59.
Smith, Virginia. 2007. *Clean: A History of Personal Hygiene and Purity*. Oxford: Oxford University Press.
Smith, Virginia. 1987. "Physical Puritanism and Sanitary Science: Material and Immaterial Beliefs in Popular Physiology, 1650–1840." In *Medical Fringe and Medical Orthodoxy*, edited by William F. Bynum and Roy Porter, 174–97. London: Croom Helm.
Thomson, Elaine. 2001. "Physiology, Hygiene and the Entry of Women to the Medical Profession in Edinburgh C. 1869–C. 1900." *Studies in History and Philosophy of Biological and Biomedical Sciences* 32 (1): 105–26.
Ueyama, Takahiro. 2010. *Health in the Marketplace: Professionalism, Therapeutic Desires, and Medical Commodification in Late-Victorian London*. Palo Alto, CA: Society for the Promotion of Science and Scholarship.
Walton, John K. 1983. *The English Seaside Resort: A Social History, 1750–1914*. Leicester: Leicester University Press.
Warner, John H. 1977. "'The Nature-Trusting Heresy': American Physicians and the Concept of the Healing Power of Nature in the 1850s and 1860s." *Perspectives in American History* 11: 291–324.
Warner, John H. 1986. *The Therapeutic Perspective: Medical Practice, Knowledge, and Identity in America, 1820–1885*. Cambridge, MA: Harvard University Press.
Wear, Andrew. 1993. "The History of Personal Hygiene." In *Companion Encyclopedia of the History of Medicine* Vol. 2, edited by William F. Bynum and Roy Porter, 1283–1308. London: Routledge.
Wear, Andrew. 1992. *Medicine in Society: Historical Essays*. Cambridge: Cambridge University Press.
Weatherall, Mark W. 1996. "Making Medicine Scientific: Empiricism, Rationality, and Quackery in Mid-Victorian Britain." *Social History of Medicine* 9 (2): 175–94.
Weisz, George. 2003. "The Emergence of Medical Specialization in the Nineteenth Century." *Bulletin of the History of Medicine* 77 (3): 536–75.
Whorton, James C. 1978. "The Hygiene of the Wheel: An Episode in Victorian Sanitary Science." *Bulletin of the History of Medicine* 52 (1): 61–88.
Whorton, James C. 2000. *Inner Hygiene: Constipation and the Pursuit of Health in Modern Society*. Oxford: Oxford University Press.
Whorton, James C. 2002. *Nature Cures: The History of Alternative Medicine in America*. Oxford: Oxford University Press.

Winter, Alison. 1997. "The Construction of Orthodoxies and Heterodoxies in the Early Victorian Life Sciences." In *Victorian Science in Context*, edited by B. Lightman, 24–50. London: University of Chicago Press.

Worboys, Michael. 2011. "Practice and the Science of Medicine in the Nineteenth Century." *Isis* 102 (1): 109–15.

Wyhe, John van. 2004. *Phrenology and the Origins of Victorian Scientific Naturalism.* Aldershot: Ashgate.

Chapter 11

From the local to the global, from the environment to the individual

Epidemiological knowledge production and changing notions of public health

Mikko Jauho

Introduction

Epidemiology is a science that studies the patterns and determinants of health and disease in populations.[1] The physical environment is one of the determinants of health. Epidemiological knowledge occupies a key position in health policy measures and illness prevention. It shapes policy decisions and guides practices to control diseases and promote health. The problems, concepts and methods of epidemiology have gone through profound changes during the long twentieth century.[2] Studying the different shapes that epidemiology has taken in different eras is crucial when thinking about the shifting relationship between public health and the environment.

This chapter illustrates empirically this change between paradigms in epidemiology. It elucidates a shift in epidemiology and public health from a holistic approach steeped in localism to a more global, targeted and individualized approach. This had important consequences for the way the environment has been thematized in public health. For lack of available space, and to make the point succinctly, the chapter concentrates on examples from only two epidemiological eras: late nineteenth-century sanitary science and post-Second World War chronic disease epidemiology. The first case acts as a contrast to highlight the features of the latter case, which belongs to the current paradigm.

The chapter draws on ideas from Science and Technology Studies, which have highlighted the *performativity* of research methods and approaches,[3] such as population surveys,[4] censuses,[5] opinion polls,[6] and epidemiological risk modelling.[7] Performativity means that the scientific assumptions, methods and models generated by experts and employed by other professional actors affect the phenomena they purport to describe. Scientific practices do not simply describe (aspects of) the world, but enact these into being. This is not an easy task, but conditional on a vast network of practices that support the facts enacted by the methods and models. In this sense, epidemiology is much more than a vehicle for representation; rather, it enacts into being its objects, such as population groups, notions of environment and the ways the latter influences the health of the former. As public health is essentially a practical science – knowledge production typically takes place in order to make a difference regarding the health status of the population – representing and intervening go together. Populations are counted and classified to make them governable.[8] This makes epidemiology "a tool of political intervention"[9] to regulate and transform populations, which are enacted in these very practices of counting and classifying.[10]

Epidemiological eras and paradigm shifts

Mervyn and Ezra Susser have provided an outline of the history of epidemiology, dividing its evolution in the last two centuries into three eras, each characterized by its own medical paradigm. In each era, the relationship to the environment is configured differently in terms of relevant ways of addressing it for the sake of public health. The first era, that of *sanitary statistics,* is characterized by the attempts of medical doctors and public health activists in the nineteenth century to account for the immense death toll of urban poverty with the help of statistical research. The key paradigm guiding these activities was the theory of *miasma*, poisoning caused by foul emanations from contaminated soil, air or water. The preferred public health measures resulting from this approach – such as the building of drainage and sewage systems, garbage collection and public sanitation, better housing, food inspection, and urban planning accentuating fresh air, sunlight and green areas – all centred on the environment. These activities were typically characterized by a social outlook, and scientific studies and reform work often went together.[11]

The second era, *infectious disease epidemiology*, emerged in the late nineteenth century and dominated the first half of the twentieth century. Its paradigm, *germ theory*, focused on bacteria, defined as necessary causes for singular diseases. This paradigm accentuated laboratory research (isolating and culturing strains, experimenting with transmission and disease reproduction), but not so much epidemiology, although experimental epidemiological bacteriology was one line of work.[12] Prevention concentrated on interrupting transmission by isolating affected individuals through quarantine and institutionalization, by vaccination and antibacterial treatments (ultimately antibiotics). Initially, the paradigm supported the old sanitary approach, since it was believed that germs thrived in unsanitary conditions, making the cleaning of the environment a crucial activity. Ultimately, however, bacteriology came to undermine the sanitary project of public hygiene, which resulted in the relative devaluation of the role of the environment vis-à-vis health, as the focus of preventive activities fastened on the capacity of individual bodies to transmit and resist infection.[13]

The third and most recent era in Sussers' model is *chronic disease epidemiology*, dominating from the middle of the twentieth century onwards. Its rise relates to the epidemiological transition, a shift in the disease spectrum from infectious to chronic degenerative diseases in the industrialized countries after the Second World War. Chronic disease epidemiology is risk factor epidemiology, as it focuses on the "risk ratio of exposure to outcome at individual level in populations."[14] Susser and Susser call the corresponding paradigm a *"black box."* Thus, strictly speaking, it is not a medical paradigm, but rather denotes the absence of one, as chronic disease epidemiology tends to relate exposures to outcomes without necessarily having any definitive knowledge of the intervening factors or underlying pathological processes. Hence, this is a truly statistical approach, characterized by the identification of potential risk factors through the correlation of exposures with outcomes in an endless calculative game. The primary mode of practice in this era is the control of risk factors by modifying either the individual lifestyle (e.g. dietary or exercising habits) or the environment (e.g. pollution or passive smoking) to protect the individual.

During these epidemiological eras, a major change in the practices of knowledge production on population health took place. More traditional data collection on different aspects of public health and healthcare was augmented by new research approaches and formal decision-making models, which relied on novel statistical methods. While vital statistics centre on calculation, mathematical statistics are analytical in nature.[15] The former focuses on describing and correlating variables extracted from statistical data with the help of averages and other simple indicators, whereas the latter designs randomized experiments and generates samples that are analysed through the concept of variation.[16] Facilitating this shift in methodology were changes in the social organization of medical research and care in the West after the Second World War.[17] The state took a more pronounced role in health policy, which increased demand for statistical information on population characteristics. The size of research institutes, hospitals, and pharmaceutical companies grew and the links between them deepened. New complex problems and issues arose, such as understanding the causes of common chronic diseases, systematically assessing the effects of the drugs being developed, and controlling and "standardizing" the work of medical professionals, which provided the concrete contexts for the methodological advances.[18]

Yet, Susser and Susser's model crucially highlights how the development of epidemiology and thus public health cannot be reduced to the evolution of research methods. The notion of paradigm[19] reminds us that the history of public health is not linear, but has gone through shifts and ruptures that have reordered the ideas, approaches and models for what constitutes legitimate contributions to the field among the involved community of practitioners. This has affected the ways the environment has been inserted into public health calculations at different points in time.

The two cases

To highlight the effect of paradigmatic shifts in epidemiology on conceptualizations of the environment in public health, the chapter focuses on two major Finnish medical studies from two different points in time: one belonging to the era of sanitary science, the other to chronic disease epidemiology. The first study is Konrad Relander's (1992) doctoral dissertation *Terveydenhoidollisia tutkimuksia Haapajärven piirilääkäripiirissä, osa 1* [Studies on Health Care in the Haapajärvi Medical District, part 1], prepared while working as a district physician in the area and originally published in 1892. He Relander presented it as the first part of a larger series of studies covering the entire medical district but a follow-up never materialized. The hostile reception given to the work probably contributed to this. One member of his dissertation evaluation committee suggested the rejection of the work due to poor scientific standards. The background to this reaction is somewhat obscure. According to Karisto and Lahelma,[20] this may have been due to Relander giving the data collection to a layperson, his focus on perceived illness rather than confirmed medical diagnoses by physicians or mortality data, or his political convictions, which were not shared by all members of the evaluation committee. It is true that the work is somewhat of an outlier when compared to mainstream public health research in Finland at the time. This research typically focused on mortality, connecting it to a limited number of factors. Methodologically, it this mainstream research was often quite rudimentary, presenting straightforward comparisons of simple ratios.[21] Neither did Relander manage to recruit many followers as a researcher. The most notable exception is Constantin Tennberg's dissertation on tuberculosis in Pietarsaari, which also focused on one locality and adopted a similar broad cultural-ecological approach.[22] Relander's study points both backward and forward. On the one hand, it is committed to sanitary science, a doctrine soon to be superseded. Some aspects of the study even echo the old German tradition of state science ("statistics"), which focused on a comprehensive description of a specific geographical area. On the other hand, it contained fresh methodological ideas, only established later, such as examining self-reported morbidity and looking for correlations. Today, it has been canonized as a landmark in Finnish health research, and it has been suggested that it would have been "a classic in English."[23]

The other example is the North Karelia Project (NKP), a community intervention project to control cardiovascular problems launched in the county of North Karelia in Eastern Finland in 1972.[24] Finland was notorious for its high levels of coronary heart disease (CHD) mortality among middle-aged men, regularly leading international statistical comparisons in the 1950s and 1960s. Peculiar to the Finnish situation was a clear east–west difference in mortality,[25] North Karelia in the east being the area with the highest numbers. Unlike previous intervention studies, NKP was directed at the whole population of the area instead of only high-risk groups. Its aim was to affect CHD morbidity and mortality by changing the culture of the local community. The primary target were three key risk factors: smoking, elevated serum cholesterol and high blood pressure. In addition, NKP promoted early detection, treatment and rehabilitation of people at risk of or suffering from heart disease in the community. Part public health intervention and service development, part epidemiological study, NKP was an "evidence-making intervention,"[26] containing a strong research aspect. The neighbouring county of Kuopio served as control in the intervention trial design. Unlike in the first case, where Relander's single monograph presented the results, NKP produced a multitude of publications, which still continue today. Also, following modern principles of teamwork, authorship is of a more collective nature compared to the first case, although Pekka Puska, the principal researcher of the project, is the key person. The initial plan was to have a five-year project, starting in 1972, but a greatly expanded and modified NKP was officially terminated only in 1997. In this chapter, I concentrate on the first phase of NKP (1972–1977), and on its evaluation report.[27]

I have selected the studies, first, based on their importance in the national context. Both occupy significant positions in the history of Finnish public health research, which means that there exists ample secondary literature on them. However, while only specialists are familiar with the former, the latter is famous both nationally and internationally.[28] Moreover, as explained in more detail below, both studies are committed to geographically limited locations, which is important when comparing different approaches to the environment. Both address a specific community, Haapajärvi or North Karelia, albeit of different size. However, while Relander looks holistically at the impact of the environmental and cultural characteristics of a geographical area on individual health, Puska and associates harness specific aspects of the environment to change a limited number of clearly demarcated individual risk factors for cardiovascular disease.[29] Relander's focus is on general morbidity, whereas Puska and associates address more circumscribed disease patterns, CHD and stroke. Puska et al. include – even stress – the role of social environment in their community intervention, whereas Relander does not account for the influence of social interaction on aspects facilitating morbidity.

Certain discrepancies between the studies are inevitable. As mentioned above, statistical methods developed dramatically from the late nineteenth century to the 1970s, in terms of both the availability and generation of data and the sophistication of analytical tools. Major changes also took place in disease spectrum, medical science and the scope and structure of health services. The latter study represents the contemporary way of conducting epidemiological research. Its approach is familiar to us, even self-evident, while the former is partly alien and belongs to a time that has already disappeared. By placing the two studies side by side, we can shed light on the specifics of what we are familiar with and unravel the obvious.

1892: The lone doctor mapping his district

Konrad Relander (1853–1936, since 1907 Konrad ReijoWaara[30]) was a medical doctor and a versatile public health activist. He was an advocate of the national cause before and after Finnish independence in 1917 and a popular educator who believed, in equal measure, in scientific medicine and Christian guidance in the realization of human health and well-being. During his career, he acted as the editor-in-chief of the first Finnish-language medical journal *Duodecim* from 1885 to 1891, as the physician at the Kymi factory from 1885 to 1887, and as the district physician in a number of areas (Haapavesi 1887–1892, Oulu 1892–1904, and the capital Helsinki 1904–1926). He served as a spokesperson for the bourgeoisie during the 1897, 1899 and 1900 sessions of the Assembly of the Estates, where he participated in the development of healthcare legislation, chairing the first Committee on Rural Health, which submitted its report in 1892. His life's work was *Terveydenhoitolehti*, a popular health education magazine, which offered advice on healthcare for the common people in their native Finnish language at a time when Swedish was the dominant intellectual language. Relander was responsible for the magazine from 1889–1920, contributing countless articles from various fields of health care and medicine.[31]

The driving force behind Relander's research was the desire to examine the health conditions of his own community where he worked as district physician. The more general quest to prevent disease and improve public health in Finland also motivated his work. According to Relander, this would require comparative data from different parts of the country to identify areas of poor health and to target measures on the most salient health determinants.

> When beginning to put into practice the principles of health care in a community, one must know the circumstances, the habits of the community, and, if possible, the general health of the people. // However, it would be necessary for similar information to be found in several other locations so that, by comparing data from different locations, it could be reliably assured as to whether the general health in one location, when compared to others, is in desperate need of repair or not, and which conditions are first and foremost to be ameliorated.[32]

Despite his local focus, Relander thus strove to generalize knowledge, so that it was comparable across sites. His "politics of knowledge" pursued a programme that would use comprehensive, systematically collected and, if possible, numerical data from across the country as a means of arguing for health policy reforms vis-à-vis those in power at both national and local level. However, as a singular example of such studies, Relander's dissertation rather attests to the problems of holistic localism for comparative purposes, as will be described below.

Relander had already started to emphasize the importance of such information production a few years earlier. From 1886, he published several articles[33] in *Duodecim* that encouraged young doctors to study the people's lives in rural areas, and record and publish their findings. He sketched out guidelines on what to look for in such a description and suggested a scholarship scheme to cover travel expenses. He also proposed that the Medical Board could hire specialized medical doctors for the task. According to him, the responsibility for producing the information ultimately rested with the district physicians, who had come to focus on treating the sick instead of their primary task: overseeing and promoting public health. District physicians were to be assisted by lay inspectors who would gather basic information under physician guidance. Relander stressed how important it was for physicians to get to know the people. In addition to being acquainted with their clientele, a political motive can also be discerned: bringing together the educated classes and the people in a spirit of nationalistic unity that would solve class antagonisms in a peaceful manner through education and co-operation. Another noteworthy emphasis was his interest in rural conditions. The countryside was often left behind on the public health agenda, because cities had more health problems and were better monitored. The model for the data collection came from Sweden, where district physician activists had presented similar projects a few years earlier. Unlike in Sweden, where the plans also featured racial measurements, Relander focused on the hygienic study of living conditions and habits. The dissertation can be regarded as a concrete example of the implementation of this programme.

Relander's approach relied on a comprehensive survey of a specific area. Following the principles of his programme, Relander hired a local layperson, the district inoculator, to collect data, performing only random checks himself. He also prepared the questionnaire used by the data collector and, in order to persuade suspicious locals to participate, a handout which explained the purpose of the study.

In the dissertation, Relander focused mainly on the relationship between housing conditions and morbidity, particularly that between bedroom volume and chronic disease or, in his terms, "long-term illness or cases of prolonged poor health and pain (*kivuloisuus*)."[34] To this end, he first calculated the number of living rooms and bedrooms available to the occupants and, in the case of bedrooms, the cubic volume and height of the rooms. He was also interested in the relationship between window size and living space, but information on this was too sparse for detailed consideration. Relander extracted from the hygiene literature minimum standards for the number of sleepers per bedroom (two adults and one child), bedroom height (2.4 m), cubic volume per sleeper ($10.5m^3$), and the ratio of the living room window size to floor area (1:12) and room volume (1:30), using these as benchmarks for the salubriousness of the housing conditions. The premise, familiar from the science of hygiene, was that overcrowding and the quality of living quarters, especially ventilation and the amount of sunlight, significantly affected individual health.

Second, Relander defined for the population of the area in question a specific "rate of poor health and pain (kivuloisuusprosentti)", which was the proportion of the population affected by chronic conditions. Among them were "prolonged heart defect (*sydänala-vika*), aches, cough, headache, or other prolonged pain (*kivuloisuus*)."[35] The study quoted but excluded acute diseases, as well as mental illnesses. The examination of chronic symptoms and poor health can be regarded as a novelty, because typically statistical health studies of the era focused on mortality or, if the subject was morbidity, on the few items listed in official disease classifications.[36]

In analysing the results, Relander used three variables to categorize his data. The most important of these was the area.

> In my calculations I have divided the municipality in 10 different areas in order to find out if there are large enough differences in bedroom circumstances and possibly in other circumstances between individual village groups of the municipality that these differences could give even hints to the causes that make the overall health position of the people in some parts of the municipality worse than in others.[37]

At the heart of each of the ten areas was one or more villages. Yet the final area division was based on a kind of overall cultural-geographical assessment of the municipality, which was of qualitative nature and required good prior knowledge of it. The study does not provide a detailed justification for the division, although it accounted for at least the wealth and cleanliness or probity of the inhabitants. The population in each area then was divided into two groups according to general housing standard, the first consisting of members of the gentry and farm owners (Group 1), and the second of crofters, cotters, and workers and servants (*huonekuntalainen*) (Group 2). The third key variable was gender. At some points, Relander also structured his data by age, distinguishing between infants (<1 year), young children (1–10 years), and adults (over 10 years).

The results revealed quite inadequate housing conditions. According to Relander's calculations, in Group 1, 42.7% of the bedrooms exceeded the norm for the number of persons (three persons), 36.9% were below the volume standard (10.5 m^3 per person), and 64.5% were below the height standard (2.4 m). For Group 2, the figures were 57.9%, 69.5%, and 88.9%, respectively. Crofters etc. lived in significantly more crowded conditions compared to members of the gentry and farm owners, but also the housing conditions of the latter left much to be desired.

Relander calculated chronic pain (*kivuloisuus*) rates by area for the different ages, genders and social groups. In the whole municipality, 17% of the population suffered from some sort of chronic condition. Women and persons in Group 2 were sicker than average, men and the better off were correspondingly healthier. Children were healthier than average; when the minors (<10 year olds) were excluded from the analysis, the morbidity increased.

The main outcome of the study concerned the impact of housing conditions on morbidity. For the purpose of analysis, Relander ranked the examined areas from the lowest per cent of chronic pain to the highest, and compared the resulting series against the proportion of the population living in crowded conditions in the areas. All three indicators for poor housing were accounted for, and the data also were analysed according to age, gender and class. In Relander's reasoning, the more similar two series were, i.e. the numbers for the different areas increased side by side in the same ranking order, the greater the interdependence between variables. Relander thought he had found such a correspondence between the cubic volume of the bedrooms and chronic pain. Although left implicit, the results suggested that providing more housing space would have a beneficial effect on people's health.

However, even with regard to Relander's main finding, the chronic pain rates were only directly proportional to the housing conditions if he ignored four of the ten areas in his analysis. In explaining these anomalies and justifying their exclusion, he utilized the other material in his dissertation. In addition to the aforementioned issues, Relander provided an overview of the geographical characteristics and climate of Haapajärvi; the grouping and construction of residential and outbuildings and the soil beneath them; the layout and physical properties of living quarters, in particular light, ventilation and heating; interior and yard cleanliness and waste management; personal hygiene; food, drink and meal patterns; and clothing, including underwear. Drunkenness, morality and sectarianism got their own chapter in the book, as did livelihoods, including wages and salaries, indebtedness and care for the poor. Relander considered that sectarianism warded off drunkenness, a major vice for a Christian health apostle, and considered the situation in Haapavesi to be quite good in this respect, as over a third of the inhabitants were "Laestadians, i.e. religious fanatics (*hihhuleita*)."[38] He used these observations to explain why some areas deviated from the relationship between overcrowding and chronic conditions. Thus, for example, in the area formed by Lehonsaari, Nevalanmäki and Kytökylä, "the population is less prone to cleanliness [...] and drunkenness is more prevalent [...] than elsewhere in the municipality,"[39] which is why the chronic pain rate was higher there than housing conditions would suggest. Relander also remarked that a large number of factors necessarily influenced complex phenomena such as chronic pain (*kivuloisuus*), so that overcrowding could not be expected to provide an exhaustive explanation.

Unlike the data on living conditions, these sections lack statistics and computation, as well as precise breakdowns by social class, gender and region. They seem to be almost of an ethnographic nature in their descriptiveness. However, they also reveal how Relander's approach rested on a deeply holistic and qualitative understanding of locality and the environment, as well as its indebtedness to the classic doctrines of hygiene.

The inventory of hygiene and local knowledge

Public hygiene was a reformist project attempting to alleviate the devastating effects of urbanization and industrialization on public health. Carried by progressive physicians, public officials and philanthropists interested in the plight of the proletariat, it believed firmly in the role of science and education in the task. Knowledge production was to elucidate the laws of health, and education would help the poor to help themselves, although more politically radical positions were not absent from the movement. In practice, following the paradigm of miasma, public hygienists concentrated on the salubriousness of the public spaces, housing and factories, working with water, air and light towards cleanliness.[40]

Philipp Sarasin has pointed out the continuities between the public hygiene of the second half of the nineteenth century and the much older tradition of personal dietetics originating from antiquity.[41] Classical dietetics focused on the so-called six non-naturals, which were health-relevant factors considered modifiable by the individual. These included air, motion and rest (exercise), food and drink, sleeping and waking, excretion, and passions (emotions). Later, as hygiene evolved into a social science that examined the determinants of population health, this outline remained the guiding framework for knowledge production and organization, albeit in an amended form. The notion of "air" was expanded to cover all environment, a new category covering all things on the body (such as clothes) was introduced, motion and rest plus sleeping and waking were fused into one category covering all types of actions of the body, and passions were replaced by/expanded to perceptions. This loose framework helped hygiene to become a general inventory of encyclopaedic proportions of all things related to health. This situation prevailed until findings provided by bacteriology changed the focus of hygiene.[42]

Although the golden age of encyclopaedic public hygiene was already starting to be over in 1890, Relander's dissertation asserts of an indebtedness to its tradition. His detailed descriptions of the various aspects of the lives of the people of Haapajärvi follow its principles. In accordance with the hygienist doctrine, he took a holistic view of the relationship between morbidity on the one hand and human habitat and ways of life on the other. Admittedly, Relander then picked out one of the many factors that may affect morbidity for a closer look, providing detailed calculations of the health effects of "cramped" bedrooms. However, he did not present this association as pivotal for better health. Rather, it was one of many aspects influencing health, but perhaps easier to calculate than some others.

Bruno Latour has drawn attention to the weakness of pre-bacteriological public hygiene: it took into account all the possible issues affecting human health and therefore failed to produce definite knowledge on just about anything. As a result, political decision-making could bypass its advice whenever considered convenient. According to Latour, the isolation of specific disease bacteria strengthened the hygiene project public hygiene by refining its gaze and refocusing its operations on more limited targets. Now the key task of hygiene was to find and destroy the bacteria causing diseases. However, this gain in strength simultaneously signalled the end of classic public hygiene. Many of its doctrines now became obsolete, since they did not have any relevance in relation to bacteria.[43]

Relander's study also gives rise to another possible explanation as to why hygiene science remained relatively weak for quite a long time. This is hygiene's *localism*, exemplified by Relander's commitment to a particular place. As discussed above, Relander limited his analysis to one municipality. In addition, he did not associate chronic pain to poor housing directly, in the entire municipality, but mediated by the division into ten areas. The association was justified by the order of the areas and not, for example, by straightforwardly proportioning the available bedroom volume per person to the degree of chronic conditions reported by the occupants. Further, the area division based on Relander's previous holistic knowledge of the surveyed municipality, which he, on the one hand, did not clearly explicate in the study, but which, on the other hand, in a sense was the subject matter of the whole study. (Remember Relander's insistence on the importance of knowing the local conditions for physicians interested in public health.) The study thus accentuated the detailed description of a small area rather than producing highly abstracted, generalizable, and easily transferable information – although the quantification of bedroom space in relation to chronic conditions did offer the latter aspect, too. I want to suggest that this localism was one aspect, which prevented the proper accumulation of hygienic knowledge. Public hygiene accentuated the particular context, which needed to be grasped in a comprehensive manner to fully understand the factors influencing health in a specific site. The situation in one location was always too complex for an immediate transfer of the insights into another context.

As a consequence, the environment took a key role in the science of hygiene. It was significant not only as a set of important factors having a bearing on health – the wetness of the soil, the harshness of the climate, the quality of the water – but also as a larger milieu, which needed to be grasped in a comprehensive and holistic manner when aiming to understand and influence the salubriousness of a specific site.

1972: Changing the culture of a whole community[44]

Coronary heart disease (CHD) emerged as a major public health problem in industrialized countries in the period post the Second World War, stirring both scientific and public imagination. Early research focused on locating the causes of the epidemic and establishing the contributing factors for CHD, eventually dubbed risk factors. At the turn of the 1960s and 1970s many experts considered the key risk factors for CHD already sufficiently established. The international research community was exploring ways to move from risk factor identification to prevention. These activities were fuelled by growing public concern about and media attention on CHD morbidity and mortality, which created political pressure to find solutions to the problem.[45]

At this point Finland, a small country in northern Europe stepped into the limelight. In the late 1940s, World Health Organization (WHO) statistics had identified Finland as one of the leading countries in CHD mortality, especially among middle-aged men.[46] This situation persisted throughout the following decades. This came into the attention of Ancel Keys, one of the fathers of the cholesterol theory in CHD causation and the driving force behind the Seven Countries Study testing it. Keys was intrigued by the fact that CHD mortality was higher in North Karelia in the eastern part of the country, where the majority of the population was engaging in physically demanding agricultural and forestry work, compared to the more affluent West. This flew in the face of the then-current idea that CHD was predominantly a condition of wealthy, urban, sedentary men.[47] As a result, Finland became involved in the Seven Countries Study, with North Karelia one of the study areas.

Preliminary information about the ten-year results of the Seven Countries Study published in late 1969 once again highlighted the poor CHD situation in North Karelia, leading to calls from the community for more concerted action.[48] The local governor, all North Karelian members of parliament, and numerous representatives of administrative and voluntary organizations in the area signed a petition pleading with the national establishment to "urgently undertake efficient action to plan and implement a programme which would organize and finance general health information to the public, necessary basic research, and individual health education to reduce this greatest public health problem" of North Karelia.[49]

This initiative was the official starting shot for the North Karelia Project (NKP), which was one of the first community prevention projects to testconcerted methods to reduce cardiovascular problems among the whole population of a specific area, instead of only high-risk groups, by changing the culture of the community. Not only answered it local calls for more efficient prevention activities but also catered for the international research community which was interested in studying the efficacy of risk-factor modification.[50]

NKP consisted of several sub-projects, supported by general programme activities. These covered primary, secondary and tertiary prevention. A major part of the activities, such as testing and case finding, counselling and health education, treatment and rehabilitation took place in the health services. Here I concentrate on the ways NKP attempted to facilitate cultural change in North Karelia. In practice, it relied on social networks and, to a lesser degree, environmental changes.

NKP adopted a three-level theoretical model.[51] The first level consisted of social relations and living conditions as well as heredity, which, however, was out of reach of intervention. These guided aspects of health behaviour, which were located on the second level. Health behavior, in turn, affected risk factors (and thus CHD) on the third level. Health behaviour included smoking, exercising, eating habits, "psychological stress," and adherence to medical treatment. These were the immediate targets of the intervention. By providing information on healthy habits and changing the normative structure of the community to support behavioural change, NKP expected to improve CHD morbidity and mortality in the area.

To mobilize social relations, project plans devised a hierarchical model that initially involved key actor groups, which then would help to reach lay people through their respective channels of influence.[52] The first group were the physicians. The second tier of key actors were other health service personnel, media representatives, teachers, leaders of public organizations, and administrative officials. Once converted into the project, these groups could then reach the common people through the channels they controlled, i.e., health services, schools, public and civic organizations and the media. Accompanying this top-down approach was a massive education campaign, which utilized every possible method and channel to disseminate the project agenda to every member of the local community. The involvement of common people thus consisted mostly of executing the changes in health behaviour stipulated by the experts and influencers, although local lay leaders were also recruited to provide links to local populace.

One NKP goal was "[i]ntroducing environmental changes that would result in behavioural changes."[53] The measures were directed at the target risk factors with a behavioural component. Smoking habits were addressed with a campaign to prohibit smoking in public facilities and vehicles. Dietary change was endorsed by introducing novel types of low-fat milk products and sausages in cooperation with local dairies and a local food company, promoting vegetable growing and use, as well as making shopkeepers aware of nutrition campaigns and getting them to promote recommended foods. The environmental measures, however, pale in scope when put against the mass of information and education activities aimed at both various key groups and the public.[54] An early project plan reveals one reason for this discrepancy. While the project affected social relations directly (through the mobilization of different actors described above), the relationship to environmental change was more indirect: changing living conditions is defined as a task of social policy and therefore falls within the remit of public administration, i.e., one of the key actor groups to be mobilized by physicians. Moreover, according to the plan, "structural changes in society cannot be an immediate objective of preventive action."[55] Structural changes targeting the social determinants of health in the area thus were not a project objective. This was an annoyance to many locals, who felt that a focus on prevention, health behaviour, and risk factors instead of treating actual diseases and their structural causes (unemployment, work stress etc.) was misplaced in terms of both priorities and resource use.[56]

Multifaceted data gathering and analysis accompanied intervention activities. The effect of the project was measured in number of ways. A baseline survey, augmented by clinical tests, provided a community analysis and established the risk-factor levels for the intervention and control populations. A final repeat survey, together with registered data and national health statistics assessed the total results of the project. Regular population surveys gauged the changes in perceived health, health habits, attitudes, and risk knowledge in the intervention area. Specific registers established according to WHO principles measured singular endpoints, such as myocardial infarctions. Official mortality data provided the information for comparisons between the intervention area and the control area. These follow the principles of modern epidemiological research, which will be discussed next.

Singular risk factors and knowledge without borders

The impetus for the development of chronic disease epidemiology was the rise of chronic degenerative diseases as causes of mortality and public interest in their aetiology, which intensified in the West after the Second World War. Extensive statistical comparisons pointed out that cancer and arterial disease had displaced infectious and deficiency diseases as the leading causes of death in industrialized countries. The reasons for this transition sparked a lively debate. One key theory pointed to aspects of western lifestyle – in the case of CHD smoking, obesity, and unhealthy eating habits.[57]

A number of large-scale epidemiological research projects attempted to define the predisposing factors contributing to CHD. The two most significant were the Framingham Project[58] and the Seven Countries Study,[59] both originating from the 1950s. The former was central in establishing the key risk factors for CHD (and, indeed, the very notion of risk factor), while the latter is credited with documenting the link between diet and heart disease in CHD aetiology. As mentioned above, Finland was one of the countries studied; and North Karelia was one of the study areas in Finland.

Together with studies on the link between tobacco and lung cancer, these studies signified a new approach to aetiology.[60] Instead of singular necessary causes, the new epidemiology identified a number of factors all contributing to the disease in "a web of causation."[61] This multifactorial disease concept was at first contested, as it diverged from established medical understanding but, since the mid-1960s, it dominated the paradigm associated with risk factor epidemiology.

Characteristic to the era of chronic disease epidemiology is the increasing standardization of research practices. Although national and local research traditions and approaches have not disappeared, contemporary epidemiological science is more international and homogeneous than in previous eras. Comparative approaches, collaborative research projects and the pooling of results to increase statistical power have facilitated the standardization of definitions, methods and interpretations. Localism has been superseded by a global approach.

Significantly, the candidate factors targeted by Framingham, the signature project in CHD epidemiology, were limited to clinical variables, while complex social variables were neglected. This is by no means a necessary characteristic of chronic disease epidemiology, but attests to the influence of clinicians to the shaping of the Framingham study. According to Gerald M. Oppenheimer, "the Framingham study, as it emerged in the 1950s, was clinically narrow, with little interest in investigating psychosomatic, constitutional, or sociological determinants of heart disease."[62] Similarly, Elodie Giroux has pointed out how chronic disease epidemiology operated with a restrictive concept, which generated "a meaning of 'risk factor' oriented towards an individualised preventive approach to CVD in medical practice."[63] In this way, the major CHD studies, together with research on the link between tobacco and cancer, facilitated the interest in behavioural modification in chronic disease prevention and the emergent lifestyle approach in public health.[64]

NKP carried this baggage of the chronic disease epidemiology. It, too, foregrounded individual-centred clinical risk factors, i.e., either physiological variables (hypertension), behaviours (smoking), or a combination of them (cholesterol/diet). While hypertension was addressed using a medical regime (and later with education on salt use), working on the two other main risk factors emphasized the role of individual behaviour. The changes in the social and material environment aimed to modify a few relatively simple practices: quit smoking or smoke less, use less fat in cooking and shift to vegetable fats. Despite the project's broad community approach, ultimately it highlighted the habits of the individual. The cultural change it advocated not only affected the norms related to smoking and eating in North Karelia and later in all Finland, but also norms on personal health care and individual responsibility.[65]

Consequently, chronic disease epidemiology, such as that embodied by NKP, employs a very specific notion of the environment. As it aims at "global" knowledge, with maximum generalizability, the specifics of each locality need to be erased to the favour of abstracted information – or, the specifics emerge as the result of the abstract calculations, as in statistical comparisons. When identifying a new, or studying the effects of a known, environmental risk factor, environment is defined as exposure, as for example, in studies on pollution's effect on health. When the interest is in modifying risk factors, as in NKP, the environment is harnessed in an instrumental manner for health behaviour modification.

Conclusion: Shifting enactments of the environment and public health

Different approaches – paradigms – enact different notions of the environment and public health. In public hygiene, the environment signified a generalized milieu relative to the specific site and health problem under consideration. In principle, in public hygiene, the influence of the environment to health could be broken down into singular – to use an anachronism – "risk factors" (e.g. the wetness of the soil, the quality of the water) but, in practice, public hygiene was not abstract enough, the description of the environment was "too thick" and comprehensive, the required outlook too holistic. In chronic disease epidemiology, the specifics of each locality emerge as the result of abstract calculations, as in statistical comparisons. These calculations concern a limited number of clearly demarcated factors. Moreover, these factors can be freely segmented and merged, and they are thus easily transferable from one context to another, unlike the knowledge of public hygiene.[66] Although public hygiene did not necessarily require it, Relander's knowledge was rooted in experience, whereas in the statistical universe of the chronic disease epidemiology information is a product of enumerative practices. In a sense, this move away from localism or "territoriality" to universalism or "globalism" results from the probabilistic sampling techniques at the core of mathematical statistics:

> The eventual realization that given developments in probability theory, sampling by random selection was more reliable led to a conceptual break with territoriality. This did not mean, of course, that prior knowledge of a field of inquiry, a global knowledge of a situation or group, would be irrelevant to the statistician. It meant only that the solution to the problem of representativeness did not depend on complete and certain knowledge of the entire geographical area under investigation. It was precisely uncertainty with which probability theory was designed to deal.[67]

Talal Asad has singled out "three developments occurring within and outside the domain of state practices [that] were especially important in the history of statistical representations: social security legislation, markets for consumer goods, and market research and national election polls." They share two characteristics. To begin with, "all of these developments produced social knowledge that is continuously and profoundly interventionist." Moreover, "they constitute social wholes that do not depend logically either on the intimate experience of a given region or on the assumption of typical social actors. They encourage and respond to individualized agents making individual choices in a variety of social situations."[68] We can add chronic disease epidemiology to Asad's list of developments. It, too, is "profoundly interventionist," although more socially orientated epidemiologists such as

Susser and Susser have complained that risk factor epidemiology is increasingly losing its connection to public health practice.[69] Moreover, while there exists an influential and vibrant minority position in chronic disease epidemiology which stresses social and environmental variables in analysing patterns of health and illness,[70] its current dominant guise highlights "individualised agents making individual choices" as part of their "health behaviour" and "lifestyle." It is food choices, exercise habits, the use of stimulants, etc. that we are today encouraged to think of as decisive for our future health. Thus, chronic disease epidemiology, too, subscribes to the "the liberal conception of modern society as an aggregate of individual agents choosing freely,"[71] with the resulting problems of individualization and responsibilization with regard to personal health care and illness.[72]

Notes

1 Susser and Stein 2009.
2 Susser and Susser 1996a.
3 For the "paradigmatic" case of economic modelling, see Callon 2007.
4 Law 2009.
5 Ruppert 2011.
6 Osborne and Rose 1999.
7 Bauer 2013.
8 Hacking 1990; Desrosières 1998; Saetnan et al. 2012.
9 Asad 1994, 76.
10 Holmberg, Bischof and Bauer 2012.
11 Susser and Susser 1996a.
12 Amsterdamska 2004.
13 Sarasin 2001; Jauho 2007.
14 Susser and Susser 1996a, 669.
15 Magnello 2002, 96–98.
16 Desrosières 1991.
17 Gaudillère 2001.
18 Marks 1997.
19 Kuhn 1970.
20 Karisto and Lahelma 1992, ix–xi. See also Mustajoki 2013, 292–93.
21 Pitkänen 1988.
22 Tennberg 1913.
23 Kaprio 1990, 194; Karisto 1981, 45–52.
24 WHO 1981; Kananen 2018; Jauho 2020.
25 Kannisto 1947.
26 Rhodes and Lancaster 2019.
27 WHO 1981.
28 See McLaren et al. 2007.
29 There is thus a certain asymmetry between the two cases: the first tries to identify factors influencing morbidity, whereas the second is an intervention study, where the relevant factors affecting morbidity in the particular case (CHD) already are considered to be known.

30 Swedish was the official language in Finland until late nineteenth century. As a token of nationalism and associated language-politics, many members of the educated classes translated or changed their family names into Finnish, Relander included.
31 Karisto and Lahelma 1992; Halmesvirta 1995; Mustajoki 2013.
32 Relander 1992, 1.
33 Relander 1886a and b; 1889, 240; 1890; 1892a and b.
34 Relander 1992, 8.
35 Relander 1992, 124.
36 See Karisto 1981; Pitkänen 1988.
37 Relander 1992, 37.
38 Ibid., 104.
39 Ibid., 144.
40 Rosen 1993 (1958), chapter 6.
41 Sarasin 2001; on classical dietetics, see, e.g. Gil Sotres 1996.
42 Sarasin 2001, 96–117; cf. Jauho 2007.
43 Latour 1988.
44 This section relies on Jauho 2020.
45 On the discussion on nutritional recommendations, see Garrety 1997; La Berge 1998; Jensen 1994.
46 Kannisto 1951; WHO 1953.
47 Keys et al. 1958.
48 Blackburn 1983.
49 Cited in WHO 1981, 4.
50 Puska 1985; Mustaniemi 2005; Puska et al. 2009.
51 For a more thorough discussion, see Jauho 2020.
52 For this purpose, the project consulted Rogers' theory of the diffusion of innovation, Puska et al. 1986.
53 WHO 1981, 45.
54 See the reported information activities in WHO 1981, 129–133.
55 Rimpelä, Matti. Luonnos yleissuunnitelmaksi verenkiertoelimistön rappeutumissairauksien ehkäisykokeilun käynnistämisestä Pohjois-Karjalan läänin alueella 6.9.1971, 11. Pohjois-Karjala-projektin arkisto, I:2 Projekti- ja tutkimussuunnitelmat ja tutkimusraportit (1971–1974), 1971, Kansallisarkisto, Joensuu.
56 Jauho 2016; 2017.
57 Aronowitz 1998: 111–44; Rothstein 2003.
58 Dawber 1980; Oppenheimer 2005.
59 Kromhout et al. 1994.
60 Berlivet 2005; Burnham 1989; Oppenheimer 2006; Parascandola 2004; Talley et al. 2004.
61 See Krieger 1994.
62 Oppenheimer 2005, 608.
63 Giroux 2013, 97.
64 Berridge 2007.
65 Jauho 2020.
66 See Bauer 2008.
67 Asad 1994, 74.
68 Ibid.

69 Susser and Susser 1996b.
70 See, e.g. Krieger 1994.
71 Asad 1994, 77.
72 See, e.g. Lupton 1993.

References

Unpublished sources

The Archive of the North Karelia Project (*Pohjois-Karjala-projektin arkisto*), the National Archives of Finland (*Kansallisarkisto*), Joensuu.

Published sources and literature

Amsterdamska, Olga. 2004. "Achieving Disbelief: Thought Styles, Microbial Variation, and American and British Epidemiology, 1900–1940." *Studies in the History and Philosophy of Biology and Biomedical Sciences* 35: 483–507.

Aronowitz, Robert A. 1998. *Making Sense of Illness: Science, Society and Disease.* Cambridge: Cambridge University Press.

Asad, Talal. 1994. "Ethnographic Representation, Statistics and Modern Power." *Social Research* 61 (1): 55–88.

Bauer, Susanne. 2008. "Mining Data, Gathering Variables and Recombining Information: The Flexible Architecture of Epidemiological Studies." *Studies in History and Philosophy of Science Part C: Studies in History and Philosophy of Biological and Biomedical Sciences* 39 (4): 415–28.

Bauer, Susanne. 2013. "Modeling Population Health. Reflections on the Performativity of Epidemiological Techniques in the Age of Genomics." *Medical Anthropology Quarterly* 27 (4): 510–30.

Berlivet, Luc. 2005. "'Association or Causation?' The Debate on the Scientific Status of Risk Factor Epidemiology, 1947 – c.1965." In *Making Health Policy: Networks of Research and Policy after 1945,* edited by Virginia Berridge, 39–74. Rodopi, Amsterdam & New York.

Berridge, Virginia. 2007. "Medicine and the Public: The 1962 Report of the Royal College of Physicians and the New Public Health." *Bulletin of the History of Medicine* 81: 286–311.

Blackburn, Henry. 1983. "Research and Demonstration Projects in Community Cardiovascular Disease Prevention." *Journal of Public Health Policy* 4: 398–421.

Burnham, John. 1989. "American Physicians and Tobacco Use: Two Surgeons General, 1929 and 1964." *Bulletin of the History of Medicine* 63: 1–31.

Callon, Michel. 2007. "What Does It Mean to Say that Economics Is Performative?" In *Do Economists Make Markets? On the Performativity of Economics*, edited by Donald MacKenzie, Fabien Muniesa and Lucy Siu, 311–57. Princeton: Princeton University Press.

Dawber, Thomas R. 1980. *The Framingham Study: the Epidemiology of Atherosclerotic Disease*. Cambridge, MA: Harvard University Press.

Desrosières, Alain. 1991. "The Part in Relation to the Whole: How to Generalize? The Prehistory of Representative Sampling." In *The Social Survey in*

Historical Perspective, edited by M. Bulmer, K. Bales and K. K. Sklar, 217–44. Cambridge: Cambridge University Press.

Desrosières, Alain. 1998. *The Politics of Large Numbers: A History of Statistical Reasoning*. Cambridge, MA: Harvard University Press.

Garrety, Karin. 1997. "Social Worlds, Actor-Networks and Controversy: The Case of Cholesterol, Dietary Fat and Heart Disease." *Social Studies of Science* 27: 727–73.

Gaudillère, Jean-Paul. 2001. "Beyond One-Case Statistics: Mathematics, Medicine and the Management of Health and Disease in the Post-War Era." In *Changing Images of Mathematics from the French Revolution to the New Millennium*, edited by Umberto Bottazzini and Amy Dahan Dalmenico, 281–96. London and New York: Routledge.

Gil Sotres, Pedro. 1996. "Regeln für eine gesunde Lebensweise." In *Die Geschichte des medizinischen Denkens: Antike und Mittelalter*, edited by Mirko D. Grmek, 312–55. München: C. H. Beck.

Giroux, Elodie. 2013. "The Framingham Study and the Constitution of a Restrictive Concept of Risk Factor." *Social History of Medicine* 26: 94–112.

Hacking, Ian. 1990. *The Taming of Chance*. Cambridge: Cambridge University Press.

Halmesvirta, Anssi. 1995. "Kansallisen vastustuskyvyn puolesta. Konrad ReijoWaara ja degeneraation idea 1880–1918." In *Historiallinen Arkisto* 105, edited by Merja Lahtinen, 13–69. Helsinki: SHS.

Holmberg, Christine, Christine Bischof, and Susanne Bauer. 2012. "Making Predictions: Computing Populations." *Science, Technology & Human Values* 38 (3): 398–420.

Jauho, Mikko. 2007. *Kansanterveysongelman synty. Tuberkuloosi ja terveyden hallinta Suomessa ennen toista maailmansotaa*. Helsinki: Tutkijaliitto.

Jauho, Mikko. 2016. "'Give People Work and the Blood Pressure will Sink': Lay Engagement with Cardiovascular Risk Factors in North Karelia in the 1970s." *Health, Risk & Society* 18 (1–2): 21–37.

Jauho, Mikko. 2017. "Contesting Lifestyle Risk and Gendering Coronary Candidacy: Lay Epidemiology of Heart Disease in Finland in the 1970s." *Sociology of Health & Illness* 39 (7): 1005–18.

Jauho, Mikko. 2020. "Becoming the North Karelia Project: The Shaping of an Iconic Community Health Intervention in Finland (1970–1977)." Accepted for publication in *Social History of Medicine*.

Jensen, T. Ø. 1994. "The Political History of Norwegian Nutrition Policy." In *The Origin and Development of Food Policies in Europe*, eds. J. Burnett and D. J. Oddy, 90–111. London and New York: Leicester University Press.

Kananen, Johannes. 2018. "Science, Politics and Public Health: The North Karelia Project." In *Conceptualising Public Health: Historical and Contemporary Struggles over Key Concepts*. J. Kananen, S. Bergenheim and M. Wessel, 174–89. Abingdon: Routledge.

Kannisto, Väinö. 1947. *Kuolemansyyt väestöllisinä tekijöinä Suomessa*. Kansantaloudellisia tutkimuksia 17. Helsinki [Kansantaloudellinen yhdistys].

Kannisto, Väinö. 1951. "Miksi Suomen miehet kuolevat ennenaikaisesti?" *Duodecim* 67 (12): 1108–12.

Kaprio, Leo. 1990. "Suomen preventiivisen lääketieteen historiaa." *Sosiaalilääketieteellinen Aikakauslehti* 27: 188–205.

Karisto, Antti. 1981. *Sosiaalilääketiede ja yhteiskunta. Katsaus suomalaiseen terveyden sosiaalisia eroja koskevaan tutkimustoimintaan autonomian ajalta 1930-luvulle.* Helsingin yliopiston sosiaalipolitiikan laitoksen tutkimuksia 3/1981. Helsinki [Helsingin yliopisto].

Karisto, Antti and Eero Lahelma. 1992 [1892]. "Konrad ReijoWaara – kansanterveystyön tulisielu ja tutkija." In Konrad Relander, *Terveyshoidollisia tutkimuksia Haapajärven piirilääkäripiirissä I*, v–xvi. Helsinki: Duodecim, 1992.

Keys, Ancel, M. J. Karvonen, and Flaminio Fidanza. 1958. "Serum cholesterol studies in Finland." *Lancet* 272 (7039): 175–8.

Krieger, Nancy. 1994. "Epidemiology and the Web of Causation: Has Anyone Seen the Spider?" *Social Science & Medicine* 39: 887–903.

Kromhout, Daan, Alessandro Menotti, and Henry Blackburn, eds. 1994. *The Seven Countries Study. A Scientific Adventure in Cardiovascular Disease Epidemiology.* Bilthoven: The Seven Countries Study.

Kuhn, Thomas S. 1970. *The Structure of Scientific Revolutions.* 2nd edition. Chicago: University of Chicago Press.

La Berge, Ann F. 1998. "How the Ideology of Low Fat Conquered America." *Journal of the History of Medicine and Allied Sciences* 63: 139–77.

Latour, Bruno. 1988. *The Pasteurization of France.* Cambridge MA: Harvard University Press.

Law, John. 2009. "Seeing like a Survey." *Cultural Sociology* 3 (2): 239–56.

Lupton, Deborah. 1993. "Risk as Moral Danger: The Social and Political Functions of Risk Discourse in Public Health." *International Journal of Health Services* 23 (3): 425–35.

MacKenzie, Donald, Fabian Muniesa, and Lucia Siu, eds. 2007. *Do Economists Make Markets? On the Performativity of Economics.* Princeton NJ: Princeton University Press.

McLaren, Lindsay, Laura M. Ghali, Diane Lorenzetti, and Melanie Rock. 2007. "Out of Context? Translating Evidence from the North Karelia Project over Place and Time." *Health Education Research* 22: 414–24.

Magnello, Eileen. 2002. "The Introduction of Mathematical Statistics in to Medical Research: The Roles of Karl Pearson, Major Greenwood and Austin Bradford Hill." In *The Road to Medical Statistics*, edited by Eileen Magnello and Anne Hardy, 95–124. Amsterdam & New York: Rodopi.

Marks, Harry M. 1997. *The Progress of Experiment: Science and Therapeutic Reform in the United States, 1900–1990.* Cambridge: Cambridge University Press.

Mustajoki, Pertti. 2013. *Mies joka hakkasi halkoja: Terveysapostoli Konrad ReijoWaara.* Helsinki: Duodecim.

Mustaniemi, Harri. 2005. *Saappaat savessa. Pohjois-Karjala projektin tuloksia tekemässä.* Joensuu: Pohjois-Karjala projektin tutkimussäätiö.

Oppenheimer, Gerald M. 2005. "Becoming the Framingham Study 1947–50." *American Journal of Public Health* 95: 602–10.

Oppenheimer, Gerald M. 2006. "Profiling Risk: The Emergence of Coronary Heart Disease Epidemiology in the United States (1947–70)." *International Journal of Epidemiology* 35: 720–30.

Osborne, Thomas and Nikolas Rose. 1999. "Do the Social Sciences Create Phenomena? The Example of Public Opinion Research." *British Journal of Sociology* 50 (3): 367–96.

Parascandola, Mark. 2004. "Skepticism, Statistics, and the Cigarette: A Historical Analysis of a Methodological Debate." *Perspectives in Biology and Medicine* 47: 244–61.

Pitkänen, Kari. 1988. *Väestöntutkimus ja yhteiskunta. Suomalaisen väestöntutkimuksen historia 1700-luvulta noin vuoteen 1950.* Suomen väestötieteen yhdistyksen julkaisuja 11. Helsinki: Suomen väestötieteen yhdistys.

Puska, Pekka. 1985. *Sydänprojekti.* Helsinki: Otava.

Puska, Pekka, K. Koskela, A. McAlister, H. Mäyränen, A. Smolander, S. Moisio, L. Viri, V. Korpelainen, and E.M. Rogers. 1986. "Use of Lay Opinion Leaders to Promote Diffusion of Health Innovations in a Community Programme: Lessons Learned from the North Karelia Project." *Bulletin of the World Health Organization* 64: 437–46.

Puska, Pekka, Erkki Vartiainen, Tiina Laatikainen, Pekka Jousilahti, and Meri Paavola, eds. 2009. *The North Karelia Project: From North Karelia to National Action.* Helsinki: National Institute for Health and Welfare.

Relander, Konrad. 1886a. "Kehoitus jalkaretkiin maassamme." *Duodecim* 2 (4): 53–6.

Relander, Konrad. 1886b. "Huomiota ansaitsevaa hygieenisellä tutkimusretkellä maassamme." *Duodecim* 2 (5): 69–75.

Relander, Konrad. 1889. "Kotimaisista matkustuksista maaseuduilla hygienisiä ja etiologisia tutkimuksia varten." *Duodecim* 5 (12): 239–46.

Relander, Konrad. 1890. "Piirilääkärilaitoksestamme." *Duodecim* 6 (11): 184–91.

Relander, Konrad. 1892a. "Terveyshoidollisista tutkimuksista ympäri koko maatamme I." *Duodecim* 8 (5): 85–8.

Relander, Konrad. 1892b. "Terveyshoidollisista tutkimuksista ympäri koko maatamme II." *Duodecim* 8 (6): 117–21.

Relander, Konrad. 1992 [1892]. *Terveyshoidollisia tutkimuksia Haapajärven piirilääkäripiirissä, osa 1.* Helsinki: Duodecim, 1992.

Rhodes, Tim and Kari Lancaster. 2019. "Evidence-making Interventions in Health: A Conceptual Framing." *Social Science & Medicine* 238. At https://doi.org/10.1016/j.socscimed.2019.112488

Rosen, George. 1993 (1958). *A History of Public Health.* Baltimore: Johns Hopkins University Press.

Rothstein, W.G. 2003. *Public Health and the Risk Factor. A History of an Uneven Medical Revolution.* Rochester and Woodbridge: University of Rochester Press.

Ruppert, Evelyn. 2011. "Population Objects: Interpassive Subjects." *Sociology* 45 (2): 218–33.

Saetnan, Ann R., Heidi M. Lomell and Svein Hammer, eds. 2012. *The Mutual Construction of Statistics and Society.* New York, Routledge.

Sarasin, Philipp. 2001. *Reizbare Maschinen. Eine Geschichte des Körpers 1765–1914.* Frankfurt am Main: Suhrkamp.

Susser, Mervyn and Ezra Susser. 1996a. "Choosing a Future for Epidemiology I: Eras and Paradigms." *American Journal of Public Health* 86: 668–73.

Susser, Mervyn and Ezra Susser. 1996b. "Choosing a Future for Epidemiology II: From Black Box to Chinese Boxes and Eco-Epidemiology." *American Journal of Public Health* 86: 674–77.

Susser, Mervyn and Zena Stein. 2009. *Eras in Epidemiology. The Evolution of Ideas.* Oxford New York: University Press.

Talley, C., H.I. Kushner and C.E. Sterk. 2004. "Lung Cancer, Chronic Disease Epidemiology, and Medicine, 1948–1964." *Journal of the History of Medicine and Allied Sciences* 59: 329–74.

Tennberg, Constantin. 1913. *Undersökningar rörande tuberkulosens förekomst i Pedersöre socken. En hygienisk-demografisk studie.* Helsinki [C. Tennberg].

WHO *Annual Epidemiological and Vital Statistics 1950.* 1953. Geneva: WHO.

WHO *Community Control of Cardiovascular Diseases: Evaluation of a Comprehensive Community Programme for Control of Cardiovascular Diseases in North Karelia, Finland 1972–1977.* 1981. Copenhagen: WHO Europe.

Chapter 12

Ultimate and proximate, genetic and environmental

History of the explanations of altruism since the 1960s

Petteri Pietikäinen and Otto Pipatti

Introduction

In 1918, George Herbert Palmer, Professor Emeritus of Natural Religion, Moral Philosophy, and Civil Polity at Harvard, gave eight lectures about altruism at the Union Theological Seminary in New York. In these lectures, Palmer described altruism as "one of the most fundamental, familiar, and mysterious of all the virtues."[1] It says something essential about altruism that Palmer's depiction is as valid today as it was 100 years ago, not that there has been any lack of research into the subject in all that time. Since the 1960s especially, there has been a growing interest in altruism and concepts related to it such as cooperation, reciprocity, and empathy. The two main approaches to the topic have been psychological and biological: psychologists and other researchers in the human sciences have focused on empathy and motivational states, while biologists – especially evolutionary researchers – have drawn on the theories of inclusive fitness (kin selection), reciprocal altruism and others which ultimately derive from a mixture of these. In addition to these major players, in what is understandably a pluralistic research field, there have been philosophical, theological, political, anthropological and various new age/spiritualist discussions on altruism. There is even an edited volume devoted to "pathological altruism."[2]

The term "altruism" was coined by the French philosopher August Comte in the mid-nineteenth century. Comte wanted to replace the Christian concepts of *caritas* (charity) and *agape* (love) by promoting a secular and empiricist conception of ethics. Central to his idea of altruism was "other-regarding behaviour" – a behaviour or action that promotes the interests of other people. The root word of altruism is the Italian *altrui*, which means "of others" or "to others." For Comte, morality signified the triumph of altruism over egoism, and he traced the origins of altruism to the social feelings of animals. He did not claim that altruistic sentiments are stronger than egoistic passions, but he believed that, as a social skill or capacity, altruism could be strengthened through education. As a result, he also believed this capacity had gradually evolved so that, within his own lifetime, humans had become more able to use their intellect for the benefit of others.[3] Comte talked about altruistic instincts and "ranked his own discovery of the innateness of altruistic instincts alongside the Copernican discovery of the motion of the earth as one of the two most important findings of modern science."[4]

Since Comte's time, altruism has become firmly entrenched in the everyday language. In the most general terms, it refers to the concern for another person's welfare without any (tangible) benefit to oneself. Yet, despite the fact that much attention has been devoted to the topic since the 1960s, a scientific study of altruism is still anything but simple. As the psychologist Helena Koppel puts it, "there has been, thus far, no general consensus as to what exactly altruism is, how it comes about, or how to best study it."[5] For a critical investigator, discussions on the nature of altruism appear to be laden with assumptions that are taken for granted, concepts that are confused, and – at the very least – radically divergent ideas about what exactly altruism is.

In this chapter, the conceptual history of altruism (since the 1960s) is examined within the framework of evolutionary and psychological ideas and theories, with an emphasis on the relationship between genetic and environmentalist approaches to altruism. Our historical approach to the knowledge production surrounding altruism as a concept is three-fold. Firstly, we examine the evolutionary approach to altruism, especially the influential behavioural and genetic theories of William Hamilton, Robert Trivers, and others. We then turn to the psychological and environmental explanations of altruism, which focus on the altruistic personality and the issues of empathy and motivation. In the final section, we discuss anthropological and historical studies in which the so-called ultimate and proximate explanations of cooperation and goodness (or competition and selfishness) are in the foreground. In all these sections, we examine how the researchers defined and explained altruism and how they described the respective importance of genetic, psychological and environmental factors to altruism.

Altruism in the history of biology

Evolutionary approaches to altruism can be clarified by distinguishing between proximate ("how") and ultimate ("why") explanations. Indeed, these are central to modern evolutionary biology, behavioural ecology, and evolutionary psychology.[6] Proximate explanations concern the immediate environmental and situational factors that trigger certain behaviours, as well as the underlying psychological and physiological mechanisms that make them possible. Meanwhile, ultimate explanations explore why these behaviours and their associated psychological dispositions exist in the first place by looking for a possible evolutionary function – for instance, why a certain trait or behavioural tendency might have been advantageous in survival and reproductive terms, and thus favoured by natural selection. Biologists and other evolutionary researchers are more interested in ultimate causes, whereas psychologists and social scientists typically study proximate causes. These different levels of analysis are often set against each other, but they should instead be seen as complementary, as both kinds of questions and answers are equally important for understanding the various manifestations of such complex social behaviours as altruism.

Altruism can be defined either by its intention or its consequences. Evolutionary biologists and animal behaviourists usually study the latter and define altruism as a behaviour which is beneficial to the recipient and costly to the actor – in terms of consequences for their survival and reproduction.[7] The technical term used to describe these consequences is *fitness* which, roughly speaking, means the lifetime reproductive success of an individual. Charles Darwin was particularly puzzled by the occurrence of self-sacrificing behaviour in nature. According to his theory of evolution by natural selection, heritable traits promoting survival and reproductive success in individuals tend to accumulate in populations over many generations, whereas traits reducing this success tend to disappear.[8] And yet Darwin saw ample examples of behaviours across many species – including humans – in which individuals act in self-sacrificing ways, sometimes risking their lives on the behalf of others. How could natural selection favour and maintain such behavioural tendencies? This was, for Darwin, "a special difficulty" and potentially fatal to his whole theory.[9] To solve this puzzle, Darwin suggested that, in some special cases, natural selection acted on a higher level than the individual, favouring traits that benefit larger units, such as groups or communities. Here, Darwin was thinking especially of social insects (such as ants, bees and wasps where worker castes are sterile) as well as early human groups where our fundamental altruistic and moral tendencies evolved.[10] Later on, this idea came to be called "group selection" and disputes over its relevance have continued to this day.[11]

Kinship as the key to altruism

After Darwin, it took nearly a century before a scientific breakthrough in the evolutionary study of altruism was made. In 1964, the young British biologist William D. Hamilton published his ground-breaking "genetical theory of altruism."[12] Hamilton's key insight was that when examining the evolution and manifestation of altruism we must turn our gaze from the individuals who perform altruistic acts to the genes that code for these behaviours. He realized that organisms not only pass their genes on to the next generation via their own offspring, but also by helping those individuals with whom they share genes via a common ancestor. Hence, natural selection may favour altruistic traits or behaviours – or rather, genes that code for these traits or behaviours – when the benefits conferred to close kin exceed any costs suffered by the actor.

Hamiltonian kin selection is thus the process by which traits are favoured due to their beneficial effects on the fitness of close relatives, and this theory predicts that altruism is more likely to occur when individuals are closely related.[13] But because helping close relatives promotes the spread of copies of one's own genes, some researchers prefer to call this form of altruism "nepotism." As such, kin selection theory is not only a biological theory of altruism, but also a major extension to our understanding of how natural selection works. In effect, it means that are selected in the evolutionary process not only because they promote the survival and reproductive success of the individual who carries these traits (direct fitness), but also for close relatives who carry copies of the individual's genes (indirect fitness). Traits or genes are thus selected and spread in a population when they increase an individual's *inclusive fitness*, which is the sum of both their direct and indirect fitness.[14] Hamilton's work thus had a number of implications: (i) it laid the foundations for a gene-centred view of evolution that emerged in the 1960s and 1970s; (ii) it had a huge impact on the study of sociality and altruism in animals; and (iii) it provided the basis for a biological theory of human family and kin relationships.[15]

In humans, kin recognition rests on environmental cues and the emotional mechanisms activated by them. Human beings are disposed to treat each other as close relatives if they have shared the same household during the childhood of one or both of the parties involved, as is usually the case with parents and offspring and with siblings.[16] For the same reason, adoptive parents become emotionally and altruistically attached to their child although they are not genetically related. Similarly, non-siblings who are raised in the same household are likely to treat each other as close relatives, and siblings who have not been in close contact with each other are less likely to do so even if they are aware of their biological bond.[17] Altruism between close kin is often mediated by emotions such as attachment and sympathy, and these psychological dispositions serve as the proximate mechanisms through which kin altruism occurs. The fact that individuals who are not genetic kin can become "psychologically" kin shows that family and kin relationships form as a result of the interaction of biological, psychological, and environmental factors.

Finally, it is worth noting that altruism can spread via kin selection even when individuals do not recognize each other as relatives, as is often the case among animals. If the offspring of the same parents continue to live in proximity to one another, altruism may be directed towards relatives without the ability to distinguish kin from non-kin. This mechanism of limited dispersal increases the genetic relatedness of individuals within a population and may also have contributed to the evolution of altruism among larger groups in ancestral human environments.[18]

Reciprocity and altruism beyond kinship

A second fundamental explanation for the evolution of altruism is reciprocity. The key figure here is the American evolutionary biologist Robert Trivers.

Inspired by the work of Hamilton in the late 1960s, Trivers became intrigued by the well-known fact that humans and some other animals display altruistic behaviour with other than close kin, which could not be explained by kin selection.[19] Indeed, as Trivers noted, biological kinship would only seem to be relevant to certain forms of human altruism:

> Humans routinely help each other in times of danger (e.g., accidents, predation, and attacks from other human beings). We routinely share food, we help the sick, the wounded, and the very young. We routinely share our tools, and we share our knowledge in a very complex way.[20]

To highlight his broader perspective, Trivers went on to define altruism as "behavior that benefits another organism, not closely related, while being apparently detrimental to the organism performing the behavior, benefit and detriment being defined in terms of contribution to inclusive fitness."[21] Trivers' solution was that altruism between non-kin could evolve when the costs suffered by the actor are compensated by benefits in return. He called this "reciprocal altruism" which, in its most basic form, can be summed up by the idiom "you scratch my back, and I'll scratch yours." Altruistic dispositions can thus be selected for when individuals are capable of recognizing each other and when they preferentially help those who have helped them in the past.[22] Trivers' theory also predicts that altruism is more likely to occur when the benefit to the recipient is high and the cost to the actor is low. Consequently, the reciprocal exchange of services and resources may produce obvious fitness benefits for both parties and would thus be favoured in the context of natural selection.

As reciprocal altruism involves a time delay between altruistic acts, such forms of cooperation are relatively rare in nature.[23] Cooperation among animals is very often mutualistic, which means that favours and services are either exchanged simultaneously or animals act in a synchronized way for immediate mutual benefit (e.g. to catch prey or drive away predators). However, chimpanzees, our closest primate relatives, practice reciprocity in exchange for grooming, food and antagonistic support.[24] There is a wide consensus among evolutionary biologists, behavioural ecologists and evolutionary psychologists that reciprocity has played a major role in the evolution of altruism and cooperation among humans.[25]

Trivers' work proved to be significant because it provided a detailed evolutionary interpretation of the emotional system underlying altruistic behaviour in humans. Trivers suggested that much of our reciprocal interactions and relationships are structured by emotional dispositions, such as affection for friends, gratitude, trust, sympathy, suspicion, moralistic aggression and guilt. The ultimate evolutionary function of these emotional tendencies is to motivate us to form and maintain cooperative social relationships, and to simultaneously protect us from being exploited by others.[26] For Trivers, humans cannot be simply split into altruists and non-altruists. It is more the case that each of us possesses both altruistic and egoistic tendencies, the manifestations of which depend substantially on our environmental and social conditions. The extent to which people act altruistically and cooperate is thus contingent upon how they perceive the prevalence of altruistic and cheating tendencies in others within their social environment. This requires there to be developmental and phenotypic plasticity in our ability to cooperate, by which Trivers meant that environmental factors have a significant impact on how altruistic and cheating tendencies will develop in each person.[27]

Because reciprocal altruism is, in fact, beneficial to both parties, some theorists have found the "altruism" in this term redundant and misleading, preferring alternative terms such as "cooperation" or "reciprocity."[28] As in evolutionary thinking in general, it is useful at this point to distinguish between the *process* by which traits may be selected and the *product* – the manifestation of altruistic behaviour which potentially reduces the actor's fitness. In other words, although the evolution of altruism via reciprocity has required the compensation of costs by return-benefits, this process may have produced behavioural tendencies which make people act altruistically (in the biological sense of the term) in different situations.

Indirect reciprocity and group selection

A third mechanism that is widely recognized as contributing to the evolution of altruistic dispositions among humans is indirect reciprocity. Whereas the direct reciprocity discussed above concerns two-party interactions, the model of indirect reciprocity, as developed by the American zoologist Richard D. Alexander in the late 1970s and 1980s, emphasizes that the return benefits of altruistic acts may also come from others than the individual aided. Indirect reciprocity is based on third-party reactions, and many evolutionary researchers believe that it is likely to have been a strong selective force as individuals prefer to cooperate with helpful partners.[29] For most of our evolutionary history, humans have lived in small-scale communities where social interactions occur "in the presence of interested audiences – groups of individuals who continually evaluate the members of their society as possible future interactants." Reputation and status are central to indirect reciprocity, and it "results in everyone in a social group continually being assessed and reassessed" based on how they interact with others.[30] The evolution of altruistic dispositions may also have occurred through punishment by third parties. To be excluded from the help of other members of the social group is potentially very costly in an environment where individuals know each other and trade information about free-riding deviants.[31]

Until the late 1960s, it was common for biologists to think that natural selection produces adaptations for the good of the group or the species. A famous case in point is the British zoologist V.C. Wynne-Edwards, who argued in his book, *Animal Dispersion in Relation to Social Behaviour*, that various altruistic behaviours have evolved because groups consisting of cooperative and self-sacrificing individuals have been more successful than groups of selfish individuals.[32] This kind of "old" group selection thinking encountered strong theoretical and empirical criticism during the 1960s and 1970s.[33] The new consensus was that, while selection at the group or population level is possible in theory, it requires such exceptional circumstances that, in practice, the influence of natural selection is much stronger at the level of individuals or their genes.

Since the 1990s, however, "new" group selection theories, commonly known as "multilevel selection," have gained ground in the biological discussions on altruism. The key idea is that natural selection operates at different levels in the biological hierarchy, from genes and individuals, to groups and populations – the relative significance of which will vary according to conditions.[34] Today, there is a heterogeneous set of approaches seeking to demonstrate the relevance of group selection for the evolution and maintenance of altruism, including gene-culture coevolution and the laboratory experiments of behavioural economics.[35] Key controversies revolve around the question of whether there are patterns of human altruism that cannot be explained as products of kin selection, reciprocity and other forms of mutually beneficial cooperation, or indirect reciprocity. As the British biologist Stuart West and his colleagues have noted, the reason that most evolutionary biologists continue to rely on these traditional approaches is that the new multilevel selection models are mathematically consistent with models based on inclusive fitness. They are, in a way, two sides of the same coin and simply offer different ways of looking at the same evolutionary process. However, individual or gene-level approaches are usually regarded as more parsimonious and with them "it is usually easier to construct models, interpret the predictions, and then apply these to real biological cases."[36] Therefore, Hamilton's and Trivers' theories continue to be central to the evolutionary study of human altruism.

Psychological and social psychological approaches to altruism

In contrast to evolutionary explanations of altruism, psychological approaches focus on the motivational aspect – on what makes us help other people voluntarily and altruistically, without asking for anything else in return. The psychology of altruism can be traced back to at least as far as English and Scottish moral philosophers of the eighteenth century – especially Francis Hutcheson, David Hume and Adam Smith. Their understanding of morality and their very endeavour to create a "science of human nature" was radical insofar as it disengaged ethical thinking not only from Christian tenets but from religion altogether.[37] These thinkers discussed altruism in terms of "moral sentiments," "sympathy," "benevolence," and "moral sense" that have since become the focus of both empirical and theoretical psychology on the subject. Even today, psychological studies concerning altruism still focus on similar phenomena, even if the precise terms referring to them have changed. Most importantly, "empathy" has become the key term in modern moral (and developmental) psychology.[38]

The altruistic personality

In psychological studies of altruism, one of the main research topics is the role of empathy as a motivating force. Empathy refers to our ability to share and understand the emotions of others. Such emotional empathy is often distinguished from cognitive empathy (or perspective-taking), which means being able to understand other people's situations and states of mind without necessarily empathizing with their emotions.[39] A number of pioneering studies on the development of morality in children have increased our understanding of the role of empathy (and sympathy) in altruistic behaviour. Key figures in this field include Jean Piaget, Lawrence Kohlberg, and Martin Hoffman. One of the most influential examples of this emphasis on empathy in the field, is *The Altruistic Personality* (1988) by Pearl and Samuel Oliner, which recounted their large-scale study of those who rescued Jews during the Holocaust. It was based on questionnaires, standard psychological tests, and interviews with 406 people who had rescued Jews in Europe. In addition, a group of controls (non-rescuers) and rescued survivors were interviewed – altogether almost 700 people. For the past thirty years, the results of this project have inspired researchers to create a kind of psychological profile for the altruistic personality.

The Oliners' project can be seen as a follow-up to the famous study on the "authoritarian personality" conducted by Theodor Adorno and his colleagues in the United States in the late 1940s.[40] Whereas the Authoritarian Personality Study explored the psychological (and psychoanalytic) aspects of fascism and ethnocentrism, the goal of the Altruistic Personality Study was to discover the main characteristics of people who risked their lives to help Jews escape the Nazis. An important criterion for determining who were rescuers was a total lack of external reward of any kind for their altruistic acts.[41]

The Oliners described their study as being rooted in a social psychological orientation that emphasizes situational factors. Thus, instead of looking for either biological-genetic or individual-psychological explanations, they focused on the ways in which the "internal characteristics of actors as well as the external environments in which they find themselves influence each other."[42] With this situational explanatory framework they tried to find out how extremely risky decisions to help the Jews were affected by personality characteristics on the one hand, and external environmental conditions on the other. A crucial external condition, of course, was the Holocaust, which totally determined the fate of Jews who were living in the areas occupied by the Nazis. The Poles, Germans, Dutch, French, and Danish (among others) who rescued them were often conditioned by their environment insofar as they despised the Nazis for what they were doing – or at least strongly disapproved of their violent persecution of Jews. However, only 17 per cent of rescuers "focused on their hatred of Nazis as even one of their reasons for rescuing Jews."[43] Thus, hostility towards Nazis probably facilitated rescue but did not, in itself, provide a sufficient explanation for it.

In the Altruistic Personality Study, the Oliners found one important characteristic in common among the majority of rescuers – they embraced universalistic ethics that emphasized the common humanity of all people. Consequently, regardless of their religious commitments, rescuers typically assessed Jews as fellow humans and rejected negative stereotypes of them. In the interviews, rescuers referred to the "whole human race," and to humanity being "one great family," as well as the need to "respect others."[44] Their sphere of altruism was not constricted to their relatives, their own community or even their own nationality or ethnicity. On the contrary, they believed that moral values should be applied universally and that all human beings are intrinsically valuable. For one group of rescuers, close contact with the Jews in their communities had sensitized them to the point that they were particularly distressed by anti-Semitic atrocities, such as *Kristallnacht* in 1938.[45]

What also characterized the rescuers was their greater receptivity to the needs of other people. Rescuers often attributed this receptivity to their upbringing: their parents had taught them to respect others and to treat people as individuals, not as members of groups, be they ethnic, religious, or political. Moreover, compared to the parents of non-rescuers, parents of rescuers seldom reverted to physical punishment, relying more often on reasoning.[46] In addition, the parents of rescuers rejected obedience as an important personality trait. Obviously, rescuers had internalized the importance of non-obedience, because to be obedient is to accept authoritarian rule. Instead, rescuers typically invoked a sense of duty and concern for equality, empathy and care as motives. What gave credibility to their attribution of such positive motives was that the "overwhelming majority (83 per cent) of rescued survivors also believed that their rescuers were so motivated."[47]

There is hardly any doubt that rescuers felt some degree of empathy towards the Jews they helped, and there is still less doubt about their helping acts – they *did* help the Jews.[48] What, however, has been unclear to many psychologists is whether their *motivation* was genuinely altruistic.

Implications of the altruistic personality study: Two viewpoints

Two prominent psychologists who have thought about the implications of the Altruistic Personality Study are Martin Hoffman and Daniel Batson. Hoffman pays attention to what he calls "empathic anger" – in his view, it is likely that feeling anger on behalf of others can lead to altruistic acts, such as rescuing Jews from the Nazis.[49] Since there were many non-rescuers who were also highly empathic, Hoffman suggests that anger could have been a contributing factor in the rescue of Jews. The non-rescuers may have avoided action during the Holocaust, either because they simply did not want to help or were afraid of the possibly lethal consequences. Another motivating factor among rescuers discussed by Hoffman is the feeling of guilt – guilt over inaction in situations of glaring injustice in which individuals or groups are treated harshly by the authorities. In addition to the Altruistic Personality Study, Hoffman refers to the American sociologist Kenneth Keniston's 1968 study of white civil rights activists, who referred to guilt as a key motive: "they would have felt guilty if they had done nothing because that would have allowed the Southern Black people's victimization to continue."[50]

In Hoffman's view, having an altruistic personality is not enough to guarantee that a person will necessarily help, especially when the cost of helping can be extremely high – as in the case of rescuing Jews during the Holocaust. Individuals who are willing to take such risks are not only empathic, they are also committed to universal moral principles that guide their actions – at times almost instinctively. In his important book that brings together the results of decades-long research on moral development, Hoffman suggests that (i) empathic morality is universal, (ii) rooted in evolution, and (iii) thus part of human nature. Empathic morality is "likely to promote prosocial behavior and discourage aggression in cultures guided by caring and most justice principles." At the same time, it "can be destroyed by power-assertive childrearing, diminished by cultural valuing of competition over helping others, and overwhelmed by egoistic motives within the individual that are powerful enough to override it." For this reason, empathic morality is fragile ("the Holocaust did happen") and it is "subject to biases that favor friends, relatives, and people similar to oneself."[51]

Like Martin Hoffman, psychologist Daniel Batson sees empathy as the necessary moral psychological foundation of altruism. His "empathy-altruism hypothesis," presented in *Altruism in Humans* (2011), claims in its strongest form that "all motivation produced by empathic concern is altruistic," while in its weaker form it "claims that empathic concern may produce other forms of motivation as well – e.g., egoistic motivation or moral motivation."[52] Batson himself supports the weaker form. In striking contrast to genetic-evolutionary theories of altruism, his psychological theory does *not* refer to altruism in terms of either "helping" or "heroic helping." Instead, he argues that altruism "refers to a particular form of motivation, motivation with the ultimate goal of increasing another's welfare."[53]

This is the crucial point of disagreement between Batson and the Oliners. In fact, Batson disagrees with all researchers who regard (heroic) helping as a basis for claiming that altruism exists, as he argues that even these "could have been motivated by self-benefit."[54] Batson claims that if we only look at the behaviour and ignore the motivational aspects, we cannot adequately answer the crucial question of *why* people (and animals) help each other, sometimes at great personal risk. If we do not attempt to answer such a question, we not only give up the attempt to contribute to the "science of human nature," but we also fail to seek the "resources that might enable us to build a more humane society."[55]

It is from this motivational perspective that Batson criticises the Oliners' Altruistic Personality Study – the Oliners do not adequately explore the *why* question.[56] To Batson, asking pre-identified altruists directly about their motives, as the Oliners did, is insufficient, because "there is no way to rule out non-material self-benefits such as anticipated guilt." Batson is careful not to deny the possibility that a risky helpful act "might be, at least in part, motivated by altruism" but just the fact that these uncommon helpful acts do exist "does not rule out the possibility that benefiting the other was only an instrumental means to reach the ultimate goal of benefiting oneself." In other words, we cannot assume that all seemingly helpful acts are altruistically motivated; Batson's empathy-altruism hypothesis argues that "empathic concern produces altruistic motivation, not that it produces helping."[57] To Batson, motivation is the alpha and omega of altruism, but – if that is the case, then the puzzle remains – how can we ever be sure that an altruistic act is *not* motivated by selfishness?

Compared to Hoffman, Batson's stringent criteria for altruism makes him more critical of biological explanations. Even though both Hoffman and Batson acknowledge the importance of evolutionary biology, Batson is quite suspicious of Hamilton and Trivers' theories being used to explain altruism in humans. True to his insistence on the importance of motivation, and on the primacy of nurture over nature, he does not see much value in the genetic explanations of altruism in humans, or even in higher mammals. Instead, he suggests that only "parental nurturance" is a plausible impulse that could be genetically "hardwired" and thus significant to a psychological theory of altruism.[58] Hoffman, by contrast, acknowledges that Trivers' theory of reciprocal altruism "is an important part of my argument for the evolution of empathy."[59]

It seems that whereas Hoffman gives credit to both ultimate and proximate explanations of empathy and altruism, Batson discounts them unless they illuminate *why* humans perform altruistic acts. In other words, Batson finds fault in the "ultimatist" approaches of Hamilton, Trivers and other "neo-Darwinians" (including the famous primatologist Frans de Waal), but he also has serious misgivings about what he calls the "proximatist" approach of the Oliners, because it fails, in his opinion, to give a satisfactory explanation for the helping behaviour portrayed in their study.

The Oliners' study has continued to play a significant part in more recent research on altruism, too: in 2010, social scientist Christopher J. Einolf published a study that "found empirical support" for the Oliners' theory that an extensive moral sense could be a cause of altruistic behaviour;[60] while in 2013, psychologists Edwin E. Gantt, Jeffrey S. Reber, and Jordan D. Hyde severely criticised psychological research on altruism for neglecting the personal accounts of those who have actually helped others, instead looking for "some unconscious egoistic processes" that supposedly reveal the real cause of their altruistic acts[61] – yet in spite of this quest for a "real" cause, altruism remained "just as 'puzzling and problematic' today [2013], as it was 15 years ago, and as it was 15 years before then."[62]

But are the self-accounts of those who rescued Jews from the Holocaust, for example, fundamentally uninformative? If they had attributed their helping behaviour to selfish motivations, would Batson and others then regard their accounts as informative and reliable? If the answer to this question is "yes," then the case is far from being closed and a serious discussion about the basic moral philosophical assumptions of psychologists should take place.

The non-linear evolution of altruism research: Biology, culture, and environment

The Oliners emphasized the importance of situational factors in understanding altruism. These factors "are the immediate external environmental conditions over which the actor has no control but that nonetheless affect a decision."[63] The impact of external environments on human social behaviour is illustrated quite dramatically in the British anthropologist Colin Turnbull's accounts of his field work with two ethnic groups in central Africa. In the 1950s, Turnbull lived with the Mbuti people ("pygmies") of the Ituri Forest in the northeast of the Congo. Deeply impressed by their culture and way of life, he wrote a Rousseau-like paean to the Mbuti that was published as *The Forest People* in 1961. He paid particular attention to what he saw as the Mbutis' profound spiritual–existential relationship with their habitat, the Ituri Forest – in his view there was something "captivating" in this relationship.[64] He was also affected by their music, effortless cooperation and highly egalitarian social structure. It is almost as if Turnbull saw the forest as a protective Mother, who was nourishing, kind and friendly to its inhabitants, whereas the outside world was "open to greed and suspicion and treachery."[65] In short, he portrayed the Mbutis as living in total harmony with the Ituri Forest.

In the 1960s, Turnbull continued his field work, but this time among another group of people in Central Africa, the Ik – a tribe of approximately 10,000 nomadic hunters living in Northern Uganda, close to Sudan and Kenya. The great difference between the Mbuti and the Ik was that the Ugandan government had displaced the Ik from their traditional mountain habitat, and had forced them to become farmers. In Turnbull's view, this change was disastrous to the Ik, who lacked experience and knowledge of farming, and who had to live in an area prone to flood and famine. As a result, they were on the brink of starvation while Turnbull was living among them – he spent the best part of 1965 and 1966 with them. In his book, *The Mountain People* (1973), Turnbull's portrait of the Ik is quite the opposite of his description of the Mbuti in *The Forest People*. While the tone in the latter was very sympathetic, in *The Mountain People* the atmosphere was Hobbesian and nightmarish. Turnbull's experiences among the Ik appeared to be so shattering that he lost his belief in the "essential beauty and goodness of humanity."[66]

Turnbull's list of things gone wrong in the life of the Ik is long and depressing: there is no sense of community, no cooperation (except for some traces of cooperative effort), no friendship, nothing resembling altruistic behaviour, not even social structure in the true sense of the term. The biggest shock to Turnbull was that family ties had been broken almost totally: parents did not care about their children, adults about their parents, husbands about their wives (and vice versa), or siblings about each other.[67] To Turnbull, the Ik had become an *un*-social people, a people who "have dispensed with the myth of altruism" and "replaced human society with a mere survival system."[68]

Turnbull did his fieldwork among the Ik during particularly hard times. Due to two consecutive droughts, the Ik were having to rely on famine relief, which must have clearly affected their community. According to Turnbull, these extremely trying situational factors had a detrimental effects on the fabric of their society, so much so that all vestiges of altruism and empathy had vanished and been replaced by extreme egoism and atomistic individualism. The measure of all was subsistence value, and their extremely individualistic and atomized lives were determined by the struggle for survival.[69] Turnbull suggests that, before they were forced to become farmers, the Ik, "much like other hunters and gatherers," were "an easy-going, loosely organized people whose fluid organization enabled them to respond with sensitivity to the ever changing demands of their environment."[70] In short, radical changes in their environment and their livelihood had turned the Ik into a group of isolated individuals who were forced to play an utterly inhuman survival game.[71]

One critic has claimed that Turnbull's observations of Ik culture were at variance with those he and his colleagues had made in 1983.[72] Indeed, it seems that Turnbull may have exaggerated the selfishness and weakness of kin altruism among the Ik.[73] Even if his highly negative account is questionable, his claim about the disastrous effects of environmental change on the social fabric of the Ik appears to be correct. The larger implication of Turnbull's contrasting accounts of the Mbuti and the Ik is that there is a correlational relationship between developments in the physical and social environment and the moral and psychological characteristics of communities, including the flourishing or exhaustion of empathy and altruism.[74]

The impact of environmental and situational factors on the moral fibre of society is also addressed by the historian Christopher Browning in his famous study of Reserve Police Battalion 101, a unit of German Order Police that was sent to Poland in 1942 to participate in the extermination of Jews. Using the official interrogations of 210 men from this unit, conducted in the 1960s, as a source material, Browning was able to develop a profile of "Ordinary Men" who became ruthless killers. As Browning laconically puts it, "[u]nknown men arrived, carried out their murderous task, and left."[75] What made this unit so interesting for Browning was that most of its members were not zealous Nazis but ordinary men, mostly middle-aged reservists from Hamburg. In Poland, they were ordered to kill Jews, and the overwhelming majority (80–90 per cent) of the men obeyed the order, "though almost all of them – at least initially – were horrified and disgusted by what they were doing." Yet, to "break ranks and step out, to adopt overtly nonconformist behavior, was simply beyond most of the men."[76] By far the easiest decision was to obey orders and shoot the Jews, many of whom were women, children and the elderly. In total, the 500 men in Battalion 101 killed no less than 38,000 Jews between July 1942 and November 1943.[77]

In addition to giving a chilly account of this "murderous task," Browning makes an effort to explain the violent behaviour of ordinary Germans with reference to social psychology experiments that have investigated obedience to authority, especially Stanley Milgram's famous experiment conducted in the early 1960s at Yale University.[78] Browning suggests that his study of the atrocities committed by the Police Battalion "render considerable support to his [Milgram's] conclusions, and some of his observations [regarding human inclination to obey the authorities] are clearly confirmed."[79] In a society ruled by the racist and extremely violent Nazi regime, and in the exceptional circumstances of war, mass murder became routine behaviour. In this situation, what was considered normal (e.g., to not kill anyone) had become abnormal, and vice versa – abnormality had become exceedingly normal.[80] Browning's poignant question at the end of the book is this: "[i]f the men of Reserve Police Battalion 101 could become killers under such circumstances, what group of men cannot?"[81]

Philosopher Paul A. Roth has discussed different explanations of perpetrator behaviour in the Holocaust. Emphasizing the primacy of situational factors, he notes that such factors "emphasize the motivational primacy of exogenous factors, e.g. peer group pressures" or "the pronouncements of presence of an authority."[82] The principal idea of such situationism is that, to a larger or smaller degree, human behaviour "becomes defined by situations." Roth argues that the "primary source of personal stability is not one's history, or one's professed values, but rather the stability of circumstances in which one finds oneself. Vary the circumstances, the individual's behavior will change."[83]

This argument is not only situationist, it is also behaviourist in that it sees the environment and the organism as essentially identical: if the social environment is strongly antisemitic and racist, then the individuals (organisms) living in this environment tend to act in accordance with, or at least conform to, racist and antisemitic tenets. For students of altruism, the question of situational factors cuts across the nature/nurture dichotomy and brings the interplay between ultimate (evolutionary) and proximate (cultural or environmental) explanations to the foreground instead. One does not have to choose between evolutionary or psychological theories of altruism, nor cling to the idea that altruism can be explained simply by our genetic make-up determined by natural selection, nor to the idea that altruism need be seen only in the context of our upbringing, education, social organization, and other socio-cultural (situational) factors. In recent decades, several moral psychologists, anthropologists and primatologists have combined evolutionary and socio-cultural perspectives in their study of morality and its evolution.[84] This synthesis of multidisciplinary research seems to offer the most promising solution to the riddle of altruism.

Conclusion

One of the main biological theorists of human kindness was the chemist and population geneticist George Price, who in 1967 moved from the United States to London to work with William Hamilton on the problem of altruism. Perplexed by the balance of cooperation and conflict that he saw characterizing so much of life, he became interested in game theory and created the so-called Price equation that bears his name. Essentially, the Price equation shows mathematically how natural selection could work simultaneously on the gene, the individual and groups of relatives. To Price, who had worked with the eminent behavioural psychologist B.F. Skinner in the United States, the key to whether altruism or spite would evolve was the environment: if goodness was to flourish and altruism to become adaptive, kindness and cooperation needed to be recognized as important. In addition to creating the Price equation to explain the passing of traits from one generation to another, we could say that Price also created the "Price maxim," which states (in the words of Oren Harman, the author of an intellectual biography of Price):

> Institutionalize cooperation and you kill competition; valorize self-interest and you penalize altruism. Virtue was already within us but needed to be helped along. Perhaps Skinner held a piece of truth after all: Create the right conditions and goodness would see the light.[85]

Arguably, what continues to make the institutionalization of cooperation a challenge is that, while norms and values conducive to altruism certainly have lip service paid to them, in reality it is self-interest and striving for individual success that counts in modern competitive societies.[86] At the same time, as moral psychologists, primatologists and anthropologists are keen to point out, humans are thoroughly social creatures who have a natural inclination to cooperate and show empathy to others. This dual nature ensures that altruism will certainly remain on the research agenda for years to come.

Notes

1 Palmer 1919, 1.
2 Oakley et al. 2011.
3 Dixon 2008, 41–44, 52; Scott and Seglow 2017, 14–15.
4 Dixon 2008, 51.
5 Koppel 2013, vii.
6 Mayr 1961; Scott-Phillips et al. 2011.
7 This standard biological definition of altruism comes from Hamilton 1964.
8 Darwin 1859.
9 Ibid., 236.
10 Ibid.; Darwin 1871.
11 Borrello 2010.
12 Hamilton 1964. For more on Hamilton's life and work, see Segerstråle 2013.
13 The key factor here is the degree of relatedness (r), which is the probability that two individuals share a copy of the same gene. In all sexually reproducing species, individuals inherit half of their genetic material from each parent. Between parents and offspring and between full siblings, r = 0.5, which means that they share 50 per cent of their genes. Between grandparents and grandchildren, between half siblings and between aunts/uncles and nieces/nephews, r = 0.25, which amounts to 25 per cent of shared genes. Between first cousins and between grandparents and great-grandchildren, r = 0.125, and so on. The degree of relatedness decreases rapidly as genetic distance increases, making altruism more unlikely to occur. For a discussion of common misunderstandings of Hamilton's theory, see Dawkins 1979.
14 West, Griffin and Gardner 2011, 232–33.
15 Dugatkin 1997; Kappeler and Schaik 2006; Salmon and Shackelford 2011; Segerstråle 2001.
16 Westermarck 1921; Lieberman, Tooby and Cosmides 2003.
17 Rotkirch 2018, 456; Price 2011, 79.
18 Hamilton 1964.
19 Trivers 1971; Trivers 2002, 5–7.
20 Trivers 1985, 386.
21 Trivers 1971, 35.
22 In evolutionary game theory, this behavioural strategy and its variants are known as *tit for tat*, in which an individual cooperates when the other party also cooperates, but stops if the other party defects. It is an evolutionary stable strategy, meaning that alternative strategies cannot be selected and spread in populations where *tit for tat* is prevalent. Axelrod and Hamilton 1981.
23 Dugatkin 1997; Clutton-Brock 2009.
24 Brosnan and de Waal 2002; Silk 2005; Schino and Aureli 2009.
25 Hammerstein 2003; Kappeler and van Schaik 2006; Sussman and Cloninger 2011.
26 Trivers 1971.
27 Ibid., 53.
28 West, Griffin and Gardner 2007.
29 Alexander 1987; Nowak and Sigmund 1998; Nowak and Sigmund 2005.
30 Alexander 1987, 85, 93–94.
31 Boehm 2012; Wrangham 2019.
32 Wynne-Edwards 1962.

33 Williams 1966; Maynard Smith 1976; Dawkins 1976.
34 Sober and Wilson 1999; Wilson and Wilson 2007.
35 Gintis et al. 2003; Fehr and Fischbacher 2003; Gintis 2011.
36 West, Griffin and Gardner 2007. See also West, Griffin and Garder 2008.
37 Gill 2006.
38 For a discussion on the differences between empathy and sympathy, see Slote 2013.
39 Preston and de Waal 2002.
40 Adorno et al. 1950.
41 Oliner and Oliner 1988, 2.
42 Ibid., 10.
43 Ibid., 144, 149.
44 Ibid., 157; see also 166–67.
45 Ibid., 165–66, 184.
46 Ibid., 178–79.
47 Ibid., 163.
48 For more on the rescuers of Jews in Nazi Europe, see also Monroe 2004 and Opdyke 1999.
49 Hoffman 2001, 101.
50 Ibid., 103. See also Keniston 1968.
51 Ibid., 282–83.
52 Batson 2011, 29.
53 Ibid., 87–89.
54 Ibid., 88.
55 Ibid.
56 For a discussion about the motivations of people who helped Jews during the Nazi occupation, see Smolenska and Reykowski 1992.
57 Batson 2011, 89.
58 Ibid., 53–55.
59 Hoffman 2001, 242.
60 Einolf 2010, 150.
61 Gantt, Reber and Hyde 2013, 20.
62 Ibid., 13.
63 Oliner and Oliner 1988, 10.
64 Turnbull 1973, 23.
65 Ibid., 159.
66 Turnbull 1973, 11.
67 Ibid., 111, 107–08.
68 Ibid., 97, 130, 239.
69 Ibid., 151.
70 Ibid., 237.
71 On the collapse of societies, including the Ik society, see Tainter 1997, 17–19, 88, 210.
72 Heine 1985.
73 For a discussion of Turnbull's book by two anthropologists who did fieldwork in Ikland in the early 2010s, see Willerslev and Meinert 2017.
74 For an overview of the current anthropological discussions concerning altruism and cooperation, see Sussman and Cloninger 2011.
75 Browning 1998, cviii.

76 Ibid., 184.
77 Ibid., 225.
78 Milgram 1975.
79 Browning 1998, 175.
80 Ibid., xix.
81 Ibid., 189.
82 Roth 2004, 215, 217.
83 Ibid., 235–36.
84 See, e.g. Haidt 2012; Boehm 2012; de Waal 2013; and Wrangham 2019.
85 Harman 2011, 209. Price, an extraordinarily sensitive person, who turned from being an atheist to becoming a devoted Christian in the late 1960s, became a real-life altruist himself, giving his possessions to the homeless drunks and beggars of London. Having become ill and depressed for personal and philosophical reasons, he eventually committed suicide in early 1975.
86 For more on this issue, see Verhaeghe 2014.

References

Adorno, Theodor, Else Frenkel-Brunwik, Daniel Levison, and Nevitt Sanford. 1950. *The Authoritarian Personality*. New York: Harper & Row.

Alexander, Richard. *The Biology of Moral Systems*. 1987. New York: Aldine De Gruyter.

Axelrod, Robert, and William D. Hamilton. 1981. "The Evolution of Cooperation." *Science* 211 (4489): 1390–96.

Batson, Daniel. 2011. *Altruism in Humans*. Oxford: Oxford University Press.

Boehm, Christopher. 2012. *Moral Origins. The Evolution of Virtue, Altruism, and Shame*. New York: Basic Books.

Borrello, Mark. 2010. *Evolutionary Restraints: The Contentious History of Group Selection*. Chicago: University of Chicago Press.

Brosnan, Sarah and Frans de Waal. 2002. "A Proximate Perspective on Reciprocal Altruism." *Human Nature* 13 (1): 129–52.

Browning, Christopher R. 1998. *Ordinary Men. Reserve Police Battalion 101 and the Final Solution in Poland*. New York: Harper Perennial.

Clutton-Brock, Tim. 2009. "Cooperation between Non-kin in Animal Societies." *Nature* 462 (7269): 51–57.

Darwin, Charles. 1859. *On the Origin of Species by Means of Natural Selection, or, the Preservation of Favoured Races in the Struggle for Life*. London: John Murray.

Darwin, Charles. 1871. *The Descent of Man*. London: John Murray.

Dawkins, Richard. 1976. *The Selfish Gene*. Oxford: Oxford University Press.

Dawkins, Richard. 1979. "Twelve Misunderstandings of Kin Selection." *Zeitschrift für Tierpsychologie* 51 (2): 184–200.

de Waal, Frans. 2013. *The Bonobo and the Atheist. In Search of Humanism among the Primates*. New York: W.W. Norton & Company.

Dixon, Thomas. 2008. *The Invention of Altruism. Making Moral Meanings in Victorian Britain*. Oxford: Oxford University Press.

Dugatkin, Lee Allan. 1997. *Cooperation among Animals: An Evolutionary Perspective*. Oxford: Oxford University Press.

Einolf, Christopher. 2010. "Does Extensivity Form Part of the Altruistic Personality? An Empirical Test of Oliner and Oliner's Theory." *Social Science Research* 39 (1): 142–51.

Fehr, Ernst and Urs Fischbacher. 2003. "The Nature of Human Altruism." *Nature* 425 (6960): 785–91.

Gantt, Edwin, Jeffrey Rebert, and Jordan Hyde. 2013. "The Psychology of Altruism and the Problems of Mechanism, Egoism, and Determinism." In *Psychology of Altruism,* edited by Helena Koppel, 1–36. Hauppauge, NY: Nova Science Publishers.

Gill, Michael. 2006. *The British Moralists on Human Nature and the Birth of Secular Ethics.* Cambridge: Cambridge University Press.

Gintis, Herbert, Samuel Bowles, Robert Boyd, and Ernst Fehr. 2003. "Explaining Altruistic Behavior in Humans." *Evolution and Human Behavior* 24 (3): 153–72.

Gintis, Herbert. 2011. "Gene–culture Coevolution and the Nature of Human Sociality." *Philosophical Transactions of the Royal Society B: Biological Sciences* 366 (1566): 878–88.

Haidt, Jonathan. 2012. *The Righteous Mind: Why Good People Are Divided by Politics and Religion.* New York: Pantheon Books.

Hamilton, William. 1964. "The Genetical Evolution of Social Behaviour, I & II." *Journal of Theoretical Biology* 7 (1): 1–52.

Hammerstein, Peter, ed. 2003. *Genetic and Cultural Evolution of Cooperation.* Cambridge, MA: MIT Press.

Harman, Oren. 2011. *The Price of Altruism: George Price and the Search for the Origins of Kindness.* London: Vintage Books.

Heine, Bernd. 1985. "The Mountain People: Some Notes on the Ik of North-Eastern Uganda." *Africa: Journal of the International African Institute* 55 (1): 3–16

Hoffman, Martin. 2001. *Empathy and Moral Development: Implications for Caring and Justice.* Cambridge: Cambridge University Press.

Kappeler, Peter and Carel van Schaik, eds. 2006. *Cooperation in Primates and Humans: Mechanisms and Evolution.* Berlin: Springer.

Keniston, Kenneth. 1968. *Young Radicals. Notes on a Committed Youth.* New York: Harcourt, Brace and World.

Koppel, Helena. 2013. "Preface." In *Psychology of Altruism,* edited by Helena Koppel, vii–viii. Hauppauge, NY: Nova Science Publishers.

Lieberman, Debra, John Tooby, and Leda Cosmides. 2003. "Does Morality have a Biological Basis? An Empirical Test of the Factors Governing Moral Sentiments Relating to Incest." *Proceedings of the Royal Society* B 270 (1517): 819–26.

Maynard Smith, John. 1976. "Group Selection." *The Quartely Review of Biology* 51 (2): 277–83.

Milgram, Stanley. 1975. *Obedience to Authority.* New York: Harper & Row Publishers.

Mayr, Ernst. 1961. "Cause and Effect in Biology." *Science* 134 (3489): 1501–06.

Monroe, Kristen Renwick. 2004. *The Hand of Compassion. Portraits of Moral Choice during the Holocaust.* Princeton, NJ: Princeton University Press.

Nowak, Martin and Karl Sigmund. 1998. "The Dynamics of Indirect Reciprocity." *Journal of Theoretical Biology* 194 (4): 561–74.

Nowak, Martin A., and Karl Sigmund. 2005. "Evolution of Indirect Reciprocity." *Nature* 437 (7063): 1291–98.

Oakley, Barbara, Ariel Knafo, Guruprasad Madhavan, and David Sloan Wilson, eds. 2011. *Pathological Altruism.* Oxford: Oxford University Press.

Oliner, Samuel and Pearl Oliner. 1988. *The Altruistic Personality: Rescuers of Jews in Nazi Europe.* New York: Free Press.

Opdyke, Irene Gut. 1999. *In My Hands: Memories of a Holocaust Rescuer.* New York: Random House.

Palmer, George Herbert. 1919. *Altruism – Its Nature and Varieties.* New York: Charles Scribner's Sons.

Preston, Sarah and Frans de Waal. 2002. "Empathy: Its Ultimate and Proximate Bases." *Behavioral and Brain Sciences* 25 (1): 1–20.

Price, Michael. 2011. "Cooperation as a Classic Problem in Behavioural Biology." In *Evolutionary Psychology: A Critical Introduction*, edited by Viren Swami, 73–106. New York: Wiley-Blackwell.

Roth, Paul A. 2004. "Hearts of Darkness: 'Perpetrator History' and Why There is no Why." *History of the Human Sciences* 17 (2–3): 211–51.

Rotkirch, Anna. 2018. "Evolutionary Family Sociology." In *The Oxford Handbook of Evolution, Biology, and Society,* edited by Rosemary Hopcroft, 451–78. New York: Oxford University Press.

Salmon, Catherine and Todd Shackelford, eds. 2011. *The Oxford Handbook of Evolutionary Family Psychology.* Oxford: Oxford University Press.

Segerstråle, Ullica. 2001. *The Defenders of the Truth. The Sociobiology Debate.* Oxford: Oxford University Press.

Segerstråle, Ullica. 2013. *Nature's Oracle: The Life and Work of W.D. Hamilton.* Oxford: Oxford University Press.

Schino, Gabriele and Filippo Aureli. 2009. "Reciprocal Altruism in Primates: Partner Choice, Cognition, and Emotions." *Advances in the Study of Behavior* 39: 45–69

Scott, Niall, and Jonathan Seglow. 2017. *Altruism.* Berkshire: Open University Press.

Scott-Phillips, Thomas, Thomas Dickins, and Stuart West. 2011. "Evolutionary Theory and the Ultimate–proximate Distinction in the Human Behavioral Sciences." *Perspectives on Psychological Science* 6 (1): 38–47.

Silk, Joan. 2005. "The Evolution of Cooperation in Primate Groups." In *Moral Sentiments and Material Interests: The Foundations of Cooperation in Economic Life*, edited by Herbert Gintis, Samuel Bowles, Robert Boyd, and Ernst Fehr, 43–74. Cambridge, MA: MIT Press.

Slote, Michael. 2013. "The Evolution of Feeling." In *Psychology of Altruism*, edited by Helena Koppel, 37–55. Hauppauge, NY: Nova Science Publishers.

Smolenska, M. Zuzanna and Janusz Reykowski. 1992. "Motivations of People who helped Jews Survive the Nazi Occupation." In *Embracing the Other: Philosophical, Psychological, and Historical Perspectives on Altruism,* edited by Pearl Oliner, Samuel Oliner, Lawrence Baron, Lawrence Blum, Dennis Krebs, and M. Zuzanna Smolenska, 213–25. New York: New York University Press.

Sober, Elliott and David Sloan Wilson. 1999. *Unto Others: The Evolution and Psychology of Unselfish Behavior.* Cambridge, MA: Harvard University Press.

Sussman, Robert and C. Robert Cloninger, eds. 2011. *Origins of Altruism and Cooperation.* New York: Springer.

Tainter, Joseph. 1997. *The Collapse of Complex Societies.* Cambridge: Cambridge University Press.

Trivers, Robert. 1971. "The Evolution of Reciprocal Altruism." *The Quarterly Review of Biology* 46 (1): 35–57.

Trivers, Robert. 1985. *Social Evolution*. Menlo Park, CA: Benjamin/Cummings.

Trivers, Robert. 2002. *Natural Selection and Social Theory: Selected Papers of Robert Trivers*. New York: Oxford University Press.

Turnbull, Colin. 1961. *The Forest People*. New York: Simon & Schuster.

Turnbull, Colin. 1973. *The Mountain People*. New York: Simon & Schuster.

Verhaeghe, Paul. 2014. *What about Me? The Struggle for Identity in a Market-based Society*. Melbourne & London: Scribe.

West, Stuart, Ashleigh Griffin, and Andy Gardner. 2007. "Social Semantics: Altruism, Cooperation, Mutualism, Strong Reciprocity and Group Selection." *Journal of Evolutionary Biology* 20 (2): 415–32.

West, Stuart, Ashleigh Griffin, and Andy Gardner. 2008. "Social Semantics: How Useful has Group Selection Been?" *Journal of Evolutionary Biology* 21 (1): 374–85.

West, Stuart A., Claire El Mouden, and Andy Gardner. 2011. "Sixteen Common Misconceptions about the Evolution of Cooperation in Humans." *Evolution and Human Behavior* 32 (4): 231–62.

Westermarck, Edward. 1921. *The History of Human Marriage vol. II*. London: Macmillan.

Willerslev, Rane and Lotte Meinert. 2017. "Understanding Hunger with Ik Elders and Turnbull's *The Mountain People*." *Ethnos* 82 (5): 820–45.

Williams, George. 1966. *Adaptation and Natural Selection: A Critique of Some Current Evolutionary Thought*. Princeton, NJ: Princeton University Press.

Wilson, David Sloan and Edward O. Wilson. 2007. "Rethinking the Theoretical Foundation of Sociobiology." *The Quarterly Review of Biology* 82 (4): 327–48.

Wrangham, Richard. 2019. *The Goodness Paradox. The Strange Relationship between Virtue and Violence in Human Evolution*. New York: Pantheon Books.

Wynne-Edwards, Vero Copner. 1962. *Animal Dispersion in Relation to Social Behaviour*. Edinburgh: Oliver and Boyd.

Conclusion

Heini Hakosalo and Esa Ruuskanen

Between the time we received the chapter manuscripts and the time we started to write the concluding chapter, a new infectious disease had emerged, reached pandemic proportions and given rise to extensive countermeasures the world over. The disease causing the outbreak is known as Covid-19 or just "corona." As historians, we are, of course, well aware that pandemics, as such, are nothing new, but that does not stop the present situation from being new. The scale of pandemics, and the multitude of the biological, social and cultural factors that go into determining their course and outlook, means that no two historical pandemics are ever exactly similar – or indeed completely dissimilar. Many things seem to have been shifted into new positions since the start of the outbreak. New issues and questions have emerged in public and academic discussions, some of the old ones have become more urgent and others have moved quietly into the background, at least for the time being.

Some of the most topical of the issues intensified by the pandemic relate to the relationship between health and the environment. For instance, given that Covid-19 (like AIDS, SARS, MERS and the avian and swine influenzas before it) is a zoonotic disease, i.e., caused by a virus that has "jumped" from animals to humans, we may well ask whether humans should reimagine and rebuild their relationship with other species if we want to minimize the risk of similar outbreaks happening in the future. The corona pandemic has also raised questions concerning the relationship between atmospheric pollution and health. Some studies suggest that airborne particles are assisting the spread of the disease, causing the virus to spread more effectively in areas with high levels of air pollution.[1] If this proves to be true, it is yet another indication of the intimate connection between the environment and human health. On the positive side of things, the dramatic drop in mobility and the use of fossil fuels seem to have given nature a respite; concentrations of air pollution are down in many parts of the world. During the first weeks of the pandemic, people were eagerly sharing images of animals taking over city streets, dolphins returning to the canals of Venice (a piece of news that was soon retracted) and the peaks of the Himalayas becoming visible for the first time in decades. One obvious question is this: if measures this drastic can be taken to combat one crisis (Covid-19), why can resolute action not be taken to avert other, potentially more destructive, crises (such as global warming and the loss of biodiversity). Major epidemics have been known to trigger major social, political and economic changes. Whether anything good will come out of the corona outbreak, it does present yet another example of the manifold ways in which health and the environment interact.

In Pursuit of Healthy Environments consists of a series of historical examples on this interaction. While the health-environment nexus is a constant presence in human history, its manifestations are truly manifold. The ways that people have construed "health," "the environment" and the relationship between the two have varied a great deal both over time and from one culture to another. It is unlikely that any general model could ever capture all these varieties. In this sense, historical case studies, partial and particular as they are, may well be the best way to approach the issue. The authors of this volume have examined the nexus under three broad thematic strands – healthy and unhealthy environments; colonial environments and health; and medical and environmental knowledge – with many connecting links between the three.

A prominent theme in the book is people's persistent need to find or construct healthy environments (i.e., places, regions and loci with the power to protect, enhance or restore health). One time-honoured tradition is to seek health from water in its different forms. Natural mineral wells, discussed by Michael Zeheter (Chapter 2), are the historical origin of the now-ubiquitous bottled table water. The history of the mineral well is related to those of sacred wells and spa towns. In Chapter 9, Kalle Kananoja discusses a mineral bath that Dutch colonists established in South Africa in the 1770s in an effort to create a healthy environment, European style. Such translations have often been unsuccessful and seem to have been so in this case as well. The notion of healing environment is also central in the history of tuberculosis, discussed by Heini Hakosalo in Chapter Four. From antiquity to the twentieth century, consumptives travelled far and wide in pursuit of healing and restorative natural locations. When the modern tuberculosis sanatorium came into being during the latter part of the nineteenth century, a certain kind of natural environment was considered essential for the therapeutic efficiency (and commercial viability) of the institution. As both demand and supply for sanatorium beds grew, the initially specific ecological requirements were relaxed. It was no longer considered necessary to find an "immune site" for the sanatorium – sunlight and fresh air were enough. In twentieth century tuberculosis medicine, the importance of the built environment increased at the expense of the natural environment, until the latter was regarded as no more than a potential source of aesthetic pleasure. What now mattered, from the therapeutic point of view, were the specific medical procedures taking place *within* the institution.

A broadly similar process of "de-placement" and commodification of natural therapeutic elements was undergone by the water cure, both external and internal. Mineral water with healing qualities initially had to be ingested *in situ*, direct contact with the healing spot and natural water source being part of the healing process. In the next stage, as Zeheter shows, the health-enhancing water was bottled, transported and sold in places far from the natural source. Eventually, "mineral" water would be manufactured in a factory, with nothing but the label and perhaps the name to link the product to its original natural site. Nonetheless, as Zeheter stresses, the product has been able to maintain its aura of "naturalness" during this historical process. Much the same sort of development can be seen in the case of the external water cure. The original water cure was available only at a healing bath, which was usually connected to a natural well or other water source. By the mid-nineteenth century, as discussed by Min Bae in Chapter 10, hydrotherapy had become a mobile and transferrable technology that consisted of baths, showers and douches that could be administered in basically any adequate facility, quite regardless of the geographical location or the qualities of the natural environment.

The book also explores the other side of the coin, that is loci that have, for a variety of reasons, been regarded as inimical to health. Marcel Hartwig's contribution (Chapter 5) discusses the experiences of an English volunteer nurse, Charlotte Bristowe Browne, in colonial America. She sailed to Northern America with the failed Braddock expedition in 1755, during the French and Indian Wars (1754–1763). Working as a matron in a military hospital, Bristowe Browne treated wounded and sick soldiers in chaotic conditions. Confronted with a hostile natural environment, and also with new diseases, she came to learn the limits of the skills and medical knowledge that she had acquired during her training in metropolitan London. A hazardous environment of a very different kind is investigated by Panagiotis Zestanakis (Chapter 3), who describes the reactions of Athenians to the toxic smog (*nefos*) that clouded the city skies in the 1980s. Zestanakis highlights the role of the media in framing the problem and in channelling environmental anxieties, exacerbated by the Chernobyl nuclear accident in 1986 and the heatwave of the summer of 1987.

Apart from their focus on hazardous environments, Hartwig's and Zestanakis' contributions share an interest in emotional responses to environmental threats. Hartwig observes them on an individual level, Zestanakis on a more collective level, with reference to concepts from the history of emotions. Their chapters also explore what it means to live in at-risk environments. In Hartwig's case, exceptional circumstances are obvious. The French and Indian War in 1754–1763 ensued from colonial power politics and mindset which created a chaotic setting in which to provide nursing care for ill and wounded British soldiers. The war led to losses and accelerated the spread of infectious diseases that made the colonial space both fluid and destructive. Zestanakis, in turn, provides an example of living in the high-risk petromodernity built on the back of cheap oil with far-reaching effects on the number of private motor vehicles, urban planning and mobility. Experiences related to *nefos* reflected social and spatial inequalities of the rapidly growing capital, and the smog, in a way, also revealed a hidden crisis of urban planning and lifestyle.

Another theme that traverses several contributions is the history of organized efforts to render harmful environments less so. Dolly Jørgensen's contribution (Chapter 1) makes it clear that such efforts are not the product of modern medicine and administration. She investigates the way in which municipal authorities in late medieval/early modern England tackled environmental hazards by means of regulations and sanctions, despite the fact that, in so doing, they had to interfere with crafts central to the urban economy. With the benefit of hindsight, the authorities' efforts seem partially misguided: recognizing environmental health hazards primarily by smell and secondarily by sight, they would overlook very dangerous odourless pollutants. A similar misconception was repeated in Lapland much later (Chapter 7), when Finnish observers self-evidently regarded Sámi dwellings as unhealthy because these seemed small, dirty and disorganized. However, it seems that the traditional nomadic lifestyle – dirt and all – was in fact more conducive to the health of the Sámi than the more "modern" agricultural lifestyle promoted by Finnish reformers (Chapter 6).

The diversity of practices and perceptions relating to the health–environment nexus emerges in clear relief in colonial contexts. Pirjo Kristiina Virtanen's and Laura Pérez Gil's contribution (Chapter 8) examines the belief system and healing practices of two indigenous peoples in Amazonia: the Apurinã and the Yaminawa. As Virtanen and Gil show, the ontological commitments that underlie these beliefs and practices set them clearly apart from the prevalent western outlook on the health–environment nexus. For the Apurinã and Yaminawa, health is a state of tranquility that depends on both human and non-human actors. They see humans not as separate from nature but rather as part of a web of animate beings. Ritva Kylli (Chapter 6) and Anu Soikkeli (Chapter 7) also look at indigenous knowledges and practices under the pressure of a majority culture. The Sámi are an indigenous people living in the northernmost parts of Sweden, Finland and Norway, and in north-western Russia. In Finland, the Sámi have been in contact with Finnish settlers and under the influence of the Evangelical Lutheran Church for centuries. For the past 100 years or so, their assimilation has been accelerated by the Finnish school system and healthcare services. However, the Sámi have also maintained parts of their traditional semi-nomadic way of life and its associated beliefs. Kylli, focusing on the pre-Second World War period, charts the way that Sámi diet and views on food were transformed as a result of the increasing influence of Finnish political, economic and cultural interests in the area. Soikkeli shows how, in the aftermath of the Second World War, the Sámi building tradition was ruptured by the centrally planned and managed post-war reconstruction projects, which were guided by ideals such as uniformity, equality, economy, modernism – and healthiness.

Turning to nineteenth-century medico-administrative efforts to manage the health–environment nexus, "hygiene" becomes a centrally important organising notion.[2] It is present in several chapters. In Soikkeli's chapter, "hygiene" emerges as an argumentative device that was used to call for the improvement and modernization of Sámi dwellings and their way of life. Min Bae (Chapter 10) tackles the definitions and implications of the concept in nineteenth-century British medicine. Mikko Jauho, discussing two phases of modern epidemiology (Chapter 11), anchors the first phase on hygiene as both a practice and an ideology. As Min Bae notes, "hygiene" had a double meaning in nineteenth-century Britain. It referred to personal cleanliness on the one hand and to public health efforts on the other. The first had strong moral overtones, and the second often had political implications. E.W. Lane, the central figure in Bae's case study, relied on the notion of hygiene in taking critical distance to the interventionist mainstream medicine of his day in favour of a more holistic approach. The political overtones are also apparent in the activities of Konrad Relander, the exemplar of the first phase of epidemiology in Jauho's account. Relander was committed to the cultural-nationalist cause and saw hygienic reform as part of the more general endeavour to uplift the common people intellectually, morally and physically.

We sometimes take it for granted that medicine and science have the last word in matters pertaining to health and the environment. One lesson that can be learned from the case studies collected in this volume is that while academic medicine and science may indeed have been the dominant sources of knowledge on health and the environment in modern western societies, they are neither monolithic nor uncontested. In present-day societies, let alone historical ones, they exist side-by-side with a wide array of lay and indigenous knowledge. Kalle Kananoja's contribution (Chapter 9) undermines the strict division between lay and scientific knowledge. The chapter follows the renowned Swedish taxonomist Carl von Linné and some of his apostles from Lapland to Surinam and South Africa, highlighting the key role of indigenous guides and informants, the "cultural go-betweens," in the production of natural historical knowledge that was subsequently attributed to western naturalists alone. The chapter also touches upon the issue of the attribution of scientific discoveries and stresses the collective nature of the scientific enterprise. Min Bae's discussion of E.W. Lane (Chapter 10), a medical graduate with heterodox leanings, shows that the nineteenth-century British medical profession was anything but unified ideologically or politically – and Lane, for one, did not think that it should be.

In discussing the production of scientific knowledge on health and the environment, the book brings the reader to the threshold of the twenty-first century. Mikko Jauho (Chapter 11) begins his exploration on the history of epidemiology from Konrad Relander's turn-of-the-century contributions and moves on to discuss the development of post-Second World War epidemiology. Post-war epidemiology has focused on chronic degenerative diseases and has highlighted the notion of exposure, outcome and risk. It has been instrumental in teaching us to think about health, and the relationship between health and the environment, in terms of cumulative risks, made visible by population statistics. As Jauho argues, this form of epidemiological knowledge, unlike that produced during the first phase, is no longer linked to a specific geographical place but transferrable and global, at least in principle. Petteri Pietikäinen and Otto Pipatti (Chapter 12) study even more recent developments in science, namely biological, medical, psychological discussions on altruism. While the focus on most of the chapters is on the construction of the natural, and, to a lesser extent, the built environment, Pietikäinen and Pipatti bring in the social environment. They discuss the way in which various research traditions – biological, psychological and medical – have sought to understand what keeps people together. Health, if we wish to examine the concept without reductionism, involves social and political as well as environmental health.

In sum, the history of the health–environment nexus is a story of variation and diversity. It would be very difficult, if not impossible, to subsume under any one model the many ways in which people have, in the course of history, conceptualized, managed and constructed their living environments to make themselves less vulnerable to disease. The human understanding of health and well-being has involved a diversity of situated notions, practices, responses and experiences. The variation is highlighted in colonial contexts, which have been meeting grounds not only for different ethnic and national groups but also for different world views, beliefs, healing practices – and germs. We have seen that the way that indigenous peoples of the Amazon approach these matters fundamentally diverges from our way of approaching them, and we have seen how the Sámi way of life was gradually adapted to pressures from the agricultural and industrializing South. Some natural and built environments have been perceived as health-inducing and others as hazardous or destructive. The belief in natural loci endowed with healing qualities seemed to become obsolete in the twentieth century, with the introduction of a host of effective biomedical means of combating disease, but may perhaps be experiencing a resurrection of sorts with the emergence of phenomena like "green care" and salutogenic architecture.

Efforts to identify, avoid or neutralize loci that make people sick are likely to be as old as humankind. For a long time, such places were identified primarily by means of odour and sight. The senses have not lost their significance in recognizing health hazards (as the case of *nefos* illustrates), but the introduction of a host of techniques for identifying pathogenic influences that cannot be detected by the senses has multiplied the number of potentially dangerous environments and made their identification a specialist task. Modern epidemiological enterprise, often referred back to John Snow (1813–1858) and a certain London water pump, has been built upon this foundation: identify the causes of ill health in the environment and in individuals and then change either or both of them. Doctors, administrators and politicians have often found it more convenient to target the latter. One of the lessons to be learned from the history of the health–environment nexus (one supported by many strands of medical science today) may be that the two cannot and should not be told strictly apart.

Notes

1   "Airborne particles may be assisting the spread of SARS-CoV-2" (2020).
2   A classic exposition of the emergence of nineteenth-century is Ackerknecht 1948.

References

Ackerknecht, Erwin. 1948. "Hygiene in France 1815–1848." *Bulletin of the History of Medicine* 22 (2): 117–55.
"Airborne particles may be assisting the spread of SARS-CoV-2. Reducing pollution seems to reduce the rate of infection." *The Economist*, March 26, 2020.

Index

For Product Safety Concerns and Information please contact our EU
representative GPSR@taylorandfrancis.com
Taylor & Francis Verlag GmbH, Kaufingerstraße 24, 80331 München, Germany

www.ingramcontent.com/pod-product-compliance
Lightning Source LLC
Chambersburg PA
CBHW060354220326
41598CB00023B/2919

9 780367 616243